Infanticide is wrong regardless, but why do the females always lose the battle, they never get a change to grow old enough to say mommy. just b/c economically they're not up the part. P.100.

Either way they're going to get rid of the girl especially if it has a defect. P.103

# CHILD SURVIVAL

# CULTURE, ILLNESS, AND HEALING

# CHILD SURVIVAL

*Anthropological Perspectives on the Treatment and Maltreatment of Children*

*Edited by*

NANCY SCHEPER-HUGHES

*Department of Anthropology, University of California, Berkeley*

## D. REIDEL PUBLISHING COMPANY

A MEMBER OF THE KLUWER  ACADEMIC PUBLISHERS GROUP

DORDRECHT / BOSTON / LANCASTER / TOKYO

**Library of Congress Cataloging-in-Publication Data**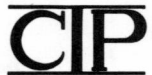

Child survival

(Culture, illness, and healing)
Bibliography: p.
Includes index
1. Child abuse -- Congresses. 2. Child welfare -- Congresses.
I. Scheper-Hughes, Nancy. II. Series
HV6626.5.C497  1987    362.7'044    87-23519
ISBN 1-55608-028-X

Published by D. Reidel Publishing Company,
P.O. Box 17, 3300 AA Dordrecht, Holland.

Sold and distributed in the U.S.A. and Canada
by Kluwer Academic Publishers,
101 Philip Drive, Norwell, MA 02061, U.S.A.

In all other countries, sold and distributed
by Kluwer Academic Publishers Group,
P.O. Box 322, 3300 AH Dordrecht, Holland.

*Dedication*

*To mothers and children at
risk, at home and abroad*

# TABLE OF CONTENTS

# ACKNOWLEDGMENTS

This volume grew out of an all day, two-part invited symposium on child treatment and child survival held during the American Anthropological Association meetings in Denver in 1984. In addition to the original panelists, several other scholars were invited to contribute to this book, and I am thankful to all of them for their patience, steadfastness and even tempers during the many revisions of their papers. Susan Scrimshaw, Margaret Clark, and Patricia Draper were incisive discussants during the original symposium. Susan Scrimshaw communicated at length with several of the contributors who benefited from her astute readings of their papers and from her experience and expertise in this field. Grace Buzaljko lent a deft hand in copy editing the manuscript at a most precarious moment. Finally, a University of California Research Fellowship and a grant from the Wenner-Gren Foundation for Anthropological Research allowed me to take a leave of absence from teaching during the fall of 1985 which made the completion of this project possible. Royalties from the sale of this book will go to the women and children involved in UPAC, the *União para o Progresso do Alto do Cruzeiro*, a twenty-year-old grassroots self-help movement in the interior of Northeast Brazil (see Scheper-Hughes, this volume) that has worked continuously to decrease the infant mortality of that community through a combination of political activism and ethno-medical ingenuity.

The poems 'Limbo' and 'Bye-Child,' from *Poems 1965–1975* by Seamus Heaney, copyright © 1966, 1967, 1969, 1972, 1975, 1980 by Seamus Heaney, are reprinted here by permission of the author and Farrar, Straus, and Giroux, Inc.

The cartoon, 'The Far Side,' by Gary Larsen is reprinted by permission of Universal Press Syndicate, and the cartoon, 'Cabbage Patch Doll Accessories,' by Tom Meyer is reprinted by permission of the New York Times Syndication Sales Corporation.

The American Anthropological Association granted permission to republish the article, 'Culture, Scarcity and Material Thinking: Maternal Detachment and Infant Survival in a Brazilian Shantytown,' which first appeared in *ETHOS*, winter 1985, Volume 13(4): 291–317.

NANCY SCHEPER-HUGHES

# THE CULTURAL POLITICS OF CHILD SURVIVAL

> Oh, children, children, how fraught with peril are your
> years!
> *Fyodor Dostoevsky*

The dialectic between fertility and mortality, reproduction and death, survival and loss, is a powerful one in the lives of most people living outside or on the periphery of the "modern," industrialized world. The pressure that biology exerts on human history is strong throughout much of the "peripheral" world, where disease epidemics and famines consign millions to an early grave, and where the "life of the species" is only marginally under human control.[1] In the world in which most of us live, however, the dialectic between fertility and mortality has lost its edge, become buried in the consciousness of most North Americans and Europeans, for whom each birth signifies new life rather than the threat of premature death, and for whom some control over fertility is assumed. Yet it was not long ago in our own "western" world (barely more than a hundred years) when reproduction was as unpredictable, and death as random and chaotic as in the contemporary Third World. In many remote rural areas and in the squalid urban slums of the 19th century, there was hardly a family that had not experienced firsthand the death of an infant or small child. Public health and sanitation, child and adult labor laws, and social welfare legislation had yet to vanquish the great uncertainties of individual human existence. A walking tour through any New England churchyard with its symmetrical rows of infant tombstones gives silent but powerful testimony to the fickleness of the natural and social orders to those people who lived and died on the threshold of modernity.

The mundaneness and ubiquitousness of child death – a fairly permanent feature of the western history of childhood until quite recently – contributed to a plethora of individual and collective defenses. Historically, one of these has been the failure to recognize childhood morbidity and mortality as a significant social or medical problem. Consequently, childhood mortality rates are often difficult to discern up through the 19th century for Europe and North America; often they were not separately tabulated from adult rates.[2] As late as 1855 the British Registrar General introduced a new subclassification of death – diseases from growth, nutrition and decay – under which adult deaths from old age and degenerative diseases were counted along with infant and childhood deaths from prematurity, congenital diseases, and from "wasting" (deaths from malnutrition, consumption and from what might be diagnosed today as "failure to thrive").[3] As Cassidy [this volume] points out, childhood malnutrition, still one of the greatest social pathogens affecting childhood survival throughout the world, was first identified as a pediatric

1

*Nancy Scheper-Hughes (ed.), Child Survival, 1–29.*

"disease" in 1933, and the more specific diagnoses of marasmus, kwashiorkor, and protein energy malnutrition (PEM) have come into clinical use only since the 1950s. Meanwhile, pediatrics, as a clinical specialization, is also of recent vintage. The British Pediatric Association was founded in 1928, and in the United States pediatric medicine developed only when women began to be accepted into medical schools and into the medical Academy at the turn of the century (Morantz-Sanchez 1986: 272).

In short, the social construction of child survival as a medical problem about which something can and should be done is fairly recent.[4] In many pockets of the western world up through the mid- to late-19th century childhood mortality tended to be viewed as an unfortunate but altogether predictable natural occurrence, and a 15% to 20% morality rate during the first year of life was not regarded as intolerable or unacceptable. For one thing, childhood mortality had a clear social class reference which allowed it to remain masked for many generations. The pernicious living and working conditions of the urban proletariat during the first half of the 19th century corresponded to the lack of social and medical concern for the mortality of working-class and underclass children. As Foucault writes, "It was of little importance whether *these* people lived or died, since their reproduction was [thought of] as something that took care of itself in any case" (1978: 126). The improvident and slovenly "Malthusian couples" who propagated without restraint, without foresight would have that devil, Nature/Biology, to pay. It would take political conflict and economic emergencies (such as the new labor requirements of an advanced phase of industrialization) to provoke state interest in the regulation and control of population, including a concern with child survival, which has recently achieved the status of a "master" social and political problem in the "modern" world.

Given the relatively recent perception of child survival in advanced industrialized nations as a social-medical problem in which the state has a clear and vested interest, it should not be surprising that this public consciousness is absent in many societies undergoing a rapid and early phase of industrialization or mired in a relatively crude form of industrial capitalism. In these Third World contexts, so often characterized by a high pressure demography of untamed fertility and high mortality, individuals themselves approach reproduction and parenting with a range of sentiments and practices rather different from our own. Parents in much of the so-called developing world (like parents in early modern Europe) understand a baby's life to be a provisional and undependable thing – a candle whose flame is as likely to flicker or go out as to burn brightly and continually. There, child death may be interpreted less as a tragedy than as a misfortune, one to be accepted with equanimity and resignation as an unalterable fact of human existence. Following from a high expectancy of loss, reproductive and child-rearing strategies may be based on a kind of thinking in sets, on the presumption of the interchageability and replaceability of offspring (Imhof 1985). Reckonings of the social, moral and economic value of the infant and small child may be measured against those of older children, adults, and the family unit as a whole. These moral evaluations are, in turn, influenced by such external contingencies as population demography, social and economic factors, subsistence strategies, household composition, and by cultural ideas concerning the nature of infancy and childhood, definitions of personhood, and beliefs about the soul and its immortality.

## MOTHER LOVE AND CHILD DEATH

Of all the many factors that endanger the lives of young children, by far the most difficult to examine with any degree of dispassionate objectivity is the quality of parenting. Historians and social scientists, no less than the public at large, are influenced by old cultural myths about childhood innocence and mother love as well as their opposites. The terrible power and significance attributed to *maternal* behavior (in particular) is a commonsense perception based on the observation that the human infant (specialized as it is for prematurity and prolonged dependency) simply cannot survive for very long without considerable maternal love and care. The infant's life depends, to a very great extent, on the good will of others, but most especially, of course, that of the mother. Consequently, it has been the fate of mothers throughout history to appear in strange and distorted forms. They may appear as larger than life or as invisible; as all-powerful and destructive; or as helpless and angelic. Myths of the maternal instinct compete, historically, with myths of a universal infanticidal impulse. Some of these contradictions and psychological projections can be found in the scholarly literature as well, so that a thorough "deconstruction" of the cultural meanings of motherhood and childhood (along with a healthy dose of skepticism) should accompany all cross-cultural and historical examinations of the quality and consequences of mothering for child survival.

In the relatively new literature on the "history of childhood", for example, it is fashionable to assume that emphatic care and benevolence toward small children have in the past been the exception rather than the rule. "The history of childhood," writes Lloyd deMause, "is a nightmare from which we have only recently begun to awaken" (1974). Edward Shorter concurs. "Good mothering," he writes in the *Making of the Modern Family* (1975), "is an invention of modernization." Writers in this genre and in the related field of psycho-history often point to such "child-hostile" and covertly infanticidal institutions as the European wet nurse, those "angel makers" and "baby killers" in Italy and France who are said to have kept infant coffin makers busily employed from the 14th through the 19th century. Wet nurses, recruited from the poorest social classes and often paid a pittance for the sale of their bodies in the servitude of mothering, were poorly motivated to lavish attention on the tiny charges entrusted to their care. Rarely were they punished for the deaths that accompanied their ministrations. In her book,

*Infanticide* (1978), Maria Piers refers to the institution of wet nursing as little more than a public license to kill unwanted and excess children in societies where active infanticide was sanctimoniously condemned by the Church and state.

It is important to note, however, that many of the infants farmed out to wet nurses were, in fact, unwanted and abandoned children to begin with. The greatest employers of professional wet nurses in the early 19th century were the foundling hospitals of Paris and London. The demand for the services of wet nurses by these institutions greatly exceeded their supply. Langer (1983: 359–360) reports that the number of infants admitted to the Paris foundling hospital during 1817–1820 represented a third of all the babies born in Paris during that period. Since it was often impossible to employ enough local wet nurses to care for the glut of abandoned infants, many of these foundlings were shipped off to the countryside to the huts of impoverished "foster mothers". The few who survived the journeys made unattended in the back of crude carts carrying other cargo often died at the breasts of their hired milk maids (Langer *op. cit.*). Yet it would be unfair to place all the blame on the class of wet nurses. Many of the foundlings arrived at the hospitals already half-dead: sickly, cold, severely neglected and nutritionally battered from the ill-conceived infant-tending and infant-feeding practices of the times. Rather than focus on the casualties produced by the social institution of wet nursing, one might point to the lives of those essentially "throw-away" children who were rescued and saved through the ministrations of these grossly undercompensated and unappreciated women.

Several contributors to Fox and Quitt's edited volume, *Loving, Parenting, and Dying: the Family Cycle in England and America, Past and Present* (1980) likewise attribute the high infant and childhood mortality in the 17th through the 19th centuries to human agency, to the insensitivity of parents (especially mothers) to the special needs and vulnerabilities of infants and small babies. Deaths resulting from careless accidents were common, and the babies of even middle class parents could be exposed to such risks as long trips away from home. Thomas McKeown has argued in *The Modern Rise of Populations* (1976) that such socially induced forms of childhood mortality served to check population growth for many centuries in western Europe.

In emphasizing the consciously or unconsciously infanticidal aspects of parenting, the history of childhood literature tends to obscure the fact that the greatest social pathogens affecting child survival in Europe from the early modern period throughout all the phases of industrialization have been poverty and female employment and not maternal inadequacies. In 19th century England among the rural poor, many young mothers were forced to leave home and join agricultural field gangs almost immediately after childbirth. They left their infants in the hands of household members unfit to work (i.e., children, the mentally and physically disabled, and the elderly) who were also generally unfit for child care as well (Phillips 1978: 160). In this population, the hand-feeding of infants was even more prevalent than either breast-feeding or wet nursing, and was also the practice "most fraught with risks to the child's health and survival" (*ibid.*, p. 165). The universal baby food in England during the 19th century was "pap", a nutritionally inadequate gruel made from water, broth or tea (rarely milk), mixed with breadcrumbs, arrowroot, cornflour, rice, or tapioca. Infants fed on pap were voracious "feeders", for they ate and ate and were never satisfied. Hence, fussy, crying, perpetually hungry infants were often quieted with opium and opium derivatives,such as a mixture of laudanum and syrup (*ibid.*, p. 162). Opium was known as a "mother's mercy" as well as a "mother's minder", for it allowed the woman to work with a modicum of peace of mind, knowing that her hungry infant was neither fretful nor dangerously awake while left alone in the house.

To attribute a kind of "infanticidal" impulse to such behaviors and practices born of exigency falls short of the mark, for it removes the locus of responsibility for child death from its true source in exploitative class relations. In addition, the idea, fostered by some of the historians of childhood, that solicitous and empathic care toward infants and young children is wholly a product of "modern" society and civilization borders on ethnocentrism and what historians refer to as presentism, the projection of our own ambivalent feelings and negative sentiments onto people whose lives are very distant and different from our own. Moreover, it minimizes the human suffering experienced by some of those parents afflicted by multiple childhood deaths. There is, for example, abundant evidence in literature and poetry, in journals and diaries, and in the popular culture preserved in prayers, proverbs, and folklore of a sometimes exquisite and doting love lavished on infants and children by parents representing all social classes, and of the pain and anguish they experienced at their children's illlnesses or death.

For example, in Michael MacDonald's (1982) careful analysis of the clinical records of a 17th century folk medical practioner Richard Napier, who specialized in mental distress, were many cases of melancholia in women and in some men attributed by the clinician to the death of a family member – especially a spouse or a small child. Among Napier's patients, for example, was one William Stoe, about whom the doctor wrote:

Much grief from time to time. . . . Had a plague in his house: two children died (MacDonald 1982).

The many cases of deep melancholy suffered by bereaved young mothers (as well as by the childless) across all the social classes treated in Napier's huge clinical practice demonstrate the fallacy of those contemporary historians who have rashly concluded that early modern parents in Europe scarce knew how to love or to cherish the lives of their children. Of the 134 cases of grief recorded in Napier's medical records, 58 were attributed to the loss of a child (*ibid*: 82). Mistress Elizabeth Foster, for example, was excessively anxious following the death of her three-month-old baby; she "trembled and said she had a sinking heart" (*ibid*). The clinician considered such grief to be a natural and appropriate response to child death. Meanwhile, mothers who *failed* to love or nurture their babies were seen as *unnatural*, unbalanced and unsavory, and women suspected of lacking in maternal warmth suffered the malicious gossip and innuendo of their neighbors. MacDonald reports:

> Mothers who abused or neglected their children were tormented with grief and were thought by others to be insane. Still despairing a year after her child's death, Agnys Nueman "took great grief that she did not tend it well." Joan Plotte fell into a suicidal gloom because she had said of her dying child, "if he die, let him die" [and] this thought troubleth her mind. . . . [Mistress] Rowley was distraught because her child smothered in bed and neighbors apparently rumored that the death was deliberate (p. 83).

Indeed, the old "rumor" of infanticidal mothers has spread even to the academy and it has since found a home among the modern historians of childhood, who have concluded (often with little evidence) that infant death by "overlaying" occurred widely from the Middle Ages through the 19th century in Europe, sometimes reaching endemic proportions (see Coleman 1974; Kellum 1974; Sauer 1978; Trexler 1973). William Langer (1974: 360–365) suggests that many poor and working-class women in the 19th century were reduced to such survival strategies as enrolling their babies in burial societies and then killing them by "overlaying" or by poison in order to collect the burial benefits. A British physician writing for the prestigious *Edinburgh Medical Journal* in 1892 attributed the "scandal" of "smothering deaths" among the poor at the turn of the century to the inferior mental and physical traits of the lower classes. The "infanticidal" parents were described as dissipated, ignorant, drunk and careless (Hansen 1979). Even the common practice of nursing mothers sleeping with their infants became suspect: co-sleeping would make it altogether too easy for desperate women to dispose of their unwanted infants by smothering them. Hence, laws were passed in some parts of England forbidding mothers from sleeping in the same beds as their infants (*ibid*.: 335).

A species of this pernicious folk belief has persisted up through the 20th century in clinical discussions of sudden and otherwise unexplained infant death where the terms "crib death" (U.S.) and "cot death" (Ireland) are often euphemisms in the medical literature for suspected infanticide until the 1960s when an alternative, bio-physiological explanation – sleep apnea – challenged the earlier view. As late as 1968 an article appeared in a medical journal (Asch 1968) attributing crib death to the "murderous fantasies" of women suffering from post-partum depression. However, Hansen (*op. cit.*) has suggested that many of the deaths attributed by historians to "overlaying" in early modern Europe were possibly deaths caused by the apneas and respiratory viruses that are today often implicated in the so-called Sudden Infant Death Syndrome.

In short, caution should be exercised with respect to second-guessing the causes of unexplained childhood death especially when this leads to assumptions regarding the motives of individuals living "long ago" and "far away" from the experiences of contemporary and middle-class people. The dangers of projection loom large, given both the historical and the social-cultural distance that separates us from the lives of those poor and working-class women who lived through the early industrialization and transformation of European society and those living today on the edge of the demographic transition of the "Third World." What still needs to be explored for these contexts, however, are the *effects* and the *consequences* of high childhood mortality on the expression of maternal sentiments and practices, including the cultural and psychological defenses that are marshalled against the pain of experiencing the loss of offspring.

Equal caution should be applied to anthropological studies of child survival, of which this venture is a part. There is a similar tendency in the anthropology of childhood literature to reconsider the nature of parenting in traditional and non-western societies in light of the child abuse and child survival preoccupations of our times. Once it was the hallmark of psychological anthropology – Margaret Mead is perhaps the best example – to extoll and celebrate the virtues of the wise and indulgent "primitive" mother who suckled her child through the fourth year of life and never gave a thought to potty training or to discipline (Mead 1928, 1930, 1935; J. Whiting and I. Child 1953; B. Whiting *et al.* 1963). Taking their cues from the social anthropologists of childhood, cross-cultural and developmental psychologists tend to wax poetic on the maternal script in technologically simple societies (Ainsworth 1967; Bowlby 1969, 1973; Konner 1976; Rossi 1977). Traditional societies were seen as creating a milieu that encouraged the "natural" expressions of maternal nurturance and solicitude. Recently, however, the characteristic benevolence of child-rearing practices in non-western cultures has been questioned and there is a new interest in the darker side of parenting. Infanticide, incest, selective neglect have once again come into the public arena of anthropological discourse (Hausfater and Hrdy 1984; Korbin, ed. 1981; McKee 1984; Rohner 1975). Where once anthropologists were interested in these phenomena only because they helped to shed light on the rules of social organization, today there is an interest and concern for the welfare of the child. The new revisionist interpretation of traditional child rearing can, however, sometimes echo the pessimism and over-statement of the social historians of childhood. For example, Robert Edgerton concludes rather sweepingly in his foreword to Korbin's edited volume on child abuse:

Throughout the history of mankind, children have only sometimes been spared the indignities, cruelties, and horrors that human beings so often inflict upon one another. At various times, in various places, children have been abandoned, starved, beaten, enslaved, sexually assaulted, and put to death (1981: vii).

While this statement is no doubt true, one could also point to the equally various times and places where children have been nurtured and cherished, suckled through the fifth year of life, almost never physically disciplined or psychologically abused, and protected from sexual assault and other forms of physical and emotional exploitation. What we need to address are *the specific conditions* under which children are more (or less) likely to be nurtured and protected than abused, battered, or exposed.

## ECOLOGICAL CONSTRAINTS ON PARENTING GOALS

In a series of provocative papers, LeVine (1974, 1977, 1980) suggested that "human parents everywhere can be seen as sharing a common set of goals in their roles as parents" (1980: 17). These include the physical survival and health of the child; the development of the child's capacity for self-reliance and eventual independence; and the cultivation in the child of cherished cultural values and attributes. The particular ecological and environmental context will often determine *which* of these goals will *most* influence parental thinking and practice, but all the goals are understood as the universal and presumptive basis of parenting everywhere.

Certainly, throughout much of human history, as in a good deal of the "developing" world today, women have given birth and have had to nurture children under environmental conditions and social arrangements that are inimical to child survival (as well as hostile to their own well-being). LeVine points out that especially in the tropics, where uncontrolled infectious disease, food shortages, and the invidious vestiges of colonial and postcolonial exploitation have interacted to make human life particularly precarious, cultural practices of infant-tending are organized primarily around *health* and *survival* goals. Under some circumstances these may translate into patterns of preferential treatment and selective neglect of those children viewed as more or less predisposed to die. In other words, selective neglect is often a manifestation of parental interventions on behalf of family *survival*.

Conversely, in societies where *economic subsistence* poses a greater risk than infectious disease or other "natural" dangers, parental childrearing stategies and goals may be organized around the eventual economic viability of children. Elsewhere I have described a pattern of vicious ridicule, a "cutting down to size" and a crippling of the aspirations of last-born, farm-inheriting sons in contemporary western Ireland so as to assure elderly parents that at least one child will remain at home to carry on the family farm through another generation. And so, the considerable psychological abuse suffered by some of these "leftover" sons may be understood as a desperate strategy to maintain the fragile economic viability of the last born son who is today, ironically enough, "disinherited" by virtue of inheriting the family farm (Scheper-Hughes, 1979, 1982).

Middle class parents in urban, industrialized societies are free of the worst risks and hazards to the physical survival and economic viability of their offspring. Hence, they can devote their energies and focus their parental goals toward maximizing those achieved and preferential traits in their children that can testify to their own cultural "superiority," such as intelligence (as quantified in school performances), physical beauty (defined in dominant cultural terms), and social skills. Only in fairly recent times and in affluent societies have most parents been able to focus on producing desired *qualities* in their children rather than on producing the *quantity* of children deemed necessary to hedge one's bets against the multiple threats to child survival and economic viability. It is possible that child abuse and battering may be one unfortunate side effect of the preoccupation of modern parents with producing "excellent" and high-achieving children. At least some of the "rejected" and abused children are those found wanting in the personal qualities or attributes necessary to compete successfully within the family, at school, or in the community at large. Insofar as these same middle class goals are adopted by poor and minority-culture parents, children who fail to achieve them may engender even greater frustration, humiliation, and rejection in parents who feel that the attainment of these attributes by their children is the *sine qua non* of class and social status mobility. Again, these feelings may reproduce child abuse.

Following from LeVine, it is hypothesized here that macro-historical, ecological, and demographic trends exert a profound influence on parental goals and on child-rearing practices. Patterns of childhood mortality (and fertility) influence child treatment, as parents adjust their behavior to conform to their collective observations about the relative fragility of human life. In this regard, Imhof (1985) has developed a framework for understanding the impact of population demography on the social history of childhood that is most useful for our purposes. Summarizing demographic transition theory, he identifies two patterns of death that separated the early modern from the modern period in Europe, as follows:

. . . the old pattern which lasted until around 1875 or so, with a structural, very high rate of infant and child mortality and then a scattered range of deaths over all later groups, with big differences from year to year; and the new pattern, "tamed" and standardized at old age, with relatively small differences in mortality from one year to another. In the past death not only occurred more frequently, but it was also less calculable (1985: 3).

This radical transition from "old" to "new" mortality pattern which occurred in Europe in the past hundred years was accompanied by new perceptions of the meaning of human life, personhood, and the relative value of the individual measured against that of the collective (family, lineage, community). New images and representations of childhood appeared (Aries 1962). Finally, the epidemiologic transition resulted in a realignment of family and social relations, including those between parents and children.

Under the old mortality pattern (the one that still characterizes much of the "developing" world), most deaths occurred during infancy. In Europe during the 17th century (as in pockets of the Third World today), it was not uncommon to encounter disadvantaged communities or sectors of the general population with a childhood mortality rate of 30% or 40%. In these circumstances each new birth was hardly an occasion for unbridled celebration, and each childhood death hardly an occasion of protracted mourning. The Irish proverb, "Sing a song at a wake, and shed a tear when a child is born," conveys the defensive guardedness with which many parents in pre-demographic transition societies armed themselves against disappoinment and tragedy. Given a world of great uncertainty about individual human life, parents may share a common understanding that subordinates the survival of the individual to the survival of the larger domestic unit, whether the nuclear or stem family or lineage. As Imhof characterizes the kind of thinking that accompanies situations of high and untamed mortality:

. . . it was not very wise, under the conditions of the old mortality pattern, to put one single person, not even their own ego, in the center of anything whatsoever on earth. This would have been too uncertain. Instead there followed a kind of thinking in roles (1985: 17).

What existed then were permanent roles occupied by individuals who were both temporary and largely interchangeable. So, for example, Imhof found in the little Bavarian village of Leimbach an unbroken succession of Johannes Hooss's, as father Johannes passed on the farm to his namesake, between 1520 to 1970. This extraordianary continuity, in light of the ravages of famine and war and the plague, was secured, in some generations, by the custom of naming each of the Hooss sons Johannes (and even some daughters) so that by means of multiple occupation of the name-place by Hooss children at least *one* might survive to continue the family name and farm. Such thinking in social roles is quite antithetical to "modern" conceptions of self and individualism. Yet, such thinking is found in many parts of the world today where human life and child survival are precarious, and where the common good is counted above that of the individual child. The mistake, as we have stressed here, is to impute an underlying and malicious infanticidal *intent* to child-rearing strategies born of the experience of repeated loss.

We might also speak (although Imhof does not) of an "old" fertility pattern, that characteristic of early modern Europe up through the 19th century as well as of some contemporary "developing" societies. The "old" fertility pattern, like the "old" mortality pattern, implies a similar lack of human autonomy in reproduction. A corollary of passive resignation to childhood death is an acceptance of a high, untamed fertility. In fact, high fertility may be a *response to*, as much as a contributing *cause of*, high childhood mortality, but this relationship is still contested.[5]

In any event, one reproductive pattern (possibly a strategy) of parents in societies characterized by the old mortality pattern is to produce a great many children and to invest selectively in each, depending on their sex, health, birth order, temperament, or other culturally significant attributes, and to trust that at least a few of the "best bets" will survive infancy. The case studies in this volume of differential treatment of children *by sex* in the People's Republic of China (Potter) and in rural north India (Miller); *by strength and temperament* among the Masai in Kenya (de Vries) and among slum-dwellers in Brazil (Scheper-Hughes); and by *physical traits and perceived deformities* among the Mexican Tarahumara (Mull and Mull) are cases in point. This pre-demographic transition reproductive strategy is especially predominant in contemporary societies and situations characterized by a dense population and often a scarcity of basic resources, as well as by short intervals between births and the expectation that many infants and small children will die. People living in pockets of poverty and ill health in modern, industrialized, capitalist societies may also conform to this reproductive pattern, as illustrated by Newman's "high risk, high risk spiral" of high fertility and high childhood morbidity and prematurity in poor, single, teenage parents in Providence, Rhode Island (this volume).

It is important to note that the "old" fertility/child-rearing pattern is not found *everywhere* in the preindustrial world. It is not characteristic of societies with a low population density, abundant resources, a subsistence-based economy, low mortality, and long birth intervals. The people of Vanatinai, Papua, New Guinea (Lepowsky, this volume), a horticultural people still living in relative isolation from the pressures and social changes wrought by world markets, cash crops, wage labor, and a money economy, have a moderate fertility rate aided by long birth intervals. Under these circumstances parents can allow themselves to invest freely and intensely in each child born. This pattern is also characteristic of traditional hunters and gatherers, such as the !Kung San peoples of the Kalahari desert intensively studied by Konner (1976), Howell (1976), and others.

Under the "old" fertility pattern, characterized by high fertility and brief birth intervals, the cultural representations of the infant and small child may reflect the ubiquitousness of childhood mortality and allow parents a certain emotional distance that is psychologically protective. First among these may be a failure to "anthropomorphize" the infant.[6] The neonate (like the fetus in our abortion-tolerant society) and the infant may be viewed, for example, as not-yet-human creatures on a par with domesticated household pets. The infant's claim to humanity must be proven over time, to some extent by the demonstration of its "wits" to survive. Deformed or physically stigmatized infants may be rejected as malevolent "witch-babies" (Sargent 1982) or as changelings. In rural Ireland up through the 19th century, deformed, sickly, or wasted infants were sometimes killed in the open fireplace or left exposed as "fairy children" (see Scheper-Hughes 1982: 143). Alternatively, frail and sickly infants may be viewed as little angels, trailing clouds of glory and anxious to return to their heavenly home, as is believed in parts of rural Mexico. Such folk beliefs allow parents to conform to situations in which they, in fact, have little control over child mortality. But they also enable parents to decide which among their babies are ill suited for surival, and they undoubtedly contribute to child death in some cases, as several chapters in this volume indicate.

By contrast, the "new" fertility pattern characteristic of modern, industrialized societies is accompanied by a different reproductive strategy: to produce few offspring and to value and invest heavily in each. This strategy is only possible once both childhood mortality and human fertility have been somewhat domesticated and controlled. What is maximized in *this* demographic context is not fertility but parental investment. What parents require of their children has also changed in the modern demographic context. In most traditional, pre-demographic transition societies children are expected to contribute to the economic subsistence of the household. Their value and status within the family are *achieved*, instrumentally-based, and usually increase with age. In the modern, industrialized world the instrumental value of children has been largely replaced by their expressive value. Children have become relatively worthless (economically) to their parents, but priceless in terms of their psychological worth: the pleasure and satisfaction they bring. This transformation carries with it risks as well as benefits to the child. The relatively strong modern ideology that *all* children are wanted and that *all* births should be intentional (given the accessibility of both contraception and abortion) means that children who are "birth control failures" or are otherwise unwanted or inconvenient may be subjected to years of psychological rejection and physical abuse by rejecting parents. By contrast, in traditional societies where individuals have been socialized to believe that fertility is in the hands of God or of fate, this kind of frustration and rage directed at excess or supernumerary children is rare and may account for the relative absence of sadistic and ideosyncratic abuse and battering of children in these societies as compared with modern, industrialized and secular societies.

The contemporary representation of children as an economic liability and burden is also an unfortunate by-product of the child's loss of productive roles in post-industrial societies. The dominant media images of children in the United States as dependent, frivolous, and voracious consumers may contribute both to parental pride in their children and their material possessions as a new form of conspicuous consumption, but may also contribute to parental rage and resentment of their "worthless", "lazy", and "greedy" children. This, in turn, may be expressed in the current "epidemic" of child abuse in North America.

### CHILD TREATMENT AND SURVIVAL

The present volume evolved out of an invited symposium on the cultural, ecological, bio-ethical and applied dimensions of child treatment and survival held at the 1984 meeting of the American Anthropological Association. The goal of the session was the application of a variety of concepts, methods, theories and approaches to understanding cultural practices and individual behaviors that have an adverse effect on child survival.

Since this volume casts the definitional net of "child" and "maltreatment" very widely to include human life from the fetus through adolescence, and practices that are culturally normative as well as those that are deviant, I must begin with a few disclaimers and explanations. First, I do not wish to suggest in the organization of this book any essentialist or universalist criteria for definitions of human life or its value, which must be understood as culturally constructed and historically situated in each instance. *Personhood* and *humanness* exist in the embryo or the fetus [see Potter, this volume], in the premature infant [see Newman, this volume], and even in the toddler [see Cassidy, this volume] as potentials to be recognized and conferred or denied and withheld, according to very different cultural understandings of what these attributes entail. Following from this, the reader should bear in mind that while I use the word "child" throughout this introduction as well as in the title of the volume to refer to the unborn fetus as well as to the neonate and the toddler, I mean only to imply the potentiality and not the actuality of that status. Similarly, reproduction and reproductive "strategy" are also used inclusively here to refer to the entire process that begins with ovulation and continues until the child is no longer dependent on others for survival, which in some instances may last twenty years more.

This volume, then, represents an attempt to situate reproduction, child treatment, and child survival within its broadest possible framework, one that takes into account bio-evolutionary, demographic, economic, moral, political, and ideological *constraints* on individual and collective behaviors toward children. In this way we are better able to pierce the alien logic that informs the traditional and normative practice of infanticide [see chapters in Part II]. Once understood in their specific ecological and cultural context we can distinguish normative forms of child maltreatment from the more deviant and idiosyncratic practices of child battering and sexual abuse [see chapters in Part IV]. The vast difference between allowing certain neonates to die for economic and ecological reasons in an *infanticide-tolerant* society, and the hostile battering of a rejected and disvalued child in an *abortion- and abuse-tolerant* society needs to be recognized and clarified. What first appears as a baffling paradox may be seen as an unfortunate outcome of the demographic transition of advanced industrial societies.

Recently Korbin (1980, 1981) offered a very useful analytic framework for the comparative study of child maltreatment. She suggested the need to sharpen the distinctions between cultural norm and individual pathology, between deviant behavior and survival strategy, between malicious intent and human exigency. In juxtaposing in this volume chapters on abortion and feticide, infanticide and selective neglect with chapters on child battering and incest, I am taking up the challenge posed by Korbin.

In this regard it is important to understand that in much of the traditional world (as in pre-modern Europe) infanticide is practiced as a form of post-partum abortion, in other words, as family planning. As such, the practice tends to be reserved for the neonate. Devereux (1967) prefers the term "neonaticide" as a more correct and less prejudicial term than infanticide. Neonaticide may be motivated by fear or by a concern to protect other vulnerable family members, especially other children and dependent elders in overpopulated households. In much of the contemporary world today the traditional practice of direct infanticide is proscribed by law, by religious authority, or both. The same end-point is reached, albeit more gradually, in the semi-covert practice of selective or "benign" neglect (Scrimshaw 1978; Cassidy 1980). A withdrawal of care and attention is generally sufficient to kill an infant or young child in poorer and tropical areas of the world, where many natural threats to child survival abound and where a constant parental vigilance is necessary to keep infants and toddlers alive. Marvin Harris (1977: 5) refers to selective neglect as passive infanticide. In keeping with this view I would classify as "infanticide-tolerant" those segments of contemporary societies in North India (Miller, this volume), Mexico (Mull and Mull, this volume), and Northeast Brazil (Scheper-Hughes, this volume) in which the gradual wasting away and death of certain infants is not identified as a social problem, nor are aggressive (or public) efforts made to rescue the vulnerable children or to chastise their parents. It is important to note that passive infanticide is difficult to recognize and identify, since it rarely exists apart from other, more "natural" threats to the child's survival (infectious disease, poor sanitation, inadequate diet, etc.). In addition, passive infanticide and selective or benign neglect involve neither direct violence nor hostility toward the child. Rather, parental expressions of *pity* for the inadequate or super-numerary infant often predominate. Parental implication in the death of their infants involves, in this case, acts of omission, rather than acts of commission, such as failing to note or respond to signs of malnutrition, dehydration and other serious threats to survivability. Deaths from selective neglect are gradual and always compounded with other exogenous causes.

While selective neglect is common in many pockets of the traditional world, what is altogether rare in pre-industrialized, "infanticide-tolerant" societies is the "classic" pattern of child abuse found in near endemic proportions in the industrialized world: the so-called battered child syndrome (Kempe *et al.* 1962). Child battering is generally done by punitive, extremely exacting and overly-controlling parents for whom the boundaries between discipline and abuse are blurred. Rejection of the child and resentment of his or her dependency and demands by emotionally immature parents can also lead to a sadism and cruelty toward the child bordering on torture. Ironically, such psychologically primitive behaviors seem to be an artifact of "advanced" industrialized societies and of western civilization. Several contributors to Korbin's volume (1981), for example, deny the existence of intentional and malicious forms of child abuse in the societies in which they conducted their research. Child battering was said to be extremely rare or absent entirely in New Guinea (Langness 1981: 26), in sub-Saharan Africa (LeVine and LeVine 1981: 38), in native South America (Johnson 1981: 58), in rural Turkey (Olson 1981: 96), and in modern Japan (Wagatsuma 1981: 120). Although reliable statistical data on the incidence and prevalence of child abuse is lacking for these societies except for Japan, the ethnographic evidence is quite telling, and the relative absence of child battering in the traditional world warrants further examination. Such research might cast light on the culture-bound dimensions of child battering in western and industrialized societies.

By contrast, what has all but disappeared in the context of "modern" and industrialized societies is the *normative* practice of direct or indirect infanticide which is regarded as highly *deviant*, indeed criminal, behavior constituting sure grounds for the termination of parental rights and the removal from the home of any other "at risk" children (*see* chapters by Handelman and by Hughes, this volume). If direct and indirect infanticide is a means of post-partum family planning in the non-western and traditional world, its counterpart in the "modern" and industrialized world is abortion. It is essential that these two practices (infanticide and feticide) be viewed as analogous and continuous – as methods of fertility control under different cultural and historical contexts characterized by different levels of medical technology. In technologically simple societies abortion is wasteful (save in the most dire circumstances), since without the appropriate technology and in the absence of antibiotics it frequently claims the lives of *both* mother and child, and this accounts for the "preference" for direct and indirect infanticide there. Meanwhile, in the United States today about one in every three fetuses is terminated by surgical intervention (*Statistical Abstracts of the United States*, 1984, cited by Potter, this volume). With the exception of "right to life" advocates (*see* Luker 1984), most U.S. citizens are neither shocked nor morally outraged by the normative practice of feticide in North American society. Sensibilities have been blunted by the cultural redefinitions of the nature and meaning of human life, personhood and individual rights, and by changes in women's roles and social status over the past few decades (*see* Petchesky 1984).

While some vestiges of passive infanticide remain in otherwise inexplicable cases of "failure-to-thrive" infants, some of whom die despite repeated rescue by child protection workers and physicians, it is clear that the emerging new threat to child survival and well-being in industrialized societies today is posed by intentional child abuse. Child battering and psychological abuse differ from passive infanticide and selective neglect in apparent motivation, social cause, expressive content, and outcome. While child abuse is certainly influenced (as is passive infanticide) by such external contingencies as economic status, household demography and composition, employment, etc., much of it cannot be explained in solely instrumental terms. Whereas infanticide, abortion, and even gradual "selective neglect" often entail a failure to recognize the fetus or the child as a human *person*, malicious child battering and other forms of child *abuse* are energized by a malicious, sadistic, and/or envious rejection of the child *as child*. In terms of the relative damage, death is only rarely the outcome for abused and battered children. The abused child in contemporary society grows up and lives, often carrying within the scars of that early experience, only to pass on the damage wrought to the next generation. While I would not want to suggest that all abused children grow up to abuse their own offspring (and, indeed, there is a good deal of evidence to the contrary) there is more to learn about the long-term effects of cruelties experienced in childhood on individual and collective ideologies, political conceptions, and world views in adults, including attitudes toward militancy, authoritarianism, and the use and abuse of power (see, for example, Suarez-Orozco, this volume). In developmental terms, we can as yet only imagine the pernicious effects of childhood scars afflicted by cruel and abusive parents on adult generativity in its broadest dimensions, including the work of "world protection, world-preservation, and world-repair" (Ruddick 1980: 346).

The chapters of this book are organized into five sections. The chapters in *Part I* examine child survival in light of the macro-level processes of population demography, "modernization" pressures, and the increasing role of the state in monitoring and controlling reproduction. We open with Sulamith Potter's astute and sensitive account of changes in state policy regarding the control of fertility in the People's Republic of China, based on original fieldwork in Zengbu Brigade, Guangdong Province, from 1979 to 1983. Potter explores two culturally valued forms of reproductive logic currently in contention: the traditional, but ultimately self-destructive, prolific fertility fostered by Chinese familism versus the new socialist logic of central planning which depends on the state's ability to curtail population growth, especially in rural areas. Three successive state policies and peasant reactions to them have produced a process of negotiated social change with both positive and hopeful potentials for Chinese parents and the health and well-being of their children. The chapter shows the limitations of applying the American rhetoric of "pro-life"/"pro-choice" to a non-western context in which neither of these ideological positions has any cultural relevance.

The chapter by Harkness and Super explores some of the potential ill-effects of "modernization" on the health and survival of children in rural Kenya, where a decrease in childhood mortality has been accompanied by an alarming increase in fertility, so that Kenya's 4% annual rate of increase (i.e., births minus deaths) ranks first in the world, and is the highest ever recorded for a single country (Mott and Mott 1980: 4). Based on ethnographic and demographic data from a rural Kipsigis community, the authors describe the socio-cultural changes – especially the adoption of bottle-feeding – that have led to a reduction in birth spacing. The new household demography of more and closely spaced children represents an emerging threat to child health, development, and survival there.

Lepowsky's analysis of the possible ecological functions of childhood food taboos on a remote island in Papua New Guinea hints at the kind of cultural arithmetic of balanced risks that may be involved in evolutionary adaptiveness for group survival. She suggests that the traditional proscription of protein foods to children under weaning age on the island of Vanatinai contributes to prevalent mild to moderate malnutrition but may also be a cultural adaptation to endemic malaria. In this particular instance (and by implication, perhaps elsewhere in the tropics as well) toddler malnutrition may actually function, in the long run, to *enhance* child survival.

The contributions to *Part II* of this volume explore the *traditional* and *normative* practices of active and passive forms of infanticide directed at particularly disvalued offspring, including costly and supernumerary female infants in patrilineal villages of rural North India (Miller) and certain sickly and deformed babies among the Tarahumara Indians of Mexico (Mull and Mull). While the practice of selective infanticide can be seen as a rational reproductive strategy designed to promote individual or group, biological or social "fitness" (*see* Dickeman 1979; Hausfater and Hrdy, eds. 1984; Trivers and Willard 1973) the more humanist and critical perspectives of the authors in this volume question the economic, ideological and political sources of the deselection process, as it were. What social institutions and cultural norms support selective infanticide, and in whose interests? Often, as in the case of North India, class, caste, or clan interests, gender hierarchies and other powerful interest groups and ideologies influence maternal behavior and responses to certain classes of infants. Understanding the instrumental sources and the cultural logic of infanticide in traditional societies need not lead to a social or political position of accepting it as morally correct or inevitable, but as the authors point out here, outside intervention on behalf of "saving" disvalued children may lead to long-term psychological abuse and other forms of maltreatment, once the child returns to his or her community.

While the chapters in *Part II* examine normative practices of institutionalized child maltreatment in relatively normal circumstances, the chapters in *Part III* look at forms of child maltreatment that appear to be the result of social trauma, including extreme poverty and deprivation, rapid culture change and cultural disintegration, and the catastrophe of famine. It is important not to confuse poverty and the unfortunate survival strategies of parents caught up in altogether desperate straits with malicious and intentional child abuse. Among the "external pressures" having an adverse effect on patterns of child treatment, Korbin earlier (1981: 5–7) identified social disorganization, the breakdown of traditional support systems, rapidly changing circumstances, and confusion about conflicting models available for childrearing. Each of the chapters included in *Part III* exemplify case studies of the effects of social trauma on patterns of child care and child survival.

Newman's longitudinal study of premature infants born to "premature" teenage mothers in Providence, Rhode Island identifies a genealogy of risk. High risk mothers (de-skilled, poor and poorly nourished, socially isolated, high school drop-outs) give birth to high risk infants (premature, low birth weight, often with multiple congenital and other abnormalities). These babies remain at high risk throughout childhood of greater morbidity and mortality, and of severe child abuse and neglect.

De Vries and Scheper-Hughes both note that biological constitution and infant temperament seem to play an important role in mothers' decisions to care or not care for their children in conditions of extreme scarcity or famine. If de Vries' analysis of Masai child survival lends support to the old folk adage that the "squeaky wheel gets the grease," then Scheper-Hughes' analysis of Northeast Brazilian child survivors similarly indicates that the feisty, the difficult, and the demanding infant and toddler may be favored by parents in situations in which differential treatment of children is sometimes necessary.

Finally, the contribution to this section by Hauswald documents the effects of rapid social change, cultural disintegration, and social disruption on the dynamics of Navajo family life and child rearing. Native Americans in the United States and Canada suffer disproportionately from alcoholism, depression, and suicide, all of which are related in one way or another to the death of their cultures (see Brody 1971). Alcoholism is a major cause of illness, injury, and general misery among native Americans contributing to their high rates of unemployment, low incomes, domestic violence, and a high incidence of identified child neglect, which Hauswald's case study illustrates for the Navajo, a people traditionally known for their benevolence toward, and love of, children.

This distinction between traditional patterns of child tending and distortions produced by social disorganization is again useful as we look at the contributions to *Part IV* of this volume on *deviant* and *malicious child abuse*. The traditional and nomadic Inuit of western Canada, discussed by Graburn, are a people who, like so many other Native North Americans, are characterized by their indulgent and extremely nurturant child rearing practices. Nonetheless, Graburn identified a traditional *but extremely rare and deviant* variant of the "battered child syndrome" (sometimes leading to the death of the child) that tended to occur in low status and somewhat marginal Inuit families and which was directed against socially inept or mentally disadvantaged children who were likely to compromise the family's already damaged prestige and ranking in the community. This idiosyncratic (but traditional) form of Inuit child abuse is to be distinguished from the more contemporary and all too common problem of severe child neglect in those *urban* and acculturated Inuit families suffering (like the Navajos, above) from social and cultural disorganization, personal alienation, poverty, unemployment and alcoholism.

The powerful chapter by Suarez-Orozco on state-sponsored and politically motivated child abuse during the Argentine "Dirty War" illustrates the dangerous and frightening end-point that can be reached when the state takes an increasingly active role in the surveillance of private, domestic life and recognizes its stake in the active "socialization" of its future soldiers and citizens.

To date, anthropological contributions to understanding child abuse (see Korbin, ed. 1981) have tended to focus on the difficulty of identifying and labeling child abuse cross-culturally. Cultures and subcultures obviously differ with respect to child rearing and discipline, the status and roles of the child at various ages, the distribution of rights *in* and *over* children, and in the recognition of the rights *of* children. Child rearing practices that might look very much like child abuse to the outside observer can often be found to make sense in the larger ecological, social and cultural context in which they are embedded. The early anthropological studies of comparative child socialization (*see*, for example, Cohen, ed. 1961; DuBois 1944; Erikson 1950; Mead 1935; Whiting and Child 1953) tended to stress the adaptiveness of the practices *and the resilience* of the child. The routine administering of severe beatings, harsh and frightening initiation rites, and normative practices of informal fosterages, child swapping, and multiple mothering have tended to be defended by anthropologists, beginning with Mead's description of weak mother-to-child attachments in the Samoan family (1928) up through Carol Stack's (1974, 1975) studies of child swapping in poor urban black communities in the United States. Only very recently have anthropologists begun to question the "goodness" and "just rightness" of such normative practices for the child, although their adaptiveness for the parents and other adults remains undisputed.

Sexual practices between adults and children in "primitive" and "exotic" cultures are another case in point. It was once the hallmark of an enlightened, liberated, and post-Victorian cultural anthropology to celebrate the "sexual lives of savages" (Malinowski 1929), including such exotic practices as infant betrothal and child marriage, the sexual initiation of young boys by their mothers or by older males, and male and female genital surgery and, in some cases, genital mutilation. Anthropologists adopted an attitude at once sophisticated and cosmopolitan, but also rather cavalier toward the uses to which the docile bodies of non-western children were sometimes subjected.

In this regard, Korbin's excellent overview of the problem of child sexual abuse in cross-cultural perspective, and Jean LaFontaine's analysis of incest cases in England (both in this volume) provide an important and convention-breaking step in the direction of correcting anthropological blindness, in the guise of an inappropriate ethical relativism, toward flagrant violations of power relations between adults and children in sexual behavior. Nonetheless, I would add a note of caution with respect to Korbin's exclusive focus on the exploitation of childhood sexuality by adults and her lack of attention to the destruction and repression of sexuality in childhood by cultural ideologies and child rearing tactics that are hostile and punitive toward various expressions of human sexuality (see Foucault 1978; Rubin 1984; Scheper-Hughes 1979; Vance, ed. 1984).

Insofar as the chapters in this volume were selected to present a diversity of anthropological approaches to and perspectives on the question of child treatment and survival, it should not be surprising that there is little agreement among these authors on the meanings, causes, and consequences of those practices that appear to affect adversely child development or survival. However, there *is* considerable agreement with respect to cautiousness in prescribing solutions or intervening on behalf of those children perceived as "at risk". The reluctance to prescribe, along with a tendency to criticize well-intentioned but misguided interventions, is not born of the scholar's natural disinclination to action, but rather from an informed understanding of the complexities of social life and of the sociogenic side-effects of a sometimes self-serving altruism. Taken together, the chapters in this volume are not so much pessimistic as they are cautious about intervention.

Several chapters in the early sections of the book raise questions about intervention. Child rescue cannot take place in a social and cultural vacuum. Miller shows, for example, that although intensive home-based visiting by health workers in the rural Punjab can reduce the number of female child deaths, such intensive public surveillance of domestic life is ethically questionable, and it cannot insure that the quality of girls' lives saved will be in any way equal to that of male children. Rather, unwanted girls may grow up to be abandoned young women, without dowries and without social support. Scheper-Hughes intervened once in the Brazilian shantytown to save the life of "Ze," and although that tale had a relatively happy ending, she decided never again to play God if she could not promise to support the life of the rescued child and his mother ever after.

An altogether similar fate seems to await those premature babies rescued by prenatal intensive care units in the United States, exemplified in Newman's case study in this volume. Although an extremely aggressive, team-oriented medical intervention can give premature, low birth weight infants a tenuous hold on life, denied such infants in most parts of the nonindustrialized world, it is debatable whether this advanced technology represents a modern medical miracle or another form of medical iatrogenesis. Newman's study indicates that such infants remain at high risk throughout childhood of illness, injury, accidents, and severe child abuse and neglect. The new biomedical mandate – a duty to survive – may mean the continuation into another generation of what Newman calls a "high risk, high risk spiral," another variant of the vicious cycle of poverty, poor nutrition, negative life chances, limited education, teenage pregnancy and maternal rejection and deprivation. The medical rescue is indifferent to the social conditions to which the often unwanted infant is returned: an environment filled with future risk and rejection.

*Part V* brings together the concerns of many of the contributors to this volume with respect to the dilemma of "child saving", a particular preoccupation of altruistic middle class North Americans. The section opens with the thorny issue of toddler malnutrition, certainly one of the greatest of childhood pathogens in the so-called Third World.

The child survival campaign presently being waged by the United Nations Children's Fund (UNESCO) as part of the World Health Organization's proposal to achieve "health for all by the year 2000" offers a case in point. During the 1950s, international development agencies promised that the "Green Revolution" would put an end to world hunger, ending the specter of childhood malnutrition in the Third World. Thirty years later international agencies are promising a "child survival revolution" based on the promulgation throughout the developing world of a simple, low-cost, lifesaving technology: mass-produced sachets of prepackaged salts to be used in preventing and treating childhood diarrhea, a major killer of small children in the tropics. Oral Rehydration Therapy (ORT) is the new magic bullet that is expected to save millions of babies and toddlers each year (Mull 1984). This kind of salvage mentality is, however, counter-intuitive to the thinking and practices of many Third World parents, who may perceive some of their babies as "wanting to die", and other babies as better off had they never been born.

Hence, despite premature announcements that the child survival revolution is underway (UNICEF 1985), and despite decades of the Green Revolution, the dominant image of the Third World child today is still the patient, expressionless, ageless face of the famine-ravaged African toddler. The chapters in the earlier parts of this volume indicate that while ORT might be able to avert a crisis of diarrhea-caused dehydration, salt packets are not breastmilk, nor are they a sufficient substitute for weaning food, clean water, attentive care, adequate housing, fair wages, free and available education and health care, and sexual equality, all of which are prerequisites for optimum child health, development, and survival. Taken together, the chapters by Lepowsky, Miller, Mull and Mull, De Vries, and Scheper-Hughes indicate the short-sightedness of technological fix thinking with respect to the complexities of child survival. These chapters belie any false promises of a child survival revolution that is not embedded in the context of a larger social, economic, and demographic revolution that can change the condition of the lives of those parents to whom the rescued – but still often supernumerary – child is returned.

Certainly Claire Cassidy's contribution to the discussion of child saving in *Part V* offers the most controversial recommendations insofar as her radical noninterventionist stance is informed by an evolutionary and bio-ecological perspective that borders on the socio-biological. Cassidy challenges North American "change agents" and development specialists with some clear cultural biases that need to be unmasked and then questioned. She notes, for example, that U.S. AID interventions on behalf of famine victims in the Third World tend to favor the needs of infants and toddlers over those of older children, and the needs of children over those of adults. This is a sound observation, with implications worthy of further exploration. However, I remain troubled by an analysis based on a free market model of population demography predicated on an assumption that childhood mortality is a bio-ecological mechanism for enhancing group survival through "pruning". Cassidy's argument is reminiscent of the kind of triage thinking so favored by the radical human ecologists such as Hardin (1974) and Erlich (1968). While Cassidy is correct in noting the resonances between the world views of some bio-ecologists and some Third World parents, both of whom agree, on a very superficial level of comparison, that it is best to allow some infants and toddlers to die, this kind of reproductive logic is the logic of the battlefield, the logic of the concentration camp, the logic that informs Hardin's "lifeboat ethics" (1974: 561). The problem is that poverty, scarcity, and famine are not natural phenomena subject to natural solutions, they are, for the most part, man-made catastrophes and therefore the social conditions that produce them can be changed. The malnourished and dehydrated infants and toddlers discussed throughout this volume are as much the victims of human greed and of international relations of production and distribution as they are of "natural" disasters. While Cassidy's arguments against mindless altruistic interventions (such as the "We are the Children" rock star extravaganza) are well taken and need to be critically discussed, there are also moral limits to radical non-intervention as well.

The remaining chapters in *Part V* question the adequacy of interventions by medical and social work professionals on behalf of abused and neglected children in the United States and Canada. With the development of every new field – and child abuse represents one such case – it is essential to examine the key concepts, generalizations, and theoretical orientations in use for their possible cultural or class bias. This is especially so in pluralistic societies where family structure, values, and socialization practices may vary considerably across class, region, and ethnic group. To date, for example, epidemiological surveys indicate that child abuse is particularly common in certain strata of society in industrialized countries. More of it has been identified in poor, single-parent, welfare-recipient, and cultural minority families. But are these findings an artifact of sampling or of cultural misunderstanding and misidentification, or are they the result of the greater surveillance and mistrust of poor, socially disadvantaged, and minority parents? Conversely, are they a manifestation of the differential stresses to which these families are exposed? These are crucial questions for clinicians, lawyers, social workers, and child care teachers who must deal on a daily basis with the identification of and intervention in suspected cases of abuse and neglect. But these questions are of equal concern to social and behavioral scientists wanting to understand the nature of parent-child interactions and their consequences for child health, development and well-being.

The final chapters by Krantzler, Scheper-Hughes and Stein, Handelman, and Hughes treat, in various ways, the problem for medical and child welfare professionals of identifying and intervening in cases of suspected child abuse. Taken together (along with the frightening chapter by Suarez-Orozco in *Part IV*) these contributions point to the risks and dangers involved in aggressive state, bureaucratic, and professional interventions in private and domestic life. Scheper-Hughes and Stein try to situate the current child abuse "panic" in the United States within its particular psycho-cultural and historical context, arguing that this "master" social problem of the late 20th century is constructed, in part, from collective and largely unconscious representations and fantasies that express a good deal of ambivalence toward reproduction and children. The current mood of toughness toward suspected child abusers serves to mask the more collective social responsibility for childhood poverty, morbidity and mortality in the United States. Furthermore, this punitive attitude plays into the unfortunate kind of victim blaming that Krantzler, Handelman, and Hughes discuss in their analyses of the mismanagement of suspected child abuse offenders.

Krantzler discusses a case in which a famous Samoan-Hawaiian healer's treatment of his daughter's diabetes is misconstrued by socially incompetent professionals as evidence of child neglect. This example of rather gross cultural insensitivity is reminiscent of an article that appeared in the *Journal of the American Medical Association* co-authored by three physicians describing the traditional treatment of the folk pediatric disorder, *caida de mollera* (fallen fontanelle) by Mexican-American *curanderas* as a "variant of the battered child syndrome" insofar as the child is turned upside down and his or her head dipped in hot water (*see* Guarnaschelli, Lee and Pitts 1972).

Handelman documents the often perverse way in which a "case" of suspected child abuse may be constructed against a lower class single mother whose fierce privacy and adamant refusal to be "helped" by social welfare professionals is the main evidence against her. Finally, Hughes discusses, from the experience and perspective of a Child Protective Services worker, the conflicts between "cultural rights" and "children's rights" in child welfare legislation and in day-to-day case management. Based on an analysis of the management of three suspected cases of child abuse and neglect in three different cultural and social settings in the United States, Hughes suggests ways in which applied anthropologists might collaborate with child welfare workers and agencies in making culturally informed and appropriate interventions.

## CONCLUSIONS

In this introduction I have tried to point out some of the common threads that unite the experiences and practices of parents, especially mothers, which bear on child survival in both the "traditional" and the "modern" world. Perhaps encoded in these pages, and in the pages that follow, is a morality tale for our times. Morality and societies evolve dialectically. On the one hand, the Judeo-Christian tradition, which put an end to the practice of direct infanticide in both the western and the non-western world that it ultimately came to dominate, was based on a great moral premise, that of the intrinsic worth and sanctity of every human life. At the same time, however, the same western tradition and civilization fostered patriarchy and other forms of male dominance, enshrined female virginity and marital chastity, and condemned various forms of sexual expression and behavior. In various times and places, western morality has condemned the practices of birth control and abortion, thus consigning a great many women to a less than happy experience of their bodies and reproductive capacities. Insofar as these moral strictures made women prisoners of motherhood, they made many unwanted children prisoners of their own childhood. The gradual lifting of some of these moral strictures in the late 20th century has enhanced female reproductive autonomy and should prevent at least some child maltreatment. At the very least, abortion is a more humane practice of family planning than infanticide and gradual selective neglect.

The accumulated wisdom of the historians and the anthropologists of childhood is that it is impossible for all parents at all times to love and nurture all their children. As Dinnage (1978: 38) has noted in this regard:

Children are weak; and the weak get hurt; and where there is hurting there are also lies, hypocrisy, rationalizations, the claim that the victim is not really human or is being hurt for his own good.

One of the greatest of these lies and self-deceptions is the denial of collective social responsibility for the welfare of parents and their children. Infanticide, selective neglect, and child battering are not in the final analysis the problems of certain demented individuals suffering from a cancer of the soul. The problems are usually social and institutional, as much as they are individual and psychological. Due to structural inequalities in the world economic order there is an imbalance in resources and in the relationships between fertility and childhood mortality. The greatest threat to child survival in the world today is the poverty of Third World mothers. The abusive and infanticidal acts of parents are often the end-products of abusive and infanticidal social structural, economic, and political relations. But this analysis awaits another time, another volume.

### ACKNOWLEDGMENTS

This chapter benefited greatly from a careful and critical reading by Eugene Hammel, and from the copy editing and helpful suggestions of Grace Buzaljko.

## NOTES

1. The high pressure demographic regimes characterized by a high fertility and high mortality that lead to the precarious balance described here may only have come into existence after the introduction of agriculture and sedentism, later intensified by the spread of labor intensive (and generally exploitative) economies from feudalism through industrial capitalism.
2. Gene Hammel suggests that while the reconstruction of these data is difficult it is not altogether impossible. Family reconstruction studies provide information on childhood mortality for France, Italy, and Germany from the 17th century onward.
3. See Peter Wright, 'Babyhood: The Social Construction of Infant Care as a Medical Problem,' in M. Lock and D. Gordon, eds. *Knowledge and Practice in Medicine* (Dordrecht, Netherlands: D. Reidel, in press); David Armstrong, *Political Anatomy of the Body* (Cambridge, England: Cambridge University Press, 1983: 54–63).
4. However, the military requirements of emerging nation States in Europe sometimes led to a public interest in keeping infant and chilhood mortality low. Austrian military surgeons were dismayed by the consequences of induced abortion in Croatia and elsewhere in Austria. (Gene Hammel, personal communication.)
5. See, for example, the following sources: H. Ware, 'The Relationship Between Infant Mortality and Fertility: Replacement and Insurance Effects,' *Proceedings of the International Population Conference* **1**: 205–225, 1977; *Infant and Early Childhood Mortality in Relation to Fertility Patterns*, World Health Organization, Geneva, 1980; A. Chowdhury, A. Khan, and L. Chen, 'The Effects of Childhood Mortality Experiences on Subsequent Fertility,' *Population Studies* **30**: 249–261, 1976.
6. In a fascinating unpublished paper, O.W. James refers to "illegitimate anthropomorphization" in infant development, by which he means the projection by parents (especially mothers) of such uniquely human attributes as the capacity for conscious intention, self-reflection, self-awareness, and human agency *to their infants*. It is coined "illegitimate" insofar as infants must *learn* to experience themselves and others as possessors of such uniquely human traits; they do not possess them at birth or in the early months of life. Under conditions of scarcity and high childhood mortality (such as existed among the mothers James studied in a community in northwest Ecuador), mothers are far less likely to "personalize" the neonate by attributing intentions and human meanings to its kicks, cries, facial expressions, and utterances. Nor are they likely to "personalize" and anthropomorphize the infant by recognizing in it its father's nose, its grandmother's mouth, and other physical attributes. James concludes that "to make either of these investments of the self, when there is such a danger that these projections and identifications of the mother will sicken and die, would be to court an intense experience of loss, and of emotional pain. Even to regard the infant as possessing human characteristics might be considered as risking a hurtful setback in these circumstances" (O.W. James, 'Diminished Maternal Anthropomorphization of Infant Behaviours in a Society with a High Infant Mortality Rate: Patterns of Mother-Infant Interaction in Northwest Ecuador,' unpublished paper, June 1980, 1, Dawson Place, London, W2, England.)
7. See Sheila B. Kamerman, 'Eight Countries: Cross-National Perspectives on Child Abuse and Neglect,' *Children Today* **4**: 34–37, 1975; 'Child Abuse, Neglect, and the Family Within a Cultural Context,' Special Issue of *Child Abuse and Neglect*, February 1978; Lesli Taylor and Eli H. Newberger, 'Child Abuse in the International Year of the Child,' *New England Journal of Medicine* **301**(22): 1205–1212, 1979.

## REFERENCES

Ainsworth, Mary
    1967 Infancy in Uganda: Infant Care and the Growth of Love. Baltimore: John Hopkins Press.

Aries, Philippe
   1962 Centuries of Childhood. New York: Vintage.
Armstrong, David
   1983 Political Anatomy of the Body. Cambridge: Cambridge University Press.
Asch, Stuart S.
   1968 Crib Deaths: Their Possible Relationship to Postpartum Depression and Infanticide.
        Journal of the Mt. Sinai Hospital 35: 214–220.
Bowlby, John
   1969 Attachment. New York: Basic Books.
   1973 Loss. New York: Basic Books.
Brody, Hugh
   1971 Indians on Skid Row: The Role of Alcohol and Community in the Adaptive Process of
        Indian Urban Migrants. Ottawa: Northern Science Research Group, Department of
        Indian Affairs.
Cassidy, Claire
   1980 Benign Neglect and Toddler Malnutrition. In L. Greene and F. Johnson (eds.), Social
        and Biological Predictors of Nutritional Status, Physical Growth, and Neurological
        Development, pp. 109–139. New York: Academic Press.
Choudhury, A., A. Khan, and L. Chen
   1976 The Effects of Childhood Mortality Experiences on Subsequent Fertility. Population
        Studies 30: 249–261.
Cohen, Yehudi, ed.
   1961 Social Structure and Personality: A Casebook. New York: Holt, Rinehart, and Win-
        ston.
Coleman, E.
   1974 L'Infanticide dans le haut Moyen Age. Annales, S.E.C. 29(2): 315–336.
deMause, Lloyd
   1974 The History of Childhood. New York: Psychohistory Press.
Devereux, George
   1967 A Typological Study of Abortion in 350 Primitive, Ancient, and Preindustrial Societies.
        In H. Rosen (ed.), Abortion in America. Boston: Beacon.
Dickeman, Mildred
   1979 Female Infanticide, Reproductive Strategies, and Social Stratification: A Preliminary
        Model. In N. Chagnon and W. Irons (eds.), Evolutionary Biology and Human Social
        Behavior, pp. 321–367. North Scituate, Mass.: Duxbury Press.
Dinnage, Rosemary
   1978 Throwaways. New York Review of Books 25(11): 37–39.
DuBois, Cora
   1944 The People of Alor. 2 volumes. New York: Harper and Row.
Edgerton, Robert
   1981 Foreword. In Jill Korbin (ed.), Child Abuse and Neglect: Cross Cultural Perspectives,
        pp. vii–viii. Berkeley: University of California Press.
Erikson, Erik H.
   1950 Childhood and Society. New York: Norton.
Erlich, Paul
   1968 The Population Bomb. New York: Ballantine.
Foucault, Michel
   1978 The History of Sexuality, vol. 1. New York: Random House.
Fox, Vivian, and Martin H. Quitt, eds.
   1980 Loving, Parenting, and Dying: The Family Cycle in England and America, Past and
        Present. New York: Psychohistory Press.
Guarnaschelli, J., J. Lee, and F. Pitts
   1972 "Fallen Fontanelle" (Caida de Mollera): A Variant of the Battered Child Syndrome.
        Journal of the American Medical Association 222(12): 1545–1546.

Hansen, Elizabeth de G.R.

1979 "Overlaying" in 19th Century England: Infant Mortality or Infanticide? Human Ecology 7(4): 333–352.

Hardin, Garrett

1974 Living on a Lifeboat. BioScience 24(10): 561–568.

Harris, Marvin

1977 Cannibals and Kings: The Origins of Culture. New York: Vintage.

Hausfater, Glenn, and Sara Hrdy

1984 Infanticide. New York: Aldine.

Howell, Nancy

1976 The Population of the Dobe !Kung. New York: Academic Press.

Imhof, Arthur E.

1985 From the Old Mortality Pattern to the New: Implications of a Radical [change] From the Sixteenth to the Twentieth Century. Bulletin of the History of Medicine 59: 1–29.

Johnson, Orna

1981 The Socioeconomic Context of Child Abuse and Neglect in Native South America. In Jill Korbin (ed.), Child Abuse and Neglect: Cross-Cultural Perspectives, pp. 56–70. Berkeley: University of California Press.

Kellum, B.

1974 Infanticide in England in the Late Middle Ages. History of Childhood Quarterly 1(3): 367–388.

Kempe, C. Henry, *et al.*

1962 The Battered Child Syndrome. Journal of the American Medical Association 181: 17–24.

Konner, Melvin

1976 Maternal Care, Infant Behavior, and Development Among the !Kung. In R.B. Lee and I. De Vore (eds.), Kalahari Hunter-Gatherers, pp. 219–245. Cambridge, Mass: Harvard University Press.

Korbin, Jill, ed.

1981 Child Abuse and Neglect: Cross-Cultural Perspectives. Berkeley and Los Angeles: University of California Press.

Langer, William

1974 Infanticide; A Historical Survey. History of Childhood Quarterly 1: 353–365.

Langness, L.L.

1981 Child Abuse and Cultural Values: The Case of New Guinea. In Jill Korbin (ed.), Child Abuse and Neglect: Cross-Cultural Perspectives, pp. 13–34. Berkeley and Los Angeles: University of California Press.

LeVine, Robert

1974 Parental Goals: A Cross-Cultural View. Teacher's College Record 76(2): 226–239.

1977 Child Rearing as Cultural Adaptation. In H. Leideman, S. Tulkin, and A. Rosenfeld (eds.), Culture and Infancy, pp. 15–27. New York: Academic Press.

1980 A Cross-Cultural Perspective on Parenting. In M. Fantini and R. Cardenas (eds.), Parenting in a Multicultural Society, pp. 17–27. New York: Longman.

LeVine, Robert, and Sara LeVine

1981 Child Abuse and Neglect in Sub-Saharan Africa. In Jill Korbin (ed.), Child Abuse and Neglect: Cross-Cultural Perspectives, pp. 35–55. Berkeley and Los Angeles: University of California Press.

Luker, Kristen

1984 Abortion: The Politics of Motherhood. Berkeley: University of California Press.

MacDonald, Michael

1982 Mystical Bedlam: Madness, Anxiety, and Healing in Seventeenth-Century England. Cambridge: Cambridge University Press.

McKee, Lauris

1984 Child Survival and Sex Differentials in the Treatment of Children. Medical Anthropology (special issue), 8(2).

McKeown, Thomas
    1976 The Modern Rise of Population. New York: Academic Press.
Malinowski, Bronislaw
    1929 The Sexual Life of Savages. Boston: Routledge and Sons.
Malthus, Thomas R.
    1926 An Essay on the Principle of Population. New York: Macmillan.
Mead, Margaret
    1928 Coming of Age in Samoa. New York: Morrow.
    1930 Growing Up in New Guinea. New York: Morrow.
    1935 Sex and Temperament in Three Primitive Societies. New York: Morrow.
Morantz-Sanchez, Regina
    1985 Sympathy and Science: Women Physicians in America. New York: Oxford University
        Press.
Mott, Frank L., and Susan H. Mott
    1980 Kenya's Record Population Growth: A Dilemma of Development. Population Bulletin
        35: (3): 3–37.
Mull, Dennis
    1984 Oral Rehydration Therapy: An Oasis of Hope in the Developing World. Journal of
        Family Practice 18(3): 485–487.
Olson, Emelie
    1981 Socioeconomic and Psychocultural Context of Child Abuse and Neglect in Turkey. In
        Jill Korbin (ed.), Child Abuse and Neglect: Cross-Cultural Perspectives, pp. 96–119.
        Berkeley: University of California Press.
Petchesky, Rosalind Pollack
    1984 Abortion and Women's Choice. Boston: Northeastern University Press
Phillips, Virginia
    1978 Children in Early Victorian England: Infant Feeding in Literature and Society,
        1837–1857. Tropical Pediatrics and Environmental Child Health (August): 158–166.
Piers, Maria
    1978 Infanticide. New York: W.W. Norton.
Rohner, Ronald
    1974 They Love Me, They Love Me Not: A World-Wide Survey of the Effects of Parental
        Acceptance and Rejection. New Haven: HRAF Press.
Rossi, Alice
    1977 A Biosocial Perspective on Parenting. Daedalus 106(2): 1–32.
Rubin, Gayle
    1984 Thinking Sex: Notes for a Radical Theory of the Politics of Sexuality. In C. Vance (ed.),
        Pleasure and Danger, pp. 267–319. Boston: Routledge and Kegan Paul.
Ruddick, Sara
    1980 Maternal Thinking. Feminist Studies 6: 342–364.
Sargent, Carolyn
    1982 Solitary Confinement: Birth Practices Among the Bariba of the People's Republic of
        Benin. In Margarita Kay (ed.), The Anthropology of Human Birth, pp. 193–210.
        Philadelphia: F.A. Davis.
Sauer, R.
    1978 Infanticide and Abortion in Nineteenth-Century Britain. Population Studies 32(1):
        81–94.
Scheper-Hughes, Nancy
    1979 Breeding Breaks Out in the Eye of the Cat: Sex Roles, Birth Order, and the Irish
        Double-Bind. Journal of Comparative Family Studies 10(2): 207–226.
    1982 Saints, Scholars, and Schizophrenics: Mental Illness in Rural Ireland. Berkeley    Los
        Angeles: University of California Press.

1984 The Margaret Mead Controversy: Culture, Biology and Anthropological Inquiry. Human Organization 43(1): 85–93.

Scrimshaw, Susan
  1978 Infant Mortality and Behavior in the Regulation of Family Size. Population Development Review 4: 383–403.

Shorter, Edward
  1975 The Making of the Modern Family. New York: Basic Books.

Stack, Carol
  1974 All Our Kin. New York: Harper and Row.
  1975 Who Raises Black Children? In T. Williams (ed.), World Anthropology, Netherlands: Mouton.

Tonkin, S.
  1975 SIDS: Hypothesis of Causation. Pediatrics 55(5): 650–661.

Trexler, R.
  1973 Infants in Florence: New Sources and First Results. History of Childhood Quarterly 1: 98–116.

Trivers, R.L., and D.E. Willard
  1973 Natural Selection of Parental Ability to Vary the Sex Ratio of Offspring. Science 179: 90–92.

UNICEF (United Nations Children's Fund)
  1985 The State of the World's Children 1985. Oxford: Oxford University Press.

Vance, Carol, ed.
  1984 Pleasure and Danger: An Introduction. In C. Vance (ed.), Pleasure and Danger, pp. 1–28.

Wagatsuma, Hiroshi
  1981 Child Abandonment and Infanticide: A Japanese Case. In Jill Korbin (ed.), Child Abuse and Neglect: Cross-Cultural Perspectives, pp. 120–138. Berkeley: University of California Press.

Ware, Helen
  1977 The Relationship Between Infant Mortality and Fertility: Replacement and Insurance Effects. Proceedings of the International Population Conference, Vol. 1. Belgium: International Union for the Scientific Study of Population.

Whiting, Beatrice, et al.
  1963 Six Cultures: Studies of Child Rearing. New York: John Wiley.

Whiting, John
  1971 Causes and Consequences of the Amount of Body Contact Between Mother and Infant. Paper read at the meetings of the American Anthropological Association, New York, November.

Whiting, John and Irving Child
  1953 Child Training and Personality. New Haven: Yale University Press.

Wright, Peter
  1988 Babyhood: The Social Construction of Infant Care as a Medical Problem. In M. Lock and D. Gordon (eds.), Knowledge and Practice in Medicine. Dordrecht, Netherlands: Reidel (forthcoming).

# PART I

# POPULATION, FERTILITY, AND CHILD SURVIVAL

> Famine seems to be the last, the most dreadful resource of nature.
>
> Malthus, 1803

SULAMITH HEINS POTTER

# BIRTH PLANNING IN RURAL CHINA: A CULTURAL ACCOUNT

The Chinese way of thinking about children is an indirect way and an oblique way. Chinese culture is far from child-centered; perhaps, with its emphasis on the formal importance of caring for the aged, one might argue that it is the very reverse of child-centered. Yet children appear to be the solution to adult problems that the Chinese take very seriously indeed. They are the means to ends which Chinese adults seek after as the thirsty seek for water: they can share the endless work necessary before prosperity can be achieved; if male, they can dignify existence by providing a sense that the family line is being carried on; but most important, they are the solution to the aching problem, "Who will ever take care of me?" In Chinese culture, being a legitimate recipient of care must be deferred until old age, because no care before that time is as valid, or as culturally appropriate, as care provided by the young for the old. By old age, the unfulfilled longing to be taken care of has grown and developed until it clamors on the consciousness, and yet a lifetime of caring for others, and deferring the wish to be cared for one's self, has provided an experience which makes people doubt if they will ever be cared for, or if it is possible to care for them enough. In having children, the Chinese see a solution to their wish for care, rather than the assumption of the responsibility to care for another. The child is born so as to be socialized into a future caretaker for the parent, and having been brought up to this purpose, the child is left with a residue of longing for care which ensures the perpetuation of the system.[1]

In discussing Chinese birth planning policy and implementation, then, the underlying questions are always deeply concerned with children, their cultural meaning, and what it signifies when they are born, or when births are prevented. But in order to discuss these matters in such a way as to convey what they mean in a Chinese context, it is necessary to work indirectly – to consider the importance of the state and of the family, the meaning of marriage, the care of the aged, the force of morality, and the impact of a rapidly changing economic context. These are of direct importance from the Chinese point of view, and the cultural meaning of having a child is integrally related to all of these aspects of Chinese social life.

The purpose of this paper is to describe birth planning in Guangdong Province in the years 1979–1983, and to present a cultural analysis of it. The data on which my analysis is based were gathered jointly by myself and Jack M. Potter during an eight month period of intensive field research in 1979–1980, and in the course of brief return visits in 1981 and 1983. Our field site is Zengbu Brigade, Chashan People's Commune, Dongguan County, Guangdong Province.[2] The focus of attention is on meanings, rather than

*Nancy Scheper-Hughes (ed.), Child Survival, 33–58.*
© *1987 by D. Reidel Publishing Company.*

numbers. Chinese birth planning can only be understood in its cultural context, and their perception of the central dilemmas involved is quite unlike our own. I have made use of explicit comparisons with the American cultural assumptions in order to clarify the striking differences involved.

Because birth planning evokes such highly significant issues, and analysis of it clarifies cultural assumptions, the process of implementing birth planning policy emerges as a drama in which the most deeply held social values are enacted. Social values find their expression in public morality. Villagers in Zengbu believe strongly that they are moral people, acting in a moral society. They believe that the social changes they have witnessed are evolving changes, taking them in the direction of greater social morality, and that the claims of Chinese society in general to be an exemplar of social morality are higher than the claims of any other society. They believe that those who act in opposition to public morality are not acting rightly. They are not open to the potential value of systems or forms of behavior unlike their own; they are not relativists, and they dislike social deviance. When they explain social action, they do it in terms of shared values and social morality. There are two levels of social structure which organize morally valid social action, the government and the family, and these structures themselves take on an intrinsic moral significance. In practical terms, people know that both the family and the government may do harm and be resented, but in terms of ideals and morality, respect for these institutions is a fundamental quality of the social order. The government must have a demonstrable moral legitimacy, and public policy is always presented and explained in moral terms. When policies are changed, or even reversed, the moral justifications for them are modified, and different principles may have the primary emphasis, but a moral justification is always made. The family, being the other important repository of social morality, has associated with it a whole complex of social and behavioral forms that are regarded as appropriate ways to demonstrate moral worth in action. Since the issue of birth planning is so important to the national government and so important to the family, the differing interests of the two levels of structure produce contradictions between two highly valued sets of moral principles.

The central government takes the position that birth planning is not only a practical but also a moral necessity, given China's inordinate population size, the impossibility of meeting the needs of such a population with the resources available, and the human suffering that will inevitably ensue if effective action is not taken at once. This position is explained and supported with statistical evidence so overwhelming that no dissenting interpretation could rationally be brought forward.[3] The central government has been at pains to emphasize the extreme importance of birth planning by labelling it a matter of "strategic significance." This is a culturally encoded political phrase meaning that birth planning is critically important to the safety and continuity of China as a whole, and that it is, in effect, a national security issue. The government's long-term commitment to the implementation of birth planning has also been emphasized, by describing it with the phrase "basic state policy." This phrase sets birth planning in a special category, above the shift and flux of interpretation and implementation that frequently characterize Chinese policy in matters regarded as less fundamental. The phrase defines birth planning as a continuing policy to be enforced over time, rather than a transitory measure. The Chinese government has chosen its strongest expressive language to convey the acuteness of the problem, its devastating implications, and the long range importance of finding an effective solution.

Chinese familism approaches the question of birth planning from a different angle. From the point of view of the family, children are the means of its highly valued continuity, the basis of its prosperity, and the only valid source of interpersonal help and care. The patrilineal Chinese family claims the right to require, with all of the mighty moral force at its command, that young women who marry in produce sons on its behalf. There must be sons, not only daughters, since daughters do not carry lineal continuity, their labor is not defined as equally valuable – in spite of the fact that they can be demonstrated to earn and produce more in Zengbu – and they marry out, to live and work in another family. There must be a large enough number of children to make it seem reasonable that they will be able to care for their parents and grandparents in their old age.

The problem of caring for the aged has two aspects, the aspect of the economic realities, and the aspect of the cultural realities, and the problem cannot be understood without considering both. From a purely economic point of view, Chinese peasants (unlike urban dwellers) have no retirement pensions. (There may be some rare exceptions to this generalization, and a figure as high as 10% for rural communes with pension plans has been quoted,[4] but even allowing for this most optimistic estimate, 90% of peasants are pensionless.) In Zengbu, instituting a pension plan seems less attractive at present than letting each family keep the use of the money that would have to be invested, although it has been discussed; under the present system, the brigade does not have the financial resources to finance a pension plan itself, without requiring contributions for the purpose. It is written into the marriage law of 1983 that all children and grandchildren are responsible for the support of their aging parents and grandparents, both patrilateral and matrilateral. So, both in practice and in law, old peasants depend on their children and grandchildren for support, with no source of support from outside the family.

If there are no children, old peasants may receive the state's "five guarantee" support. In 1979–1980, old people in Zengbu on "five guarantee" support lived in pitiable circumstances, in decrepit dwellings, with barely enough to eat, a tiny allowance of a few yuan a month (3 ¥ = $1) from their teams, and tattered and inadequate bedding. They were dependent on the goodwill of their neighbors for water from the well and fuel to burn. The introduction of the production responsibility system and the weakening of the team could only reduce this already exiguous support system. The inadequacy of the "five guarantee" system is officially recognized, and a provincial level official commented, "We want to intensify our work on this problem." But in any case, the recipients of "five guarantee" support feel humiliated in accepting it, and ashamed of the inability to work which forces them to do so, because being unable to work suggests that one has no right to receive. One old lady said, "I do not like to accept this; I have my conscience, and other people are working hard." It is felt that the only right and appropriate way for the aged to receive care is in their own homes, from their own sons. When Happy Homes for the Aged were tried in Chashan Commune during the Great Leap Forward (1958) they were a failure, and the reason was that the old people were miserable in the role of the recipients of care given by outsiders.

This idea of the appropriate care of the elderly is a cultural construct of the most complex kind: that it *should* happen is taken for granted; when it fails to happen, it is a matter of great sorrow; and the meaning of it, when it does happen, is replete with the expectation of happiness, the burden of obligation, and feelings of ambivalence and despair. The needs of aging parents are great. Indeed, they are conceived of as virtually insatiable. This sense of the insatiability of a parent's needs is traditional, and can be confirmed by reading the *Book of Filial Duty* (trans. Chen, 1909). In this text, a series of sons make superhuman efforts to meet parental needs which have no limits and no end: sometimes they are unable to meet these needs without supernatural aid. Furthermore, the moral force of a parent's needs supersedes all other considerations, however urgent. It is felt that the satisfaction of parents' needs would be impossible without extraordinary human resources. This is why no finite number of sons seems like enough, and the village proverb says, "The more sons, the more happiness." The happiness implied by many sons is a particular kind of happiness, a happiness based on knowing that appropriate care will be provided in one's old age; this is a happiness which signifies an economically secure, culturally approved state of recipient dependence. Children, especially sons, are the means to this most desired end.

The idea of limiting the number of children, or contenting one's self with daughters rather than sons, raises the possibility that in purely practical terms, the aged will not receive their basic needs. At the same time, it raises the possibility of moral failure, a moral failure that would be very deeply felt. In cultural terms, when a family has many children, security and happiness are possible for them, because the manpower and the resources to care for the aged will not fail. But a family with a limited number of children is less likely to find the kind of happiness they seek. If they fail in practical terms, they fail in cultural terms as well, and their sense of security cannot be solidly grounded.

The villagers make the assumption that it is the old, rather than the young, whose need to be cared for is most legitimate, and that the young are the ones who bear the obligation to care for the old. The Western assumption that parents bear an important moral obligation to be a source of security for their children is reversed, and children are thought of as the source of future security for their parents. When one looks at human dependency as dispassionately as possible, it seems clear that care is most needed in childhood and in old age, but in the West, the moral emphasis is on the importance of caring for children, and in China, the moral emphasis is on the importance of caring for the old. Child care is a means to an end, a form of long range self-interest. The contrast between Western and Chinese values can be brought out clearly using literary sources, in the comparison between the *Book of Filial Duty* and the *Pirates of Penzance*. In the *Pirates of Penzance*, even people so lost to conventional morality as pirates nevertheless sympathize with the plight of an orphan, deprived of care by the untimely death of both parents. In the *Book of Filial Duty*, there is an analogous story about a group of bandits. Even these bandits display some remnants of moral decency, however, because they are moved by the plight of a poor old lady who will be left helpless in the world if they kill her only son. In these two stories, the weight of sympathy is distributed analogously, but in opposite directions. To have children is to be protected from the pitiable situation, analogous to being orphaned, of being left without care in one's old age. When villagers speak of having children so that old people may be taken care of, they are invoking a whole complex of cultural ideas embodying a definition of happiness resting on dependent security. This cultural complex is inseparable from the family system itself. In examining this complex, the relationship between family structure and cultural assumption, as they work in an integrated way to become social organization in process, is easily seen.

When an idea exists at the level of a cultural assumption, it exists pervasively, and appears at every level of society. The people who are the central government policymakers are cultural beings and family members, as well as administrators with a clear interest in seeing the importance of national issues, and the interests of the nation as a whole. It is inevitable that central policy will draw on cultural assumptions, and it does so, producing a confusion of direction that tends to affirm the importance of the family point of view, and to weaken, however unintentionally, the stated position of the state. One very clear example of the primacy of culture over political theory is to be seen in the system of production responsibility by households. This system is plainly based on the traditional cultural assumption that the peasant family, with all of its members working together, is a wholesome economic unit likely to produce prosperity. (Chinese history provides considerable evidence that this is not necessarily the case.) Although, in formal terms, the policy comes from the central government, actually, it draws on the assumptions of familism, and is congruent with the belief that more children provide more labor, and thus contribute directly to prosperity. The household responsibility system is a policy that makes population increase appear to be the social solution it traditionally was, rather than the social problem it now is. It has been implemented at a time when the central government is most acutely aware that in the wider context, and from any point of view larger than that of the family, more children, and the cumulative population increase that they imply, nullify hard won economic gains and make prosperity impossible in the long run. So, the central government's overt message stands in opposition to the covert message implied by an economic policy based on the cultural assumptions of traditional familism. The policymakers are the bearers of their own culture, and cannot stand aside from it, in spite of the unambiguous logic of their own analysis of the significance of China's rising population.

Peasants also perceive both points of view simultaneously. However narrowly familistic they may feel inclined to be, they have seen the private plots become smaller over the years, as Zengbu's limited land is redistributed among increasing numbers of villagers. Some villagers have concluded that they should have more children, so that their families can control more of the tiny plots, an involutional solution that intensifies the problem it recognizes and tries to solve. The villagers have seen available house land built over, so that new houses must be built in undesirable outlying locations; the deliberations of the committee that assigns housebuilding land are tense. Everyone can clearly see the intrinsic opposition between the interests of the villagers considered as a whole, the limited resources available, and the legitimate needs of the family as the family understands them. It is plain that these urgently felt needs and interests are incompatible.

In this social context, where the claims of the family and of the government are so pervasive, the private interests of the husband or wife, or of the couple together, have never been regarded as important; indeed, they are scarcely relevant. Marriages in Zengbu are not formed on a basis of personal emotion, and children are not born to provide their parents with emotional fulfillment. An emotional rationale for such important social actions would strike the villagers as flimsy and insubstantial at best, indecent at worst. Rather than emphasizing the relationship between husband and wife, people think of marriage as the taking of a daughter-in-law to help continue the family line, and the husband's parents, rather than the bride and groom, are congratulated at the wedding. Marriage is to create family continuity, and the explicit purpose of marriage is to have children: this is the pattern of human existence. When a child is born, its importance lies in its social relationships. It exists in relation to the family, as one who is carrying on the line, if male, or as one who will help to carry on the line of another family, if female. The child also exists in relationship to society at large, and so the government's interest in births, which is based on the aim of administering morally so as to produce prosperity is understood as a direct and legitimate concern. But a child is not thought of as having validity or importance in isolation from its social context. Social experience is valid experience; isolated experience is insignificant experience. The social aspects of the person are relevant; the separate aspects of the person are not relevant. Valuing a child as a "human life," in isolation from its significance to the family and to society, is a senseless abstraction when considered in terms of Chinese ideas about what it means to be a person.

For these reasons, it is clear that the Chinese do *not* have a concept of birth as legitimately the personal decision of a woman about her body. They are not "pro-choice;" rather, the importance of a birth to levels of society greater than the individual legitimizes the intervention of these levels in the process. It is interesting to make the comparison between Chinese assumptions and the U.S. Supreme Court decision in Roe *v*. Wade, January 22, 1973. According to the decision,

We recognize the right of the individual, married or single, to be free from unwarranted governmental intrusion into matters so fundamentally affecting a person as the decision whether to bear or beget a child. That right necessarily includes the right of a woman to decide whether or not to terminate a pregnancy.

In Chinese thinking, primacy is given to the fact that the birth fundamentally affects the family and the state, and whether it fundamentally affects the person is a less important consideration. By contrast, the U.S. Supreme Court regards the fact that birth fundamentally affects the person as the validation for superseding the claims of the state, and by implication, in the phrase "married or single," of the family as well. Yet, the fact that the Chinese are not "pro-choice" does not at all imply that they are "pro-life." Both the family and the state understand a birth in purely instrumental terms, as it affects the welfare of the family unit or of the polity. The idea of valuing an unborn life in and of itself, without regard for its social significance, is alien and irrelevant in Chinese social thinking. So, the paired opposition, "pro-choice" vs. "pro-life", reflects specifically American cultural concerns. Attempting to impose these categories on Chinese birth planning leads only to misunderstanding.

The people of Zengbu, living a social life based on these assumptions, inhabit a social world in which no normal adult remains unmarried, for the social meaninglessness of single life is unthinkable, and no married couple remains childless by choice, for a childless marriage is a tragic inability to fulfill cultural expectations, rather than a personal sorrow or a private decision. In 1979, when we began to work in Zengbu, these cultural assumption existed in conjunction with the general principles on birth planning formulated by the upper levels, and with specific regulations implemented by the brigade. At this time, birth planning was not yet a matter of strategic significance or a basic state policy, but it had been explained by Chairman Mao, and was clearly understood as a goal of appropriate social change. As Women's Federation leaders from the county level said, "We are instructed by Chairman Mao himself that birth planning is closely connected with the national economy, the Four Modernizations, health, the development of science and culture, and prosperity. It protects women's health, and liberates them from the burden of having too many children. It also protects children's health and education, and helps to nurture them well." In this formulation, the emphasis is primarily in terms of the nation, and secondarily in terms of the people whose exploitation is legitimized by the traditional family system – the women, urged to produce child after child in order to fulfill the wishes of their husbands' parents, and the children, brought into the world as means to the end of the future comfort and satisfaction of others, rather than as beings with important claims or interests of their own. Mao's formulation links the interests of government with the interests of those exploited by the traditional family.

More specifically, policy was, as it had been for several years, to encourage one birth, strictly control second births, and resolutely prevent third births. But this gnomic formula was variously interpreted and implemented by the different levels of government. Furthermore, its significance and implications were quite different in rural and urban areas. It must be remembered that "rural" and "urban" are birth-ascribed statuses belonging to differently organized social and economic sectors of society, and that the distinctions are not merely analytical, but are legally maintained and enforced (Potter, 1983). In urban areas, the policy was implemented as the "one child family." There is not, and has never been, a one child policy implemented in Zengbu. It is solely for urban residents. In rural areas, like Zengbu, policy was filtered through a complex bureaucratic process which produced entirely different regulations. Tracing the different interpretations of policy from level to level demonstrates the kinds of modifications that are made as the policy moves farther from theory and closer to implementation; it also illustrates the extent to which the lower levels are bound, and the extent to which they are free to act independently. Any preconception of Chinese society as a series of subordinate levels carrying out with unthinking obedience the fiats they receive from above is a considerable distortion of Chinese political process.

There were several important regulations bearing on birth planning being implemented in Zengbu at this time. The first of these concerned the required late age of marriage. Peasant men were not permitted to marry until they reached the age of 25, and peasant women until they reached the age of 23, unless hardship could be demonstrated. A legitimate hardship would exist, for example, if the parents of an only son were extremely old and infirm, and could be better cared for with the help of a daughter-in-law. In no case could a marriage take place if the man was younger than 20, or the woman younger than 18. This regulation was not the administrative responsibility of the brigade, but of the Civil Affairs Office at the Commune headquarters, one level up, which issues marriage licenses. According to their figures, 93% of all marriages in the commune were between men over the age of 25 and women over the age of 23. The relationship between this regulation and birth planning is that it tended, in the long run, to reduce population by lengthening the time between generations. It was an acceptable regulation, rather than a hateful one, because it involved no direct intervention, and imposed a wait to bear children, rather than a prohibition. It was consistent with the interests of the families of adult daughters, because these women are prodigious earners in Zengbu, and since their earnings were paid to the head of household, their families retained control of a significant economic contribution. The young women themselves preferred to marry late because the life of a daughter-in-law is indubitably harder and less pleasant than that of an adult daughter.

The brigade level was responsible for enforcing the other regulations affecting birth planning. They received general principles from the higher levels, rewrote them into specific regulations taking "local conditions" into account, and transmitted them to the villagers. "Local conditions" can be decoded as the tremendous pressure of traditional familism to have many children and hope for many sons, and the degree to which this exerts its influence on the brigade's capacity to implement and enforce. The regulations bearing on birth planning in 1979 stated that each married couple in Zengbu Brigade was allowed four births in the attempt to have at least one son without paying any penalty at all. Each child would receive a ration of grain at the artificially low state-supported price of 9.80 ¥ per 100 catties (5.9¢ per pound), rather than having to pay the normal off-ration price of 25 ¥ per 100 catties (16.6¢ per pound). So the rule was actually providing a life long food subsidy to up to four daughters per couple. This rule is in dramatic contrast to the "one child policy" applied in urban areas; when it is remembered that 80% of the Chinese are classified as peasants, the impact of such rules as this is enormous. It is interesting, also, to compare this rule with the position of the Catholic Church in favor of births: the Catholic Church makes a moral case for having children, but it also provides alternatives to marriage, and it does not provide life long food subsidies for up to four children of parishioners under parallel conditions. Such subsidies as this importantly modify the relationship between a family's economic circumstances and a decision to have more children. They reduce the economic deterrents to having children by having society, rather than the family, shoulder the cumulative financial burden, which, in capitalist systems, remains the family's own.

When we expressed surprise at this rule, the women's leader of the brigade, who is the person responsible for birth planning work, said that "local conditions" were an important factor. She added, "If people here were not allowed to try for a son, there would be trouble." If a couple had children after the fourth daughter, or had more than two children including at least one son, these children would not be subsidized, but rice would have to be purchased for them at the unsupported price. Versions of this rule have been misunderstood by the Western press in China because lack of access to a ration of subsidized grain has been interpreted to mean that excess children would receive no grain at all, rather than that they would have access to unsubsidized grain instead. In any case, from the local point of view, the rise in the price of rice for children over the subsidized number was not a deterrent. The women's leader said, "Most families think it is worth it."

Another rule regulated the spacing of births. The first child could follow immediately upon marriage, and almost invariably did. Subsequent children were supposed to be born at intervals greater than four years. If the interval between children was less, grain for the child was to be purchased half at the subsidized price, and half at the unsubsidized price. Such complex compromising rules as this, in which a situation with two aspects (that the child was within the permitted number, but violated the permitted spacing) is dealt with by a regulation with two aspects (grain shall be half subsidized and half not subsidized) are entirely typical of local level administration in Zengbu. There are many parallels to be found: the calculations of payment for work, for example, or the formulae for selling pigs fatter than the required quota to the state. Such rules were also used historically in the distribution of lineage resources. From the point of view of the villagers, these rules are a fair way of dealing with factors that are present simultaneously and have conflicting implications.

In order to make it possible to observe these regulations, it was expected that all couples of childbearing age should practice some form of birth control. The women's leader was responsible for providing birth control supplies to all the married women in the brigade. She knew which methods were used by each of the 701 couples still in their childbearing years in the brigade. The methods were as follows:

| Method | Women | Men | Couples |
|---|---|---|---|
| Pills | 101 | | 101 |
| Sterilization | 19 | 2 | 21 |
| Ring-shaped loops | 424 | | 424 |
| Injections | 3 | | 3 |
| "Own methods" | | | 69 |
| Legitimate non-users | | | |
|   a. Recently married | 57 | | 57 |
|   b. Recently gave birth | 26 | | 26 |
| | | | 701 |

We asked what "their own methods" would mean in practice, and the women's leader replied austerely, "I never asked them." It is most likely that this category includes the methods for which the husband is directly responsible, condoms and withdrawal, about which a women could not appropriately ask; in Zengbu, these matters cannot be discussed between people of opposite sexes.

Abortion was used as a back-up method of birth control if other methods failed, and there were modest incentives – 15 days rest, 30 ¥ ($10), and continued work points while resting – to encourage the use of abortion to end an unplanned pregnancy, rather than letting the child be born by default. If these incentives did not appear sufficiently attractive, the pregnancy could continue, and the penalty would be in the price of rice.

So, birth control methods were a subject of public record. This may be resented as an intrusion inimicable to the family's interests, but it is not thought of using the Western category, "invasion of privacy." It is felt to follow logically from the legitimacy of the state's interest in births. In similar fashion, the husband's parents are felt to be legitimately concerned in a couple's decisions about birth control. For example, one commune level women's leader commented, "If there are only two daughters, the husband's mother will not agree to birth control for the daughter-in-law." This shows clearly how decision making, if it is not in the hands of the state, is in the hands of the family, and not in the hands of the individual. Because the individual interests of the husband and wife are not defined as socially significant in Zengbu, the concept of privacy, which validates these interests in the West, does not exist to be invoked. Indeed, as the distinguished Chinese thinker Zhao Fusan has pointed out in a more general context,[5] the concept of privacy is impossible to translate into Chinese without conveying connotations of crass lack of respect for the needs of others and the claims of society as a whole. Attempts to act on a concept of personal privacy would appear antisocial in a Chinese cultural setting. Since the concept does not exist, it is not present in people's thinking, and when birth planning policy is resented, the resentment is conceptualized in other terms.

As well as being the person to implement policy into practice, the women's leader also had the job of educating people about the importance of birth planning from a more general perspective. She tried to make people see the importance of population control in principle, and urged the villagers to limit themselves to two children. (She herself had had two children, a son and a daughter, and then underwent a tubal ligation.) Her message was generally received as an irksome and uncongenial matter of little practical importance, since it was not enforced; people did not like hearing the subject discussed. They tended to think of her as the personal agent of policy, so she was the recipient of considerable criticism, some silent, and some overt. Since she is herself a villager, extremely concerned with behaving rightly, and finely attuned to the social pressure applied by her fellow villagers, bearing the criticism was a bitter form of labor that was part of the job. It was an added source of difficulty to have one's mother-in-law as one of the silent critics. The women's leader indicated that, should her mother-in-law become a vocal critic, it would be impossible to continue doing the job and also maintain a sense of being a culturally appropriate daughter-in-law. The more vocal critics in 1979 would say things like, "If you want to have just two children yourself, that's fine, but why don't you let other people be, so they can do what they want?" But she defended herself on ethical grounds, affirming that, in her opinion, population control was of first importance to the country as a whole. In her social role as the structural mediator between levels, she was criticized by familistic fellow villagers, and defended her position by citing the importance of the needs of the country. In dealing with the upper levels, she was called upon to state the other point of view, and explain that "local conditions" made it impossible to enforce regulations more stringent than the ones in place. She was unable to satisfy either side with these explanations. She carried out an extraordinarily demanding social role, and in 1979, she carried it out alone. In terms of practical support, and in terms of political emphasis, other issues were regarded as primary. This could be gauged by the attention devoted to birth planning at the Three Level Meeting, a political ritual of affirmation and reintegration which is held twice a year. Leaders of the commune, the brigades, and the teams attend the meeting. People compare the bad old past with their bright hopes for the future, and publicly bear witness to the experience of good which their beliefs have made available to them. (The quasi-religious quality of these meetings cannot be missed.) The Three Level Meeting is also the time for introducing and explaining new policy measures. At the Three Level Meeting in Fall, 1979, birth planning received a single mention in passing on the third and final day, as a state goal which would, it was to be hoped, be achieved successfully in the indeterminate future.In spite of the theoretical importance of birth planning, in political context it was not, in 1979, the central focus of attention it was shortly to become, and no particular resources beyond the personal dedication of women's leaders were allocated to the process of implementation. There was a clear disparity between the formal importance of birth planning, and the actual degree of attention given to it at the local level. It was an issue that local level leaders preferred to handle as little as possible, unless they were required to intervene. In 1979, with "local conditions" being given the greatest consideration, and with the subsidization of four daughters per couple, it was clear that birth planning policy was dramatically pronatal in practice, and that the forces of traditional familism were well in the ascendant.

By June 1980, however, concern with birth planning had intensified, and the brigade put out a new set of regulations. As before, these regulations were formulated in specific terms at the brigade level, on the basis of general principles handed down from above. The regulations were based on economic incentives and penalties which were intended to be more significant than the previous penalties related to the price of rice. The incentives were stated first. Couples who agreed to limit themselves to one child would receive an incentive of 100 ¥ ($67) annually. No couple in the brigade regarded this as a rational choice. The brigade was unable to offer the further incentives that are offered to one-child couples in urban areas, such as special high-quality schooling, free child care, and access to better jobs, because these benefits do not exist in the countryside, and are not available to peasants. Another urban incentive, more living space, was meaningless in the countryside, since peasant houses are privately owned and built. The negative economic sanctions were to fine couples who had a third child 250 ¥ ($166) annually; there was a retroactive fine of 150 ¥ ($100) for couples who had already had a third child. Generally speaking, village families could afford these fines. The brigade also stated that no private plots, litchee trees, or collective income were to be distributed to children born in excess of the rules. Under the collective economic system in use in 1980, this would be a serious loss of future income, and it would require the family rather than the collective to absorb the economic disadvantages of population increase. Furthermore, no housebuilding plots would be provided to the parents of supernumerary male children on their behalf. (Housebuilding plots are not provided for female children in any case.) This too was a serious sanction. Since houses are privately owned in Zengbu, much of a family's economic efforts go to accumulating the money necessary to build a house for each son on a building plot distributed by the collective. The house is the most important form of village property, and young men without houses have difficulty in finding marriage partners.

The brigade also ruled that people who did not observe the required interval of four years between births would be fined 10 ¥ ($6.67) per month until the interval was up. These fines, and all other fines, were to be paid to the teams. The "combined teams," the new administrative unit equivalent to the natural village, would adjudicate violations. Finally, the concluding rule stated, "Everyone is equal under these regulations." This rule reflected the villagers' concern that if Good was to be Limited, as George Foster(1965), would put it, no one should receive an unfair advantage. This is a crucial element of the villagers' definition of justice. They will accept an unpopular policy if the hardship appears to be equally shared. However, if they think that some people are receiving privileges denied to others, they will resent it so much as to threaten the possibility of enforcing the policy.

Early in 1981, a series of important changes took place which altered the institutional constraints on birth planning, and introduced new elements. First, and most importantly, the new system of production responsibility by households was brought into use. This system distributed economic resources to households in a way that made the brigade's economic sanctions of the previous June meaningless, since families now had a lasting claim on resources, rather than receiving distributions that were re-evaluated from year to year. The economic power of the brigade was vitiated, and its political power as well. The production responsibility system provided apparent advantages to households with larger numbers of laborers, and this increased peasant motivation to have more children.

At the same time, the national marriage law was changed. Although the language of the law was to raise the minimum age for marriage, it imposed no legal delay on marrying, and at the local level, late marriage policy was no longer enforced. As a result, the effect of the change was to *lower* the permissible age of marriage for peasants to 22 for men, and 20 for women. Everyone who became eligible to marry under the new law married as soon as possible. In the long run, this would have the effect of increasing population by shortening the length of time between the generations. Coming into effect when it did, it enlarged the category of young people eligible to marry just as an unusually large demographic cohort was entering that category. As a result, the number of births that were culturally imperative because they followed new marriages also increased. The brigade, in a renewed effort to find an effective economic sanction, announced that it was planning to raise the penalty for having a third child to 400 ¥ ($266) annually. In the light of this, some peasant families concluded that they should try to have another child immediately, rather than waiting for the approved interval only to pay a higher fine.

At this time, early in 1981, a new birth planning policy was introduced by the upper levels. It was based on using abortion as a means for preventing excess births, rather than continuing to rely on the economic sanctions that were ineffectual in practice. Under the terms of this policy, as it was implemented at the brigade level, couples who already had two children including one son were called upon to have an abortion if the wife became pregnant again. If both children were daughters, the abortion was not urged. In order to understand this policy, it is important to understand the cultural meaning of abortion in China, and in order to do this, it is necessary to stand aside from the emotionally powerful connotations that abortion has in American society, particularly at the present time. The American association of abortion with sex, guilt, violence, and the question of the relationship between being female and the necessity to assume the social role of motherhood are profoundly beside the point to the Chinese. Devereux has pointed out in his book, *A Study of Abortion in Primitive Societies* (1979) that "we are culturally conditioned to assume that an abortion is an extralegal act, whose purpose is to conceal the dereliction of a woman" (p.133). He adds that "we may hope to overcome our ethnocentric bias . . . most effectively by examining in detail those instances of abortion which are imposed upon the women . . . in a more or less *public* and *legal* manner." Chinese policy is certainly such a case. The use of abortion has a long history in China. According to Alan F. Guttmacher (1973), "The earliest medical manuscript extant, a Chinese herbal 5000 years old, recommends mercury as an abortifacient" (p. 164). It is reasonable, then, to assume that abortion is indigenous and traditional. The current cultural view of abortion was put as follows by a county level leader. She said, "In our opinion, abortion is not cruel. It would be much more cruel to let the population continue to grow, and to let the future generations suffer. If we don't stop the population from growing, there will be what we call a human explosion calamity. People will be reduced to eating people. There will be no land and no houses." She is thinking of abortion in pragmatic and instrumental terms. It is seen as a trivial evil compared with the horrors of mass starvation. And starvation is not an abstract concept in this context; every villager in Zengbu over the age of forty has actually seen people starve, and younger people have known shared hunger.

The second point that needs to be understood is what it means to be "called upon" to have an abortion. In this non-relativist system, people either share the system's values or are defined as incorrect, and the solution is to persuade them to change their minds by the use of example, explanation, and discussion. This is a traditional solution, rather than an innovation since 1949, as Jerome Cohen and Sybille van der Sprenkel have shown (Cohen, 1968, p. 98). Persuasion of this kind is considered an appropriate and legitimate way of dealing with an erroneous outlook. Family visits are made by local level leaders to carry out persuasion; if repeated visits fail to change a person's mind, leaders of higher and higher rank are brought in. This simultaneously respects the importance of the dissenter, and makes the social system one in which dissent is more and more difficult to sustain as the process continues. At the same time, fellow villagers begin to fear that the dissenter will succeed in avoiding the sacrifice that they themselves have already been required to make. They apply social pressure by indicating the resentment they will feel if the sacrifices are not clearly equal. The cumulative social pressure is so strong as to be virtually irresistible. However, a distinction is made between social pressure and physical force, the use of which would be wrong. Indeed, the Chinese Communist Party Central Committee sent out a letter, dated September 25, 1980, reminding local level leaders engaged in birth planning work to "avoid any forceful methods." A county level leader explained the position by saying, "A good leader won't force an abortion. They rely on education. An effective leader would repeatedly educate a person who was in violation of the rules. Leaders at the brigade, commune, and team levels would come again and again to the person's house, and yell at her constantly. If they discovered a person trying to escape, they would mobilize all of her relatives [to help persuade her], and check out all her sisters. Usually nothing can be done if the woman absolutely refuses. They just fine her." This shows the intensity of persuasion permitted, as long as it remains verbal, and the way in which the person's relatives are drawn into the persuasive process, rather than being defined as separate. The reason for checking out the woman's sisters is that, in this strongly patrilineal society, they will have married out, and be difficult to trace, so it is easier to conceal one's self among them or other matrilateral relatives. Her remarks also indicate that the failure to persuade, or the use of physical force, implies failure of leadership.

In implementing birth planning policy then, local level leaders were permitted to apply persuasive social pressure and forbidden to apply direct force. Fellow villagers would apply social pressure as well, as long as the policy was seen to be fairly applied and effectively carried out, but if the policy was perceived as variably enforced, the villagers would cease to pressure for universal compliance, and start to pressure for the chance to be one of the exceptions. This gave the holdouts a tremendous political significance, and presented local level leaders with almost insoluble problems. In Zengbu, the brigade women's leader was now being helped in her task by the other ten brigade level leaders, rather than working alone as before. This was a clear indication that the importance of birth planning was much greater than it had been. From the point of view of the women's leader, the problem lay in implementing an unpopular policy in a way that would be perceived as perfectly fair. She emphasized to the villagers that there were to be no exceptions whatsoever, "even leaders." At first, villagers were not sure if the policy was really firm. Some families resisted the pressure to have an abortion in the hope that they might outwait the leadership. The political significance of these families was very great. If villagers were told that they were being called upon to have abortions, and yet saw that others, who refused to comply, were allowed to bring their pregnancies to term, the policy ceased to have any meaning. The women's leader said, "With these pregnancies, neighbors pressured the couple, and watched them, and gossiped. The gossipers said, 'If the leaders allow this birth, why can't *we* have more children?' We decided that either we had a policy, or we didn't."

One woman who was pregnant at this time described the effect of policy on her as follows: "I preferred to have two sons and one daughter, and I was trying for a second son. Well, actually, I was using an IUD, but it failed. I chose to be fined and have the third child. But then the campaign started at the upper levels, and the local level leaders had to follow. The women's leader said, 'Now the campaign has come. You have one son and one daughter, you must go get an abortion.' At first, I refused her request. Later, the head of the Women's Federation at the commune level came to see me. She told me not to give birth. She said it was unfair of me to try to have more children than other people. She said, 'You must carry out the abortion. If you refuse to do so, and try to give birth, leaders of higher and higher levels will come to educate you, and you will be fined.' I didn't want to be fined 400 ¥ for the third child, so I got an abortion.'

In Zengbu brigade, there were two of the crucial test cases in which the pregnant women and their husbands' families did not concede to mounting social pressure. One case involved a couple from the village of Sandhill, who had one son and one daughter when the wife became pregnant again. Leaders tried to persuade this couple to have an abortion, but they refused. They left the village and concealed themselves among the wife's matrilateral relatives. The Zengbu leaders sealed up their empty house and went to look for them, but could not find them. The woman gave birth to a daughter away from the village. When she returned, the brigade leaders imposed a fine of 1000 ¥ ($667) and 400 ¥ ($267) annually for life. This was reduced to 200 ¥ ($134) annually when she agreed to have a tubal ligation. The woman's leader commented that the initial 1000 ¥ did not even cover the cost to the brigade of the unsuccessful search. Public reaction to this case was to call the woman twice a fool: first to give birth to a daughter rather than a son, which is culturally defined as being her own fault, and second, to give birth at all when the penalty was to pay such an exorbitant fine. Yet this case also raised the possibility that people who could hide successfully would not be bound by the same rules as the others.

The second test case involved a woman from Louhs' Home Village. She and her husband had two daughters and one son already. She would not agree to have the abortion, in spite of efforts to convince her to do so by the brigade women's leader and other leaders from levels as high as the county. Ten days before the baby was due, the couple left the village in hopes of giving birth elsewhere. The brigade leaders closed up their house and nailed a sign to their door. They urged the husband's brothers to get the couple back. They said that in three days the husband's brothers' houses would be sealed as well. This reflects the cultural assumption that the acts of family members can be thought of as linked and inseparable, and that it is reasonable for a man's brothers to share in his punishment. The brigade leaders met with the wife's mother and the wife's mother's brother. (The latter was the traditional mediator in cases involving conflict between the lineage and a woman who married in.) In meeting with these relatives, the leaders made the cultural assumption that the couple were likely to have turned to the wife's matrilateral relatives. In this meeting, the brigade leaders told the wife's relatives that the land which had been distributed to the couple would be taken back, both private plots and production responsibility land. This would leave the couple with no share of the village resources with which to make a living. At 8 P.M. on the second day, in time to avoid having the husband's brothers' houses sealed, the couple returned. The abortion took place on the following day, using the injection method. The brigade women's leader explained that the injection method would not necessarily kill the baby at once. She said that if the child was born alive, it wouldn't live more than two or three hours. In this case, they didn't pay any attention to the child or take any measures to save it; the child died as a result of deliberate inattention to its perinatal distress, which was presumably the result of the method of abortion. The women's leader could not tell this story without evident distress of her own, even after an interval of two years. She repeated the justifications for the brigade's actions: "Everyone in the village was watching this case. The leaders felt that if she had her baby, the whole policy would become unenforceable. If we had let her go freely, it would have had a very bad effect on everyone else." In spite of the validity of these justifications in her mind, her distress indicated that the presence of another point of view, the family's point of view, existing simultaneously, and recognized as valuable. Several years earlier, in explaining her reasons for becoming politically active, the women's leader had described the extreme poverty of her bleak childhood, and the abusiveness within her family that was the direct result, in her opinion, of the economic circumstances of the surrounding society. Her idea of socialism was that it would provide prosperity and economic justice, and that as a direct result, there would be social justice and harmonious family life as well. Socialism was the natural, complete, and far-reaching solution to the problems of family life, and the exploitation, particularly of women, inherent in the family structure. Her political goals included the presupposition that it was important to make family life less sordid by making it closer to cherished ideals. What was socialist and what was most valuably and validly Chinese were linked in her way of thinking. Her own social idealism, and her ways of being kind and considerate to others, were expressed using the formulae of socialist theory. Now, by carrying her principles through to their logical conclusion, she served her goals in the long run, but in the short run, she injured the family interests of some fellow villagers. Respect for the principles of the state conflicted with respect for the principles of the family, with the essentially tragic result that people on either side of the question could no longer define themselves as essentially good, because they were inevitably in conflict, if not with one, then with the other aspect of their own valued principles.

This second test case demonstrates that letting the neonate die is regarded as socially legitimate when the reasons are compelling. In this case, the compelling reasons were those of the state. But the question can also be raised, under what circumstances might it seem legitimate to the family to let the neonate die? Clearly, given the importance of a male rather than a female child, families would be more motivated to let a female neonate die. Female infanticide existed in traditional China. It has been reported and deplored in the national press as an immoral act; the state takes the position that all children appropriately and legitimately conceived should be protected. It is only if they violate the legal restrictions on giving birth that they can be allowed to die. According to the brigade women's leader, there has been no infanticide of female babies in Zengbu, in spite of the clearly displayed assumption that males are more important and more fully human than females. Since all pregnancies are monitored and their results known, the statement of the women's leader is to be accepted. Families, although wishing strongly for sons, are not experiencing sufficient desperation to make female infanticide seem legitimate. Women's leaders at the commune level say that there has been no female infanticide in Chashan Commune, although they have heard that it does sometimes happen in "remote areas." The phrase suggests that it is more characteristic of people in less civilized areas, and, by implication, that it is not really a civilized thing to do. At the county level, birth planning leaders report one case of attempted infanticide in their experience. (It should be remembered that the population of the county is more than one million.) In this case, a young woman tried to abandon her female baby "on the hillside" but her fellow villagers found it and brought it back. At the provincial level, a birth planning leader reported that infanticide exists in certain remote islands along the coast that are difficult to control. Presumably, limitations on pregnancy are also difficult to implement in such areas, so stringent policy enforcement and female infanticide would not logically be linked. The leader affirmed the official position that once appropriately born, the child must be protected. She said that in her opinion, the amount of infanticide in Guangdong Province must be negligible, since the sex ratio for newborns is well within the bounds of the normal. According to Li Chengrui, the Director of the State Statistics Bureau, as quoted in an article 'Sex Ratio of China's Newborns and Infants' in *Women of China* (August, 1983) a normal sex ratio for newborns is defined as "about 100:105, with a margin of 103 to 108" for males outnumbering females (p. 11). Li gives Anhui Province as an example of a locale with an abnormal sex ratio; there, there are 100 girls to 111.12 boys. It is interesting to compare these modern figures with historical ones. For example, under the old regime, in the village near Shanghai studied by Fei Hsiao Tung, the sex ratio was 100 girls to 135 boys (1939: 34). So it would not be reasonable to suggest that state birth planning policy has precipitated female infanticide by families in the part of Guangdong Province we studied, and probably elsewhere as well.

The villagers did not like the policy using abortion as the focus of birth planning implementation, and by comparison with it the former policy, which had been disliked in its day, appeared preferable. We asked one male villager, "What did the people think about the leadership calling on them to have abortions?" and he said, "The attitude of the villagers is that leaders should fine people, rather than requiring them to have abortions." However, if the policy were to exist at all, public opinion supported universal enforcement. In the second test case, for example, they supported the leadership's actions on the grounds that it would have been unfair to permit the couple to have their baby when other people could not.

We also asked the women's leader about the feelings of the women who had the abortions, and she said that if the child would have been a son, the women were really upset, but not if it would have been a daughter. This exchange reflects, in the question, the Western assumption that an experience takes its meaning in an important way from the emotions of the person having the experience. In the answer, it reflects the Chinese assumption that a person's response to an experience will reflect its social implications – in this case, the importantly differing significance of having a son rather than a daughter.

The policy based on abortion can be understood more clearly if it is looked at in perspective, and in the light of some interesting comparative figures. In evaluating the degree of completeness with which the policy was implemented, it is worth noting that according to the provincial level, in 1982, in the province as a whole, 19% of all births were third or higher order births. This bespeaks a very considerable gap between policy and implementation, suggesting that many areas had leaders whose efforts were weak or ineffectual in comparison with Zengbu's leaders, and that many supernumerary pregnancies were brought to term. Rather than suggesting a high degree of successfully enforced compliance, the figure, on the contrary, indicates that in the province as a whole, carrying out policy took place with a wide disparity between theory and practice. This does not surprise the leadership, since they think of policy as a goal, an ideal to be approached, rather than a law. As Vivienne Shue puts it, in discussing the Land Reform period (1949–1956), "they were prepared for only partial fulfillment of goals . . . they did not expect or insist on perfect compliance . . ." (1980, p. 5). This distinction between policy and law is critical and complex, and produces a socially specific and distinctive attitude to social control.

In considering the qualities of the policy in comparative perspective, it has been easy for the uninformed to assume that such a policy would produce a number of abortions that could be considered excessive or shocking in international terms. A comparison with abortion figures for the United States is surprising and instructive. Using the format of the *Statistical Abstracts of the United States* produced by the U.S. Census Bureau (1984), abortion figures are quoted in terms of the numbers of abortions per 1000 live births. In the U.S. as a whole, in 1980 (the most recent figures available), there were 428 abortions per 1000 live births, in a range between Utah's 97 and the District of Columbia's 1569. In New York, the figure was 780, and in California it was 598. In Guangdong Province, in 1982, using figures provided by provincial officials, there were 523 abortions per thousand births. (Leaders provided the most recent complete figures for an interview in August, 1983, and did not rehearse the data for earlier years.) In Dongguan County, in 1982, there were 816 abortions per 1000 births. In Chashan Commune, in 1981, there was a ratio of 727 abortions per 1000 live births, based on actual figures of 656 births and 477 abortions. In 1982, 605 births and 370 abortions yielded a ratio of 612 to 1000. In 1983, for the first six months of the year, there were 213 births and 96 abortions, yielding a ratio of 450 abortions per 1000. The average for the entire $2\frac{1}{2}$ year period is 640 per 1000. In Zengbu brigade, where the women's leader provided figures showing 150 abortions and 257 births in the $2\frac{1}{2}$ year period, the ratio is 584 per 1000. These figure indicate clearly that at the height of the policy emphasizing abortion as a method of population control, the figures remained well within a range currently found in the United States.

The policy relying on abortion only yielded temporary results, since a woman who had an abortion under the policy might soon become pregnant again. Its cost was high: financially, in terms of funding many abortions, in stress, because it forced people between the jaws of two conflicting sets of principles and then required them to act, and in administrative difficulty. Under this policy, only the people whose refusal to respond to the claims of the wider society was most adamant, determined, and wily, would be rewarded with a supernumerary child. The policymakers raised the issue that repeated abortions were harmful to the health of women, signaling a change in the official attitude, and the policy was discontinued. It was necessary to construct a new policy that would be exquisitely fair in equalizing the sacrifices, that would be effective in reducing population growth, and that would be within the capacity of local level leaders to enforce.

In 1983, the state formulated a new policy for peasants, requiring those who had given birth to two children and were demonstrably at risk for having a third, to undergo sterilization. This policy was intended only for the rural areas, not for the cities, where the "one child policy" was the rule. As one provincial level leader explained, "There is no sterilization policy in the city, where people have only one child. We will never ask couples with one child to undergo sterilization, because that would prevent them from having another if their child died." The sterilization policy for peasants with two children was a state policy, and provinces were encouraged to adopt it, but it was not mandatory. Rather, provinces which adopted the policy would sum up their experiences and a mandatory policy would be formulated later. Guangdong Province and four other densely populated provinces – Sichuan, Hebei, Shandong, and Henan – adopted the policy. Guangdong Province leaders spelled out the meaning of the policy from their point of view in great detail. Peasant families could give birth to a second child if and only if the first was a girl, which would, it was felt, constitute a hardship in household based agriculture. But one son, or two children if the first was a girl, was, from the province's point of view, to be the limit. Exceptions were carefuly described. A deformity or defect complete enough to make the child incapable of working in later life would permit the birth of another child to compensate for the incapacity. Families in debilitating occupations, such as mining or fishing, could have extra children. So could people in remote mountain areas or small islands, and minority peoples. A remarriage renewed the right to have children; a provincial leader said, "We must remember that the purpose of marriage is to have children." Children born in multiple births resulting from approved pregnancies were unquestionably legitimate exceptions to the ordinary limitations. In effect, the policy rationed the right to have children. Because of this, it became important to prevent people from exceeding their ration. Sterilization was to be the means whereby this was to be ensured, and it was to be used in cases where the risk that a couple would exceed the ration was apparent. Thus, if a couple had two children already, and the wife became pregnant again, she was to have an abortion, and one member of the couple was to be sterilized. (If the wife was over forty, however, sterilization was not required, on the grounds that her fertility was almost over in any case.) If the couple had two children and were not using any contraceptive method, one of the couple was to be sterilized. If the couple had violated the four-year spacing rule by having two children since 1979, one of the couple was to be sterilized. Finally, if the couple used contraception, but the wife had

had an abortion since 1979, indicating contraceptive failure, one of the couple was to be sterilized. The decision to turn to sterilization as a method was the result of a long term experience of repeated contraceptive failures. A provincial level leader said, "In the countryside we've had a lesson. Contraception is not effective. The peasants are not used to condoms, the side effects of contraceptive drugs are strong, the rings and other IUDs have many failures, and repeated abortions harm the health of women." In conjunction with the sterilization policy, there was a new propaganda emphasis on raising a "healthy superior child." This new emphasis marks an attempt to make an important shift in underlying attitudes: the shift from the expectation of large numbers of children, with the failure to thrive of one or another of them a matter to be endured, to the expectation of fewer children, each more important, and each to be nurtured with resources formerly spread thin.

The sterilization policy differed from previous policies in that it required a permanent rather than a temporary measure to be taken. It also differed from previous policies by requiring a measure that has extremely serious cultural implications. Traditional values attribute far more horrifying significance to sterilization than to abortion. (By comparison, in the United States at the present time, there is significant religious feeling that abortion is a wicked and immoral procedure, yet there is no comparable outcry urging the prevention of sterilization procedures on moral grounds.) According to these traditional values, the social worth of a person depends on the ability to work and the ability to carry on the family line. These abilities are believed to be linked, and men are believed to possess them to a higher degree than women. The assumption is made that people who are sterilized have their capacity to work permanently damaged, and this, as well as the loss of the capacity to reproduce, damages the meaning of their relationship to the family. Because work, reproduction, and the family are as one and inseparable, sterilization is understood as damaging all three. Sterilization is regarded as even more damaging to men's greater capacities than to women's lesser ones, and many people regard the idea of a vasectomy with horror. Tubal ligation for women is thought of as the less damaging alternative, so, faced with the choice, many women accept sterilization themselves, rather than letting their husbands be sterilized. It is a reasonable inference that this policy would not have been implemented, or even formulated, if the provincial leadership did not think of it as the only remaining possibility in a situation where the consequences of failing to act were worse than the consequences of acting.

The county level modified this policy in such a way as to permit more children. A county level leader said, "Central policy is that, if you have a son first, you have to stop, but our county lets the peasants have a second child, even if the first child is a son." This decision freed 100% of peasant couples to have two children, instead of limiting 50% of them to one child; in so heavily populated a county (the population is over a million) the practical implications of this decision are very great, and would produce a much higher birth rate than if provincial level policy were followed as formulated. But, a county level leader said, "While the upper levels were scolding us, we agreed to what they said, but when they had gone, we did what we thought was right." Nonetheless, the county level's liberalized policy was still painfully restricted by peasant standards.

At the commune level, at a Three Level Meeting devoted to the topic, in May 1983, the local leaders heard the policy explained, and found themselves confronted with the problem of implementing the sterilization of everybody who fell into the categories called the "four yardsticks." The four yardsticks measured couples who already had two children and defined which of them must now be sterilized. As at the provincial level, the commune required sterilization if the wife was pregnant again, if the couple was not using any form of contraception, if the second child had been born after an interval of less than four years, or if the wife had had an abortion since 1979. Couples who had used contraception effectively would not have to be sterilized, a powerful implicit incentive for future contraceptive use. In implementing this policy, the commune emphasized that the force of example was even more important than persuasion, and the local leaders were told that, if they fell into the categories, they had to be sterilized first. The women's leader of the brigade said, "When the leaders heard this, they couldn't understand it in their minds. They looked around at one another. They were told, 'If you don't take the lead in this drive, how can you get the peasants to follow you?'" Both of the brigade level leaders from Zengbu who fell into the categories underwent vasectomies. In its social context, this was undoubtedly impressive. Only when the vasectomies had taken place did the brigade present its own modified version of policy to the villagers.

Brigade policy respected the urgency of the cultural preference for a son by saying that couples with two daughters, who would otherwise have fallen into the four categories, were not required to be sterilized. This modification reduced by 25% the number of couples who would otherwise have fallen into the commune's category for required sterilization. There was a clear implication that later on, these couples could have a third child in trying for a son, and pay a fine. Brigade leaders felt that their ability to implement the policy at all hinged on this crucial provision, and that without it, they could not succeed in getting the villagers to comply. The brigade also announced that, since they had not previously enforced the four-year spacing rule, they would not sterilize couples who had violated it. Brigade leaders felt that the sterilization of couples who violated the four-year spacing rule would leave those couples unable to replace children who might not be viable; children born since 1979 were still too young to make it reasonable to assume that they would survive, it was argued. The argument shows that at the brigade level, people still lived in the expectation of high infant mortality. However, the brigade announced that it would enforce the four-year spacing rule in future.

The villagers' reaction to the policy was predictably strong. One man commented, "We preferred abortion to sterilization, because then, if a child died, it could be replaced." Another man said, "I oppose it! You *must* have a son to carry on the family name. If you don't have a son, you won't have anyone to worship the dead parents' souls. [This in spite of the fact that ancestor worship was forbidden from 1949 to 1981.] It will cut the generations, there will be no ancestors. You raise sons, sons support you in your old age. It is impossible for daughters to take care of the aged, because they marry out. The men believe that the strength of the man is in his sperm. They fear the weakening of the body through sterilization. The men must go out to work. If the man dies, the family will be destroyed." A male leader, speaking of his daughter-in-law's sterilization, said sadly, "It is easy to agree to the necessity for sterilization in an open meeting, but it becomes very hard when it is a member of your own family."

In order to make the situation as acceptable as possible, commune level leaders hired more highly qualified doctors from the medical school in Guangzhou, so as to allay fears that the operations would not be competently performed. The brigade offered financial incentives to those who had the operations immediately. The incentive was 200 ¥ ($134). There were 216 couples in the brigade who fell into the brigade's sterilization categories. In the two weeks following the announcement of the policy, 187 sterilizations, including 8 vasectomies, were performed. This took place in the second two weeks of May, 1983. The rest were to be sterilized in June, or, if they were ill, in September. In August, 1983, the brigade women's leader said, "At first they didn't understand. But no one refused the operation, and no one ran away. Their thinking changed. In the beginning, they shouted at us. Everyone was watching the main trend. They saw the others were doing it, so they got caught up." By using the force of example, explanations, incentives, the hiring of special doctors, and the momentum of social pressure, the leaders succeeded in implementing their version of the policy.

Over the short span of four years, Zengbu Brigade had seen four birth planning policies: first, refusal to subsidize supernumerary children, second, the imposition of fines, third, the policy relying on abortion, and fourth, the policy relying on sterilization. These policies had evolved from partial subsidization of traditional values toward a comparatively active and painful rejection of these values. Yet by December, 1984, there were signs that policy was retrenching. Provincial level officials had been told that there should be more emphasis on research, and less on the practicalities of implementation and enforcement. Some leaders had lost their jobs in the wake of the 1983 campaign. The conflict continues between the values of familism and the necessities of a nation burdened with the most overwhelming population on the face of the earth. There is a recognition that the cherished values embodied in familism have become agents of destruction to China as a whole. Yet it is overwhelmingly difficult to reject beliefs as beloved as they are dangerous, even in the certain knowledge that such a rejection is the only possible alternative. If the extraordinary pronatalism of traditional culture is overcome, then what it means to have a child in China, and to be a child in China, will change completely, yielding dramatic new cultural and structural forms. There will be the resources to provide decently for those who are born, and to care for them so that they can indeed be healthy and superior. If the extraordinary Chinese pronatalism is not modified, future generations of Chinese children will suffer increasingly until they are destroyed by the weight of their own numbers.

## ACKNOWLEDGMENT

The generous support of the Wang Fellowship Program in Chinese Studies facilitated the analysis and data presentation set forth in this chapter.

## NOTES

1. My formulation of these points differs from that of Richard H. Solomon, in *Mao's Revolution and the Chinese Political Culture* (1971) yet his work is relevant and important, and of interest to anyone who wishes to pursue these topics further.
2. Funding for the writing up of these field materials was provided by a grant from the Wang Institute of Graduate Studies' Fellowship Program in Chinese Studies.
3. For recent studies of China's population as a whole, in demographic terms, see, among others, H. Yuan Tien's 'China: Demographic Billionaire,' *Population Bulletin*, Vol. 38, No. 2, April, 1983, and Nathan Keyfitz's 'The Population of China,' in *Scientific American*, Vol. 250, No. 2, February, 1984.
4. Reported by Deborah Davis-Friedmann at the Regional Seminar in Chinese Studies, University of California at Berkeley, October 27, 1984.
5. Zhao Fusan, personal communication, January 17, 1980.

## REFERENCES

Anon.
    1909 The Book of Filial Duty, trans. Ivan Chen.
Anon.
    1983 'Sex Ratio of China's Newborns and Infants,' *in* Women of China, August, p. 11.
Cohen, Jerome Alan
    1968 The Criminal Process in the People's Republic of China 1949–1963: An Introduction. Harvard University Press, Cambridge, Mass.
Devereux, George
    1979 A Study of Abortion in Primitive Societies. International Universities Press, Inc., New York.
Fei Hsiao T'ung
    1939 Peasant Life in China. Kegan Paul, Trench, Trubner & Co., Ltd., London.
Foster, George
    1965 'Peasant Society and the Image of Limited Good,' *in* American Anthropologist 67 (2): 293–315.
Guttmacher, Alan F.
    1973 Pregnancy, Birth, and Family Planning. Signet, New York.

Keyfitz, Nathan
    1984 'The Population of China,' *in* Scientific American 250 (2): 38–47.
Potter, Sulamith
    1983 'The Position of Peasants in Modern China's Social Order,' *in* Modern China 9 (4): 465–499.
Shue, Vivienne
    1980 Peasant China in Transition: The Dynamics of Development Toward Socialism. University of California Press, Berkeley and Los Angeles.
Solomon, Richard H.
    1971 Mao's Revolution and the Chinese Political Culture. University of California Press, Berkeley and Los Angeles.
Tien, H. Yuan
    1983 'China: Demographic Billionaire,' *in* Population Bulletin 38 (2): 2–42.
United States Census Bureau
    1984 Statistical Abstracts of the United States. Washington, D.C.

SARA HARKNESS AND CHARLES M. SUPER

# FERTILITY CHANGE, CHILD SURVIVAL, AND CHILD DEVELOPMENT: OBSERVATIONS ON A RURAL KENYAN COMMUNITY

Social change over the last century has had varied and dramatic effects not only on populations as a whole, but also on the survival and growth of individual children. On the one hand, improvements in medical technology and health care have reduced death rates, which in developing countries are particularly high for infants and young children. On the other hand, changes in habitat – for example from rural to urban – have had less uniformly positive effects on the environments of children and their families.

Rapid population growth in particular has been associated with a number of negative changes, some of which are discussed elsewhere in this volume: a decrease in available food resources for families, rises in unemployment, and shortage of living space, to name only a few. For children, in particular, rapid growth of the population will inevitably lead to a scarcity of services such as education and health care, essential to successful development in a changing economy.

Kenya is outstanding among countries characterized by high population growth. The most recent estimates put Kenya's rate of annual population increase at over 4 percent, with a projected doubling of the population in 17 years (Digest, 1984). Although much of Kenya's growth can be attributed to declines in mortality, demographic research also suggests that fertility is increasing even over previously high levels (Faruquee *et al.*, 1980). At present rates, women in Kenya are giving birth to an average of more than 8 children over the course of their reproductive careers (Digest, 1984).

The balance between people and resources is an equation made at the societal level. Rapid population growth, however, is also reflected in the micro-environment of the family. Reduced infant and child mortality, in this context, leads to larger families. Likewise, higher fertility may be expressed at the family level in earlier marriages, closer birth spacing, or more prolonged childbearing. It is this micro-environment, the "developmental niche" of children in rural Kenya, which is the focus of the present discussion. We will suggest that fertility changes, which can be observed at the community as well as the national level, are associated with changed patterns of childbearing that create a new set of risk factors in the treatment and survival of children in this sociocultural setting.

## THE KIPSIGIS PEOPLE AND THE COMMUNITY OF KOKWET

Our observations are drawn from one ethnic group, the Kipsigis, and specifically from one community where we carried out field research from 1972 to

*Nancy Scheper-Hughes (ed.), Child Survival, 59–70.*
© *1987 by D. Reidel Publishing Company.*

1975. The Kipsigis are a Highland Nilotic people who inhabit the Western Highlands of Kenya, a green and fertile area elevated between the Rift Valley on the east and the lowland plains south of Lake Victoria on the west. Together with their close relatives the Nandi, Marakwet, Elgeyo and others, the Kipsigis form an ethnic cluster known as the "Kalenjin," which follows in population size the two major ethnic groups of Kikuyu and Luo. The Kipsigis have followed a middle course in adaptation to Western-introduced social change. A relative abundance of land has allowed them to maintain traditional family economies based on farming and keeping cattle, rather than leaving to seek salaried work in the towns and cities as is more common among most other groups; yet they have participated in the growing national economy through production of cash crops and cash dairy farming.

The community of Kokwet, where we carried out field research from 1972 to 1975, is a Kipsigis settlement of 54 households established on land repatriated from the British at national independence in 1963. As a government-sponsored "settlement scheme" Kokwet was in the early 1970s intentionally modern in some respects, but the community remained traditional in many significant ways: most adults had little or no schooling, few men worked at salaried jobs away from the homesteads, cows were still used for the customary brideprice, and virtually all adolescents still chose to undergo the traditional circumcision ceremonies.

## TRADITIONAL REGULATION OF FERTILITY

Childbearing in Kipsigis traditionally followed the "natural fertility" pattern typical of many sub-Saharan African cultures, whereby couples do not change their reproductive behavior in response to the number of children already born (Lesthaeghe, Ohadike, Kocher, and Page, 1981). It should not be concluded, however, that families in Kipsigis were "unplanned" or that the culture placed no constraints on fecundity. Several aspects of traditional social organization and customary behavior limited the beginning and end of women's reproductive careers, as well as the spacing of births.

First, a lower limit on age of marriage for women was maintained by the required completion of the female circumcision ceremonies. These ceremonies, which included the physical ordeal of clitoridectomy and removal of the outer labia without benefit of anesthesia, were necessary before a girl could be considered a woman ready to bear children. The intensity of this belief is underscored by the fact that infanticide, otherwise unknown in the culture, was prescribed in cases where a girl gave birth before undergoing the ceremonies (Peristiany, 1939). Because of the severity of the circumcision ordeal and the importance of performing bravely, parents might hold their daughter back from undergoing the ceremonies until they felt she was sufficiently mature, as we observed on several occasions in Kokwet.

[Once married and having born her first child, a Kipsigis woman's fertility was moderated by the customs of extended lactation and post-partum sexual abstinence. It was in this area that the conscious part of fertility control was exercised. Short birth spacing was considered a threat to the health of the baby already born, who would be deprived of milk as the mother stopped breast-feeding when she became pregnant again. To avoid this problem, "new mothers" were not supposed to have intercourse with their husbands for a number of months. The practice of post-partum abstinence was supported in turn by the institution of polygyny, such that men could co-habit with their wives by turns. Since it was often the case that wives might live in different areas far removed from each other, the husband of a "new mother" might be absent for a long period of time while she remained at home with her infant.]

It seems probable that birth spacing was traditionally prolonged beyond what would have been achieved by post-partum abstinence through the biological effects of lactation. Babies in Kipsigis, as in other East African cultures, were nursed on demand, and kept in close contact with their mothers both night and day. At night, mothers slept in skin contact with their babies, who could nurse easily as they awoke. During the day, the baby was carried either by the mother or by a child caretaker who would be near the mother in case she were needed. Under these circumstances, nursing frequency was high. Studies of other African cultures where mothers breastfeed frequently have shown an association between nursing frequency and ovulatory function (Delvoye and Robyn, 1980; Konner and Worthman, 1980; Ojofeitimi, 1982), and the relationship between lactation duration and birth intervals has been documented at the population level (e.g. Bongaarts, 1976).

[Finally, although large families were valued, women's childbearing was probably also limited in their later years by a decline in coital frequency due to the husband's greater attention to his younger wives.]Thus, although childbearing continued to a later age for Kipsigis women than is customary in Western societies, nevertheless it tended to decline before the physiological limit of childbearing. It is worth noting, however, that these constraints on fecundity were social and cultural, rather than physiological in origin. In contrast to some African populations, secondary sterility due to venereal disease was not present to any appreciable extent.

[In summary, fertility in traditional Kipsigis culture was a function of two complementary strategies, one favoring the production of as many children as possible and the other favoring the survival of each child.]Although fertility was high, it was limited by traditional customs which defined the beginning and end of childbearing within somewhat narrower limits than the full span of fecund years, and which tended to ensure adequate spacing between births. Given the other constraints of traditional Kipsigis life, including high mortality in infants and young children as a result of diarrheal and infectious disease, a pattern of birth spacing that supported the infant and young child in these vulnerable first years of life was an important element in the niche for development.

## FERTILITY TRENDS IN KENYA AND KOKWET

Although the measurement of fertility in Kenya is made difficult by the lack of written records or cultural attention to birth dates, demographic researchers generally agree that fertility in Kenya has been high in the past and that there has been a trend toward even higher fertility. According to the results of the Kenya Fertility Survey, conducted in 1977–78, the estimated total fertility rate of women was 8.1 births (Digest, 1984). Analyses of these data as well as other surveys suggest that fertility is positively associated with some aspects of what is commonly called "modernization" (Dow and Werner, 1976; Mott and Mott, 1980). Thus, for example, women with some education had higher fertility than women with no education, and women in monogamous marriages tended to have higher fertility than those in polygynous marriages. Younger women were found to be having children at shorter intervals than older women. These trends are typically ascribed to the lack of acceptance of modern contraceptives (which were used by only about 6 percent of married women surveyed) coupled with a breakdown of traditional constraints on childbearing.

### Data Sources

The data on fertility in Kokwet come from a census taken at the beginning of our stay in the community and maintained over three years. There were no written records of birthdates for many of the children, nor for virtually all of the mothers; nevertheless, fairly reliable estimates for children born during the previous ten years were made using a combination of field methods, for these ages were of direct concern to our research on child development (Super, 1985). In our census interviews, mothers were asked the date of their own birth and the dates of birth of all their children, including those who had died, in chronological order. We were assisted by a local mother, who was able to help our respondents remember births and place dates in relation to other events. A review of birth histories given by the mothers suggested that some of the older mothers probably omitted some births, either because these children had died or because they had grown up and moved away; the present analysis of fertility therefore is limited to women of childbearing age (15 to 45; $n = 87$). The other data presented here come from three sources: ethnographic knowledge based on our three years of residence in Kokwet, including participant observation and informant interview; a structured interview with all mothers in Kokwet during 1973–74 (including grandmothers, visiting married daughters, etc.; $n = 76$) that included questions on family planning and related topics; and finally, specific quantitative studies of developmental phenomena, e.g. child language, which are published and described more fully elsewhere.

## Data Analysis

Given the fact that demographic trends have already been established at the regional and national level by large-scale surveys, the purpose of analyzing fertility trends for a single community needs to be briefly explained. Our interest here is to establish whether trends evident in large-scale samples can also be seen to a significant degree at the community level, and if so, then to examine the relationships between fertility measures and the other quantitative and qualitative data which are available for this community. Our presentation of fertility data from Kokwet is in two parts. First, we describe fertility patterns in Kokwet and demonstrate their resemblence to patterns found in larger Kenyan samples. Second, we use a specially constructed sub-set of mothers in the community, and analytical procedures from inferential statistics, to address the question of whether there is a tendency toward shorter birth intervals in the younger mothers.

## Results

Fertility patterns in Kokwet resemble those of the "high fertility" areas of Kenya, including patterns for larger Kipsigis samples. There were no women in the community aged 25 or over who were not mothers; and average age at first birth for mothers 25 to 45 was 18.1 years. Mothers aged 25–29 had an average of 4.5 children, with family size increasing to 6.0 children for women aged 30–34, 7.4 for women aged 35–39, and 7.7 for women aged 40–44. Birth intervals reported by the mothers averaged 28 months, compared to a national average of 30 months (Digest, 1984). The timing of childbearing for these women followed the "broad peak" pattern which characterizes much of sub-Saharan Africa, with births occurring over a relatively long span of years by comparison with Western industrialized societies. Older as well as younger mothers seemed to be producing large families through a steady pace of childbearing, starting in the late teens and continuing into the late 30s or early 40s.

Examination of the data on age at first birth for women of different age groups suggested no general trend toward either earlier or later childbearing. In order to see whether there was a tendency for the younger mothers to reproduce at shorter intervals, as has been found in large-scale studies, the following procedure was devised. First, all the mothers (except for five)[1] with at least two children (and therefore at least one birth interval to measure) were ranked by age and divided at the median age at 30 years, yielding two samples of "older" and "younger" mothers (total $n = 46$). The average age of the younger mothers was 26.4 years, and that of the older mothers was 37.0 years. The mothers were then paired on the basis of age at first birth, by rank order within each group. All but two of the 24 pairs were matched within one year of age at first birth, and none was as much as two years apart. The average birth intervals for the younger mothers were computed for the total number of children they had at the time of our last census. Average birth intervals for the older mothers were computed using the birth intervals corresponding in order and number to the matched younger mothers; thus, if the younger mother had four children at the time of our census, the average birth interval for the matched older mother was computed from her first four children. By this method, the average birth interval for the younger mothers was found to be 2.16 years (or 26 months), compared to 2.55 years (or 31 months) for the older mothers; this difference is statistically significant ($t = 1.99$, $df = 22$, $p = 0.03$ one-tailed).

## SOCIOCULTURAL DETERMINANTS OF FERTILITY

The shorter birth intervals typical of the younger mothers logically must be due to changes in parental behavior that have shortened the "post-partum non-susceptible period" – the time after giving birth when, for social or biological reasons, a woman does not become pregnant. Like most women in Kenya, the women of Kokwet did not use modern methods of birth control, although these methods were not unknown in the community. In interviews, only 5 percent of the women indicated they had ever used "family planning," even though more than half of them had attended at least one government-sponsored meeting on the topic, and almost two-thirds thought young women should go to the meetings. Twenty-three percent of the women indicated they might someday use modern contraception, but most expressed the desire to have as many children as possible, or as many as God should give them. Family size was not considered a topic that should be discussed between husbands and wives, though the women suggested that their husbands wanted even more children than they did themselves. Thus, the length of birth intervals in this community continued, as in the past, to vary as a function of post-partum sexual abstinence and the effects of lactation on fecundity. Of these two, post-partum sexual abstinence had been reduced to a period of only a few months – in many cases, two or three months, according to interviews with some of the women in the community.

Breastfeeding was universal and babies were fed on demand at close intervals – only a little less frequently than once an hour, day and night, at least up to the age of eight months (the oldest age monitored: Super and Harkness, 1982b). It appears, however, that lactation amenorrhea is quite sensitive to the interbout interval (see Konner and Worthman, 1980), and the rate of daytime nursing probably declined near the end of the first year. Most of the mothers in the community (70 percent) also stated that they had used bottle feeding at least on occasion, as well as breastfeeding, for their most recent baby. The bottle was seen as a useful device to extend the period a sibling caretaker could remain in charge of the baby, especially after 6 months or so. Weaning was typically initiated after the child could walk, or shortly into the next pregnancy: the median age of weaning was 15 months. It is not known whether the women had begun to create shorter birth intervals by weaning their babies earlier, or whether despite the high frequency of nursing episodes in the early months after childbirth, the use of bottle feeding or other changes in feeding routine had led to a shorter period of lactation amenorrhea and earlier resumption of ovulatory cycling.

The reasons for changes in both post-partum sexual abstinence and feeding practices seem related to larger aspects of social change. Women reported in interviews that bottle feeding seemed "modern." Post-partum sexual abstinence was becoming shortened due to pressure from husbands, especially those who did not have other wives. In Kokwet, average birth intervals tended to be slightly shorter for women in monogamous marriages, women whose husbands were more strongly Christianized, and more educated women, although these tendencies were not statistically significant.

## BIRTH INTERVALS, INFANT MORTALITY, AND CHILD DEVELOPMENT

The shortening of intervals between births, in Kokwet and other communities like it in Kenya, is cause for concern about the health of mothers and particularly of infants. A recent study based on the World Fertility Survey has suggested that there is a substantial increase in the risk of mortality for infants born after an interval of less than two years following the previous birth (Hobcraft, McDonald, and Rutstein, 1983). The increased risk was ascribed to uterine depletion in the mothers, maternal malnutrition leading to insufficient lactation, and lack of time and energy for the mother to care for two babies at the same time.

Infant deaths in Kokwet had many proximate causes, including complications of labor and delivery and tetanus infection for newborns, and infectious disease and diarrhea for older infants. During our three years in Kokwet there were nine infant deaths before the first birthday, the period during which risk factors related to short birth intervals would be expected to be most strongly in evidence. A comparison of birth intervals preceding the births of these babies who died with the larger sample of surviving children born in the community showed that the former were typically born after very short intervals: 1.64 years on average (s.d. = 0.72), compared to 2.43 years for the rest of the sample (s.d. = 1.10), a statistically significant difference ($t = 2.12$, $df = 263$, $p = 0.04$). In fact, of the nine babies who died, only three were born after intervals of two or more years.

Birth interval was also related to the physical, social and cognitive development of the next to youngest children, that is, those who were *followed* by younger siblings born soon after them. As has been described elsewhere (Harkness and Super, 1982, 1983), the transition from infancy to early childhood in Kokwet was defined primarily as a function of the birth of the next baby. Mothers reported in interviews that if they became pregnant while breastfeeding, they would wean the baby. A shortened birth interval would thus contribute to earlier weaning, with possible effects on the nutritional status of the child and vulnerability to diarrheal and other infectious diseases.

With the birth of the next baby, there were also other changes in the role of the next to youngest. From a favored position in the mother's bed, the child was now moved to sleep with the other children or at the mother's back. During the daytime, the child was no longer carried by the mother, but was expected to join the older children's playgroup.

The nature of the changes in children's social and cognitive environments that ensued with the birth of a younger sibling has been charted by a cross-sectional study of child language socialization in Kokwet (Harkness, 1977; Harkness and Super, 1982). Some of the children in the study had younger siblings, while others did not. Comparisons of the observational data for second-to-youngest versus youngest children indicated that those who had a younger sibling spent significantly less time interacting with adults ($r = -0.56$, $n = 19$, $p < 0.05$) and more time with other children ($r = 0.53$, $p < 0.05$). The children who had younger siblings also were also talked to less ($r = -0.72$, $p < 0.01$). and did less talking themselves ($r = -0.52$, $p < 0.05$). The amount of time the children were observed talking was related in turn to their mean length of utterance (a measure of language development): with age controlled by regression analysis, children who were observed talking more had a higher mean length of utterance ($r = 0.70$, $p < 0.01$). Thus, in general the birth of a younger sibling entailed, for the second-to-youngest child, a decline in attention from adults, with implications for the rate of language development. Our own personal observations of these children was that they tended to be quiet and shy, in contrast to the more self-confident and talkative demeanor of children who were still the youngest members of their families.

## FERTILITY AND THE DEVELOPMENTAL NICHE

In considering the structure of environments for infants and young children in Kokwet, and the nature of the changes associated with culturally defined developmental stages, the "developmental niche" is a useful organizing framework (Harkness and Super, 1982, 1983, 1985; Super and Harkness, 1981, 1982a, 1982b). Briefly, the developmental niche is conceptualized in terms of three basic dimensions. The first consists of the physical and social settings which the child lives in, including for example where he or she spends different amounts of time, in whose company, and engaged in what kinds of activity. A second dimension consists of culturally regulated customs of child care and rearing, or the repertoire of techniques which parents and other caretakers call on in meeting the needs of children. Bottle-feeding, carrying the infant on the back, innoculation with live vaccines, circumcision, and hiring strangers as babysitters are such customs routinely sanctioned, or not, by the culture. The third dimension of the developmental niche is the psychology of the caretakers, or the beliefs and values which inform the ways parents and others structure children's experiences and respond to their behavior.

One of the purposes served by this approach to children's environments is to make visible the multiple connections between childrens' day-to-day lives and the larger culture. The economic, social, and value systems in which parents function influence their fertility behavior: in the present case, we have suggested that shorter birth intervals are among the outcomes. The implications of shorter birth intervals for the developmental niches of infants and children in Kokwet were striking. The daily lives of children with younger siblings were different from those of others the same age, perhaps close neighbors or even half-siblings, who were still the youngest members of their families. Caretaking strategies for these children also differed, as we have noted. The organizing principle behind these differences is to be found in the third dimension of the niche: the cultural meaning of the birth of a child for the second-to-youngest child. In essence, the birth of a baby in Kipsigis, as in many other sub-Saharan African groups, provided the mechanism for the transition from infancy to childhood for the second-to-youngest child. Thus, for the Kipsigis, the child who became the last-born in his or her family was seen as inadequately socialized and likely, even as an adult, to be "spoiled," self-indulgent and thoughtless of the needs of others: "babies" in spirit if not in body.

Within the constraints of the larger Kipsigis socio-cultural environment, the traditional pattern of births spaced two-and-a-half or three years apart was well suited to the developmental capacities of infants and young children. Infants benefited from intensive care by their mothers, as well as by older sibling caretakers. Two or three-year-old children were, by the time a younger sibling was born, at least able to interact verbally with their parents, and to begin assimilating the roles of mother's helper and member of a semi-independent children's peer group. Given the prescribed roles of both infants and second-to-youngest children, however, the shortening of birth intervals to two years or less tended to have negative consequences for children in either position. For the second-to-youngest child, a short birth interval necessitated a social transition for which the child was developmentally unready; because this transition was likely to be problematic, the infant's place in the family became difficult. For the infant, birth after a short interval increased the risk of morbidity and even mortality. In short, birth spacing was a crucial element in shaping the developmental niches of both infants and children in Kokwet.

## SUMMARY AND CONCLUSIONS

In this chapter, we have discussed the implications of large-scale demographic change for the survival and development of infants and young children. Current increases in fertility in Kenya, we have suggested, are creating new issues in the treatment and survival of children in rural areas. The interface between these large-scale changes and the outcomes for infants and the children is the "developmental niche," or micro-environment of the child as it is shaped by the culture.

It has often been argued that families in traditional cultures do not perceive the adverse effects of rapid population growth on the family economy, since the benefits of having many children to help with the work of the household and to support the parents in their old age outweigh the disadvantages of dividing the family's resources, such as land, among a growing number of users. The importance of child spacing for the health of mothers and babies, on the other hand, has traditionally been appreciated in rural Kenyan cultures, whose customs played a role in balancing the parental goals of having many children and having healthy ones. As with many aspects of culture change, the current trends in fertility in Kenya have brought unintended changes for the survival and development of children and their families. It is to be hoped that a heightened awareness of the relationships between fertility and the developmental niches of infants and young children in Kenya will enable parents to mobilize traditional values to preserve favorable child spacing as they confront an emerging risk factor for child survival and development.

## ACKNOWLEDGMENTS

A preliminary version of this paper was presented at the 1984 meetings of the American Anthropological Association. The research reported here was supported by the Carnegie Corporation of New York, the William T. Grant Foundation, the Spencer Foundation, and the National Institute of Mental Health (grant no. 33281). The authors would like to thank Martin G. Larson and Joseph Potter for their helpful comments and criticisms on earlier versions of this chapter. All statements made and views expressed are the sole responsibility of the authors.

## NOTE

1. In the analysis of fertility change using matched pairs of older and younger mothers, one mother (and her matched pair) were removed from the sample. This woman had 11 years of schooling (more than any of the other women in the community) and had grown up in close contact with Western influences as she lived with an American family while attending an American missionary school. She was monogamously married to a man of the same Christian

sect as herself. She had five children (after which she had had a tubal ligation – the only woman in the community to have done so), and an average birth interval of 1.62 years, one of the shortest of the community. This woman was an apt illustration of the social trends associated with shortened birth intervals, but at the age of 34, she fell into our "older" age group. We justify her removal from the sample for this analysis on the grounds that she was atypical of the women as a group. Including her and a matched younger mother in the sample for this analysis produces an average birth interval of 2.5 years for the older women (compared to 2.55 years for the sample excluding her), with a slightly lower significance level for the difference with the younger mothers ($t = 1.78$, $df = 23$, $p = 0.04$ one-tailed). Three other women were excluded from all the analyses reported here because of clearly inadequate or suspect fertility data.

## REFERENCES

Bongaarts, J.
  1976 Intermediate fertility variables and marital fertility rates. Population Studies 30(2): 227–241.
  1982 The fertility-inhibiting effects of the intermediate fertility variables. Studies in Family Planning 13: 179–189.
Digest.
  1984 *In* Kenya, modernization, drop in breastfeeding and low contraceptive use bring rising fertility. International Family Planning Perspectives 10: 131–133.
Delvoye, P., and Robyn, C.
  1980 Breast-feeding and post partum amenorrhea in Central Africa. 2. Prolactin and post partum amenorrhea. Journal of Tropical Pediatrics 26: 184–189.
Dow, T.E. and Werner, L.H.
  1976 Family size and family planning in Kenya: Continuity and change in metropolitan and rural attitudes. Population and Development Review 2: 321–366.
Faruquee, R. *et al.*
  1980 Kenya: Population and development. Washington, D.C: The World Bank.
Harkness, S.
  1977 Aspects of social environment and first language acquisition in rural Africa. *In* C. Snow and C.A. Ferguson (Eds.), Talking to children: Language input and acquisition. Cambridge, England: Cambridge University Press.
Harkness, S., and Super, C.M.
  1982 Why African children are so hard to test. *In* L.L. Adler (Ed.), Cross-cultural research at issue. New York: Academic Press.
  1983 The cultural construction of child development: A framework for the socialization of affect. Ethos 11: 221–231.
  1985 The cultural context of gender segregation in children's peer groups. Child Development 56: 219–224.
Hobcraft, J., McDonald, J.W., and Rutstein, S.
  1983 Child-spacing effects on infant and early child mortality. Population Index 49: 585–618.
Konner, M. and Worthman, C.
  1980 Nursing frequency, gonadal function, and birth spacing among !Kung hunter-gatherers. Science 207: 788–791.
Lesthaeghe, R., Ohadike, P.O., Kocher, J., and Page, H.J.
  1981 Child-spacing and fertility in sub-Saharan Africa: An overview of issues. *In* H.J. Page and R. Lesthaeghe (Eds.), Child-spacing in tropical Africa: Traditions and change. New York: Academic Press, pp. 3–21.
Mott, F.L. and Mott, S.H.
  1980 Kenya's record population growth: A dilemma of development. Population Bulletin 35: 1–43.

Ojofeitimi, E.O.
  1982 Effect of duration and frequency of breastfeeding on post-partum amenorrhea. Pediat-
       rics 69: 164–168.
Peristiany, J.G.
  1939 The social institutions of the Kipsigis. London: Routledge & Kegan Paul.
Super, C.M.
  1985 The use of multidimensional scaling techniques to assess children's ages in a field setting.
       Unpublished manuscript.
Super, C.M., and Harkness, S.
  1981 Figure, ground, and gestalt: The cultural context of the active individual. *In* R.M.
       Lerner and N.A. Busch-Rossnagel (Eds.), Individuals as producers of their develop-
       ment: A life-span perspective. New York: Academic Press, pp. 69–85.
  1982a The development of affect in infancy and early childhood. *In* D. Wagner and H.
       Stevenson (Eds.), Cultural perspectives on child development. San Francisco: Free-
       man, pp. 7–19.
  1982b The infant's niche in rural Kenya and metropolitan Boston. *In* L.L. Adler (Ed.),
       Cross-cultural research at issue. New York: Academic Press.

MARIA LEPOWSKY

# FOOD TABOOS AND CHILD SURVIVAL: A CASE STUDY FROM THE CORAL SEA

## INTRODUCTION

Traditional feeding practices which restrict or prohibit animal protein foods for children under weaning age have been reported from widely separated areas of the tropics. The indigenous explanation is often that the forbidden foods would cause a very young child to fall sick or die. Scientific observers and medical personnel who have described these food proscriptions or analyzed their implications in a particular area have emphasized their apparent deleterious effect upon the nutritional status of a particularly vulnerable group, young children aged about six months to three years. Due to the synergism between undernutrition and many infectious diseases, the food proscriptions may contribute to greater morbidity and mortality among young children in populations which adhere to them. Therefore writers describing these traditional child feeding practices have often recommended intervention by health workers, particularly nutrition education programs emphasizing the dangers to child health.

Animal protein food proscriptions for young children have been labeled a form of child neglect by several observers, usually with the qualifications that parents in these societies do not consciously intend to be abusive or neglectful of their children, that the practices are ordained by custom, are the prevailing community standard, may be adaptive for the overall population, or that the adults believe the proscriptions protect the child's health. Scrimshaw (1978) describes "infant feeding patterns" which "lead to increased morbidity and mortality in infants." She notes in this respect that "(m)any foods considered unsuitable for infants in some cultures are those richest in protein." She sees these "infant feeding patterns" as a form of "underinvestment in children" and "a form of 'neglect' (which) may be facilitated by cultural norms about child care that reflect subtle responses to population pressures or . . . familial desperation with existing conditions" (Scrimshaw 1978: 392–394). Langness (1981: 16), in a survey article on child abuse and neglect in New Guinea, describes "cultural practices in New Guinea (which) would be seen as abusive or neglectful by Western standards," although they may be practiced "for the purpose of improving the child's health or beauty." Citing Lewis's 1975 research on the Gnau of the Sepik River area of northern Papua New Guinea, he observes that, "Sometimes children are malnourished as a result of certain food taboos even though the taboos are ostensibly for their protection." Similarly, Cassidy (1980) describes proscriptions on giving animal protein

71

*Nancy Scheper-Hughes (ed.), Child Survival, 71–92.*
© *1987 by Reidel Publishing Company.*

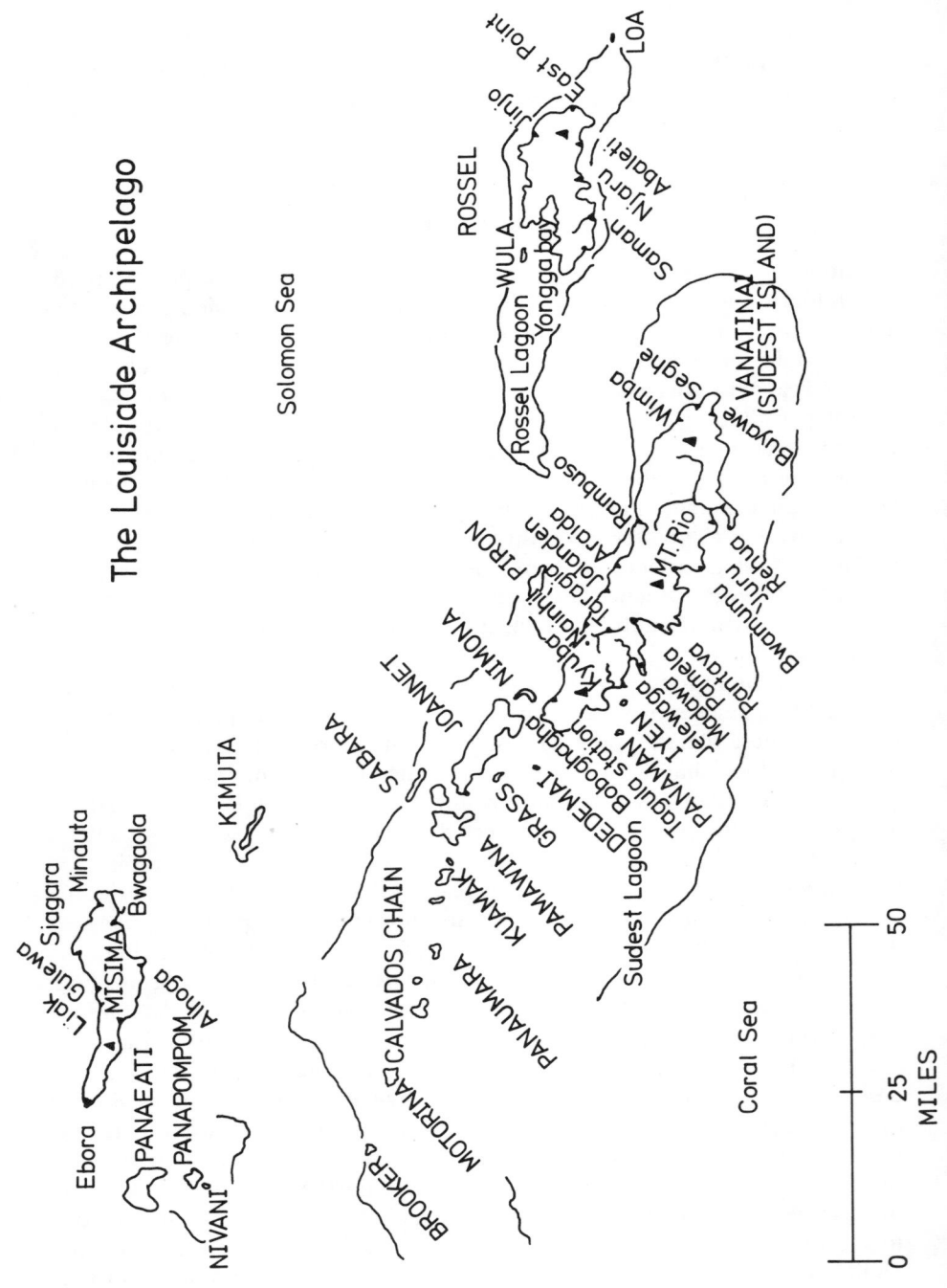

The Louisiade Archipelago

Solomon Sea

Coral Sea

MILES
0          25          50

foods to young children in various parts of the world and argues that these cultural practices are a form of culturally sanctioned "benign neglect" (see below).

This chapter examines the cultural and ecological context of child treatment, particularly infant and child feeding practices, on a remote island in the Coral Sea, 225 miles southeast of mainland Papua New Guinea. It analyzes the traditional food taboos which prohibit giving animal protein foods to children under weaning age, that is, until about three years of age, in terms of the cultural logic of these taboos and their possible adaptive significance. The conclusions drawn from this case study may be relevant to the study of child health and nutrition in many parts of the lowland tropics. They also indicate the necessity of detailed analysis of the costs and benefits of traditional child treatment practices such as food taboos for the individual and for the population before these practices are labeled as child neglect or as detrimental to child health.

## ENVIRONMENT, SUBSISTENCE AND CULTURE ON VANATINAI

The island, called Sudest or Tagula on maps and charts (see map), is the largest island in the Louisiade Archipelago of southeastern Papua New Guinea.[1] At fifty miles long by about ten miles wide, it is the largest piece of land for 200 miles. The indigenous name for the island, Vanatinai, means both "motherland" and "mainland." Vanatinai is inhabited by 2075 people, giving it an extremely low population density of about four persons per square mile. Early reports by British visitors indicate that the population has been stable for at least 100 years (see Lepowsky 1981). A central mountain range rises steeply from the sago swamps and runs the length of the island, rising to a height of 2645 feet at Mt. Rio, which is believed to be the home of the spirits of the dead. Vanatinai is encircled, along with the adjacent small coral islands of the Calvados Chain to the northwest, by one of the world's largest lagoons. The infrequent and difficult to find breaks in the barrier reef and the treacherous patches and shoals in the shallow lagoon discourage motor vessels from visiting the region and contribute to the island's lack of integration into the world cash economy. Many families obtain no cash at all in a year, and per capita income in the region is well under $20 per year.

The people of Vanatinai grow yams, taro, sweet potato, manioc, and bananas and pineapple in their gardens. They also process sago starch from the trunk of the mature female sago palm (*Metroxylon sagu*), which grows abundantly in the island swamps. They keep pigs, which are fed sago pith and allowed to forage in the rainforest. The islanders also gather substantial quantities of edible wild nuts, legumes, tubers, leaves, ferns and fruits in the forest. Both men and women hunt for possums and marsupial fruit bats, and men hunt wild pig, crocodile and monitor lizard with spears.[2]

The streams, coastal mangrove swamps and fringing reefs of Vanatinai provide a rich environment for fish, shellfish and marine animals which are collected by men and women. These include freshwater shrimp and eels, oysters and crabs, dugong, turtle, giant Tridacna clams, and a wide variety of fish. Pelagic fish such as tuna and barracuda are found farther out in the lagoon.

The islanders produce a sufficient surplus of yams, sago starch and domestic pigs to trade to the people of the Calvados Chain, Panaeati, Misima, and even Ware Island, 175 miles to the northwest. Vanatinai and the other islands scattered off southeastern Papua New Guinea are linked in a traditional trading and ceremonial exchange network which was first described in detail by the famous anthropologist Bronislaw Malinowski (1922) based upon his field research in the Trobriand Islands, 300 miles northwest of Vanatinai. The islanders continue to travel in their outrigger sailing canoes to visit trading partners up to hundreds of miles away to exchange foodstuffs and locally manufactured household goods such as clay cooking pots, wooden platters, sleeping mats and coconut-leaf skirts as well as highly prized ceremonial valuables, including shell-disc necklaces, *Conus* shell armlets (in the northern part of the region), greenstone axeblades, ceremonial lime spatulas of wood and tortoise-shell, and shell currency pieces (in the Vanatinai and Rossel Island area). This exchange system is called *kula* in the northern area and *kune* or *ghune* in the southern.

The primary impetus for a trading expedition is an upcoming obligation to contribute food and valuables at one of a series of feasts which commemorate the death of each individual. Although the customs of the mortuary feast sequence vary among the different linguistic and cultural groups which comprise the region, the valuables circulate throughout as a result of far-flung individual trade networks of men and, in the southern area, of women as well (see Lepowsky 1983 for a detailed account of trade and exchange on Vanatinai and Leach and Leach 1983 for an overview of exchange throughout the region today). As Malinowski himself noted in a later publication (1935), the importance of food exchanges among islands with different resource bases as a motivation for inter-island exchange was not sufficiently stressed in Malinowski's classic study, *Argonauts of the Western Pacific*. The climactic mortuary feasts found throughout the region typically feature the exchange of large quantities of yams, sago, pigs, and other foods, as well as ceremonial valuables.

## CHILD MALNUTRITION

In this environment of seemingly abundant food resources, with ample garden land, large tracts of sago palms, wild game and vegetable foods, one of the world's richest fishing grounds, and sufficient food surplus to support an inter-island exchange system and elaborate feasts, it seems improbable that large numbers of young children should suffer from malnutrition. But the

Papua New Guinea National Nutrition Survey, made public in June of 1978, reported that a majority of the children aged one to five in the Vanatinai (Sudest Island) census division and the neighboring East Calvados census division suffered from mild to moderate undernutrition, with their weight for age less than 80% of the Harvard reference standards.[3] The issue of the appropriateness of using anthropometric standards derived from measurements of Euro-American children will not be discussed here, because the same standards were used for children throughout Papua New Guinea in 1978, and certain districts of the Louisiade Archipelago showed a mean weight for age dramatically lower than adjacent districts and well below the Papua New Guinea national mean.

The National Nutrition Survey report caused surprise and consternation among government and health personnel in Milne Bay Province, the political division which is comprised of the southeastern Papuan islands and the adjacent tip of the main island of Papua New Guinea. The reported prevalence of child malnutrition for the Vanatinai region was double the Papua New Guinea national mean of 35% in this age group, despite adequate garden land, rich marine resources, and a traditional subsistence diet rather than the store-bought diet which has wreaked nutritional havoc in recent years in Papua New Guinean towns and plantation communities. The provincial government then carried out its own survey using middle upper arm circumference as a criterion (Lewis and Henton 1979). In the provincial survey about 60% of Vanatinai children between one and five were below the 14 cm cut-off value used internationally as an indicator of child malnutrition. Furthermore, 92% of Vanatinai children between one and three were below the cut-off value. The adjacent East Calvados Islands had a malnutrition rate of over 78% in this survey, the highest in the province. A subsequent survey by the provincial nutritionist using weight charts from Maternal and Child Health Clinic records to ascertain weight for age found that 96% of the Vanatinai and East Calvados children between one and five were below 80% of mean weight for age of Harvard reference standards, with 14% of these below 60% of the reference standards, indicating more severe malnutrition (Leonard 1980).

The other surprise in the data collected in the national and provincial nutrition surveys was that the reported patterns of child malnutrition did not follow environmental or ecological patterns but cultural ones. The Louisiade Archipelago is comprised of both high, continental islands and low, coralline islands, with the latter having poorer soil and water resources and a traditionally greater reliance upon exploitation of marine resources. Yet the coralline islands of the Calvados Chain, whose environmental resources are virtually identical, showed a marked disparity between the East Calvados and the West Calvados census divisions, which are culturally and linguistically distinct. The East Calvados had high rates of reported child malnutrition (78%), while the West Calvados had the lowest reported rate in the province at 16%.

Adjacent Panaeati and Misima Islands, culturally and linguistically the same as the West Calvados, had reported child malnutrition rates which were almost as low, 23% and 30% respectively (see Lepowsky 1985).

As an anthropologist residing on Vanatinai and carrying out the first research on the island's culture (Lepowsky 1981), I had been asked by Dr. Colin Lewis, then the Provincial Health Officer of Milne Bay Province, to undertake an investigation for the health department of cultural factors which might affect health and nutrition of people on this remote and culturally conservative island, particularly mothers and children, and to write and submit a report on the findings (Lepowsky 1979). The high prevalence of child malnutrition in the region indicated in the national and provincial nutrition surveys subsequently emphasized the urgency of Dr. Lewis' request. It also presented an intriguing research problem with significant practical implications: the reported presence of large numbers of malnourished children in an area with an apparent surplus of food and the patterning of the reported malnutrition in congruence with cultural rather than ecological boundaries.

I therefore collected extensive data on subsistence, its seasonal variation and its changes in the last few generations, diet and food habits, food beliefs and proscriptions, infant and child care ideology and practice, and ideology and practice related to health, illness, healing, pregnancy and childbirth. I intend to make quantitative assessments of food intake and production, nutritional status, morbidity and mortality during my next period of research on Vanatinai and nearby islands.

## FERTILITY AND THE VALUE OF CHILDREN

Children on Vanatinai are highly prized. Many islanders are concerned about their low population, fearing government-sanctioned resettlement of Misima islanders on their territory, and children are eagerly sought in adoption by community members. The present low population density of four persons per square mile on Vanatinai over the last one hundred years is apparently not the result of a significant population decline following exposure to infectious diseases brought by Europeans (see Lepowsky 1981 for a discussion of the historical evidence). By contrast, Misima Island, a high island about 70 miles to the northwest, has one-fifth the land area of Vanatinai and four times the population, about 8000, giving it a population density of 80 persons per square mile, 20 times that of Vanatinai, where the population is 2075. Because of this population pressure, people from Misima migrated to the small coral islands of the East Calvados chain, "so that we could eat fish," they explain, long enough ago to develop their own language which, although closely related, is not intelligible to Misima speakers. Misima-speaking people have more recently settled the low islands of Panaeati Lagoon and of the West Calvados chain.

In 1978 the average number of living children, including adult children, per woman aged 18 or older in the Jelewaga Village, Vanatinai, census division (which includes outlying hamlets for a total population of 219) was 2.27. About 10% of women between 18 and 45 were childless. There were nine living children in the largest family.

Vanatinai people attribute their own low population to their island's notorious sorcerers, who are blamed for almost all deaths and serious illnesses, and to the women's use of traditional herbal contraceptives and abortifacients (see Lepowsky 1981). Vanatinai traditional child spacing ideology and practices clearly influence completed family size. People say that another child should not be born "until the first is already running around and playing with its friends." This would be at about three years of age. Children are customarily breastfed until the age of three. There is also a postpartum sex taboo until the child is weaned. If this taboo is violated, it is said that the child would become sickly and might die. This taboo is probably frequently violated, judging from the village gossip which often blames an infant or child's illness upon the parents' not being "able to control themselves." The parents are supposed to sleep at opposite sides of the house or on separate sleeping mats. The presence of the taboo undoubtedly cuts down the frequency of parental intercourse during the first years of a child's life and thus the likelihood of conception.

The prolonged period of breastfeeding also contributes to child spacing. Vanatinai women say that they normally do not begin to menstruate until about one year after the birth of a child. They may also be anovulatory during much of this period. Long-term lactation may also cause the mother's percentage of body fat to decline and thus depress fecundity (cf. Frisch 1975, Frisch and McArthur 1974, Hamson, Boyce and Platt 1975).

Childless individuals on Vanatinai are pitied, for it is said that they will have no one to care for them in their old age, to fetch water and firewood for them and to cook their food. The birth of girls is welcomed in this matrilineal society, for they will grow up to give birth to new members of their natal kin group. Boy babies too are welcomed for their future contributions to family subsistence, such as making sago. Vanatinai has an ideal postmarital residence pattern of bilocality, with a married couple residing alternately throughout the year with the kin of each spouse and aiding each group with their subsistence activities. The parental or lineage group "investment" in childcare for both boys and girls therefore "pays off" when both sexes mature and contribute their labor to their natal families. Loss of the labor of females after marriage has been suggested as a contributing factor to "selective neglect" of female offspring, female infanticide, and a resulting imbalance in the sex ratio in some patrilineal, virilocal societies with dense populations (Scrimshaw 1978, Wyon and Gordon 1971, Miller 1981).

Infanticide was traditionally practiced on Vanatinai for abnormal offspring or when the mother felt that she already had too many children. The newborn would be abandoned, unwashed and with its umbilical cord still attached, by being placed by someone in the branches of a tree near the hamlet, where it would die of exposure unless it was retrieved by another person who wished to adopt it. I was told of three living men, all in their sixties, who had been abandoned and adopted by other women in this way. It is not clear whether female infants would be less likely to be abandoned or whether they would, if so abandoned, be less likely to be adopted by others.

Adoption is common on Vanatinai, as in many Pacific Island societies (Carroll 1970). It serves as a further mechanism for the absorption of children from households with larger families. Childless couples and individuals, grandparents and elderly kin of either spouse, and families with children of only one sex are extremely interested in adopting an infant or older child.

Adoption is called *vaghan*, which literally means, "to take and feed." The islanders say that any woman who has previously borne a child can begin to lactate again if she puts the child to her breast. Infants are often not adopted until about age two, when they are weaned early and given to the adoptive parents. Adopted children retain their natal kin group membership and rights to inheritance within their natal family.

Infants whose mothers die in childbirth and/or who are unable to nurse are fed green coconut water, and the prognosis for their survival is poor unless a wetnurse is found. Only a member of the mother's matrilineage will nurse the child of another woman.

Accurate statistical information on infant and child mortality is not available for the Louisiade Archipelago, as census figures of deaths in a given year rarely include the deaths of neonates or infants younger than one or two.

### INFANT AND CHILD TREATMENT

The people of Vanatinai are loving and indulgent parents whose philosophy of child rearing is extremely permissive. This seems to be characteristic of New Guinea societies (Langness 1981: 23–25). Vanatinai parents say that it is dangerous to leave an infant crying, "or it may become angry and leave us," or in other words, it may die.

Scheper-Hughes (this volume) describes the "maternal detachment" of Northeast Brazilian women living in conditions of extreme poverty, crowding, and appallingly high child mortality rates. These women take a guarded attitude toward infants, extending the greatest amount of their affection and parental care toward children who are physically strong and who survive the first couple of years of life. On Vanatinai it is not customary to name a child until a few weeks after birth, and the ritual presentation by the mother's family of shell currency necklaces or greenstone axeblades to the father's kin to "thank him" for siring a new member of the mother's matrilineage does not take place for about six months. Presumably these delays assure that naming and "childwealth" exchanges are only performed for children who are expected to survive. But in distinct contrast to the women of Northeast Brazilian shanty-towns, parents on Vanatinai lavish the greatest amount of overt affection and attention upon very young infants, who are perceived as being close to the ancestor spirits and perhaps ambivalent about remaining in the human world. Extreme parental indulgence lessens gradually as the child grows, and older children are expected to defer to the cries and demands of very young siblings.

Vanatinai culture is marked by a high degree of respect for the autonomy and the will of individuals of all ages. Idiosyncratic behavior is attributed to the force of the individual's personality. This laissez-faire attitude is backed by supernatural sanctions: the infant has a spirit with its own strong will, and adults are believed to have the power to kill through sorcery and witchcraft if they are angered by others. Children too are protected by the fear of sorcery carried out by an adult relative, just as they may be victims of adult sorcerers seeking revenge on the child's adult kin.

Young children are allowed to manipulate firebrands and sharp knives without remonstrance, and injuries are rare. They do occur though: one four year old girl had accidentally amputated parts of several fingers on her right hand by playing with a bush knife (machete) used in gardening (contrary to Sorenson's 1976 contention that Fore children of the Eastern Highlands of New Guinea, similarly allowed to play with fire and knives, never injure themselves).

Children are rarely punished for any kind of misbehavior, although they may be scolded after they reach the age of three, particularly if they are bothering a younger sibling. Children under three are permitted to grab food from the portions of older siblings and adult family members as long as the food is not of the prohibited category.

The word *tabwa* means both "fat" or "plump" and "to grow." A fat baby is considered to be a healthy and attractive one. Bottle feeding is completely unknown on Vanatinai. Supplemental foods such as premasticated taro or mashed yam, sweet potato, manioc, banana or pumpkin are given at about six months of age in gradually increasing amounts. Children eat pieces of boiled vegetable foods from the adult meal from about one year of age (see Lepowsky 1985 for a detailed discussion of infant and child feeding practices). Breastfeeding continues on demand until age three.

## FOOD TABOOS

Traditional food proscriptions on Vanatinai prohibit children under weaning age from consuming any of the foods characteristically described as *love*, which means both "sweet" and "greasy." These include all animal protein foods such as fish, pig, fruits, greens, and storebought foods (the latter being rarely consumed by anyone). The only exception to this rule is that coconut cream, in which tubers and other vegetable foods are normally boiled to make *tamja* (literally, "squeezed food"), the daily staple, may be eaten by young children even though it is *love*. These food taboos are rigidly followed because, parents say, "otherwise the child will fall sick and die." One mother explained, "We must take good care of our children, for we are living very far from hospitals." The food taboos are described as part of *taubwaragha*, "the way of the ancestors."

These food taboos are adhered to in the Vanatinai and East Calvados regions, where there is a reported high prevalence of child malnutrition which is particularly dramatic among children aged 1–3, the same age at which the food taboo has a demonstrable impact upon the diet (the nutritional status of children less than one was not measured). Similar taboos were previously followed in the Misima, Panaeati and West Calvados regions, which have much lower reported prevalences of child malnutrition, but they are largely ignored nowadays due to intervention by government, mission and health personnel, all based at Misima, which has been the government and mission center of the entire region for almost one hundred years.

It seems therefore that the presence of traditional food taboos against feeding animal protein and other foods to children under three in the Vanatinai and East Calvados regions accounts for the reported prevalence of child malnutrition, mostly of a mild to moderate level, in areas with seemingly abundant food resources. The observance of these food taboos in some cultural groups and not in others would also account for the reported pattern of child malnutrition, which follows cultural rather than ecological boundaries.

The question which then arises is why such seemingly maladaptive food taboos, which negatively affect the nutritional status of young children, should be found and adhered to in a society which highly values children and which does not suffer from overpopulation. The synergism of malnutrition and many infectious diseases has been well-documented (Scrimshaw, Taylor and Gordon 1968, Taylor 1985). Presumably then the malnutrition of children in the Vanatinai region should contribute to their mortality risk.

Similar food taboos prohibiting all or some animal protein foods to infants and young children have been reported from many parts of the world, including West Africa (Hendrickse 1966: 344, Ogbeide 1974: 213–5), East Africa (Gerlach 1969: 392), India (Jelliffe 1957: 131, 134), Malaysia (Wolff 1965, Bolton 1972: 791–2) and New Guinea (Van Der Hoeven 1958: 74, Lewis 1975). In most cases the food proscription is accompanied by a statement that a child fed such prohibited foods will sicken or die.

Scientific observers and health personnel writing about these food beliefs usually discount parental concerns for the child's health. Bolton (1972), points to what he calls "an element of greed" in aboriginal Malay restrictions of prized protein foods to adults, particularly adult men. At best the belief that the food proscriptions are for the child's health are seen as misguided or based on ignorance. Virtually all observers recommend intervention and nutrition education to improve the nutritional status and the health of local children. As Taylor (1985: 289) points out, understanding of the synergism between undernutrition and certain infectious diseases has become apparent as improved nutrition improved the health of tuberculosis and typhoid patients, and "(a) major justification for nutritional programs became that they could help control infections. Infectious disease specialists also claimed that their programs would improve nutritional status." Thus intervention in areas following these food proscriptions has commendable intentions for improving health and alleviating suffering.

Cassidy (this volume), who has written extensively on similar food taboos and toddler malnutrition in cross-cultural perspective, points out that interpretations of the significance of these taboos or of resulting child malnutrition depends upon the worldview of the observer. In an earlier paper (1980) she describes the toddler malnutrition which arises from this and other causes as a form of culturally sanctioned "benign neglect," a term which she distinguishes from "malign neglect," where parents intend to injure or to withhold care from their children. She argues that the practices which result in this malnutrition may be detrimental to the health and the survival of the individual child but beneficial overall to the group as a form of population control, as a natural selection mechanism, and as a means of adapting more "fit" individuals to the conditions of food scarcity which they must face as adults. Cassidy's argument would thus label the Vanatinai food taboos a form of "benign neglect."

The insufficient diet in terms of quantity or quality fed to some children in a number of societies cross-culturally has been labeled "selective neglect" by Scrimshaw (1978). She suggests that unwanted children, due to their sex, poor health or high birth order, suffer from parental "underinvestment in some children," including poorer diet and less attention to the child's health, leading to higher mortality among the children at risk. As Taylor (1985) notes, the synergism of malnutrition and infection is highly correlated with sex and socio-economic status, with poor children and female children being at greater risk in many societies.

The Vanatinai food taboos affect all children equally and are thus not a form of selective neglect. Selective neglect would more likely be found in an area of high population, poor economic conditions, or low value of female children (e.g., Scrimshaw 1975, 1978, Scheper-Hughes 1984 and this volume, Miller 1981).

The intense concern which Vanatinai parents show for their children's health and the high quality of care which island children receive overall led me to wonder whether there was any benefit to the individual child in the traditional food taboos prohibiting animal protein and whether the parental explanation that the child might sicken or die if fed the prohibited foods had any basis in fact. One consequence of the animal protein taboo is the emphasis in the child's diet upon breastmilk as a high quality and digestible form of protein. The fatty, prohibited foods would not be easily processed by the infant's immature digestive system and might cause diarrhea, which can be a danger to life in very young children (Jelliffe and Jelliffe 1978, Ogra, Fishaut and Theodore 1980, Carlsson, *et al.* 1980). Consumption of breastmilk also proportionally reduces the child's consumption of water, which on Vanatinai is often contaminated by the feces of pigs or dogs or by the human excrement washed into streams by torrential rains (the islanders normally excrete in certain areas of the forest near the settlement or on certain sections of beach). Breastmilk also contains maternal antibodies which protect the young child against a number of infectious diseases, and as noted earlier, the mother's prolonged period of lactation decreases the likelihood that she will conceive a child who would displace its older sibling from the breast at a vulnerable age and contribute to its risk of mortality.

The traditional proscriptions on consumption of animal protein foods by young children may also adapt the child to a low-protein diet. Most adult Papua New Guinean diets are notably low in protein, and nutritional researchers have been struck by the apparent health and vigor which these Papua New Guineans nevertheless maintain (e.g., Macpherson 1963, Ferro-Luzzi, Norgan and Durnin 1978, Norgan, Ferro-Luzzi and Durnin 1974). Vanatinai adults eat surprisingly little animal protein despite their island's rich marine resources, perhaps because of their traditional inland settlement pattern and subsistence orientation (see Lepowsky 1985). Children eating a low-protein diet will be shorter in adult stature but require less protein to maintain health in later life (Stini 1979). The amount of protein necessary to maintain health in humans is presently the subject of considerable research and discussion by nutritionists, with some authorities suggesting, on the basis of clinical research, substantial reductions in international standards of adequate or minimum protein intake.

The following section suggests an additional way in which proscriptions on consumption of animal protein foods may benefit the individual child on Vanatinai and in many other parts of the Old World lowland tropics.

## MALARIA, FOOD TABOOS AND CHILD SURVIVAL

Malaria is one of the greatest worldwide threats to human health and to child survival. About 100 million cases occur each year. Estimates of malaria mortality range from nearly one million annually, mostly of children under fourteen (Wyler 1982) to two to four million fatalities per year (Kolata 1984).

Malaria is a parasitic disease caused by one of four species of the *Plasmodium* protozoan which affects humans. The parasite is transmitted by *Anopheles* mosquito species. Vanatinai is an island with extensive tracts of brackish and freshwater swampland in which three species of *Anopheles* mosquitoes and *Plasmodium falciparum* and *P. vivax* malaria are endemic (Spencer, Spencer and Venters 1974: 23, Parkinson 1974: 12) *P. falciparum* is a potentially fatal disease to which children between the ages of six months and three years are particularly susceptible. Younger infants are protected by fetal hemoglobin and by maternal antibodies (Maegraith 1967, Pasvol et al. 1976), and individuals who survive malaria attacks may become partially immune to the disease, with their degree of immunity increasing as they reach adulthood (Molineaux and Gramiccia 1980, Nardin et al. 1979). The child death rate from malaria on Vanatinai is unknown, but in parts of lowland Papua New Guinea, "20 percent of infant deaths have been attributed to malaria" (Black 1972: 682).

Malaria is not only a potentially lethal disease. It suppresses host immunity to other infectious diseases, causes host malnutrition as manifested by hemolytic anemia and low weight for age and height, increases the rate of miscarriage and contributes to low birthweight in infants, lowering their viability (Burnet and White 1972, Katz 1982). The prevalence of malaria on Vanatinai probably contributes significantly to the island's low birth rate and small population relative to other islands of the Louisiade Archipelago which have less swampland and fewer species of anopheline vectors.

Scrimshaw, Taylor, Nevin and Gordon's (1968) landmark volume on the interaction of nutrition and infection uses evidence from human and animal studies to document the synergistic relationship between malnutrition and many kinds of infectious diseases. But their survey of case studies and experiments on the relationship between nutrition and malaria indicates that in over half the cases, the interaction of either overall nutritional status or of deficiencies of particular nutrients was antagonistic. The individual human or animal host with poorer nutritional status had less severe symptoms or did not manifest the disease at all. They conclude that the Plasmodium may be more susceptible to nutrient deprivation than the human or animal host and be unable to replicate optimally (see Eaton 1976, Wyler 1982). Beisel (1982: 749) observes that, "Malaria may be considered an illustration in humans of an antagonistic interaction between severe malnutrition and a parasitic disease" (cf. Weinberg 1978, Carmichael 1985).

Overall mild to moderate malnutrition and deficiencies of protein, iron, vitamins A, C, E and several of the B vitamins, as well as the presence of an all-milk diet have been correlated with greater resistance to malaria and lowered risk of mortality from the disease (Scrimshaw, Taylor and Gordon 1968). The human or animal host may have similar nutrient needs to the Plasmodium, and the low availability of nutrients necessary for plasmodial growth and reproduction may cause the parasite to "starve" before the host does.

The evidence for an antagonistic relationship between malaria and malnutrition comes from a variety of sources. For example, experimental data using animal hosts show that mice on a vitamin E-deficient diet had less severe infections of Plasmodium berghei than mice receiving a vitamin E-supplemented diet (Eaton et al. 1976). Animal experiments have also indicated that folate deficiency is associated with lessened severity of plasmodial infection (Katz 1982: 805). Rats fed a high-protein diet had a correspondingly high level of plasmodial parasitemia (Targett 1981).

Severe malnutrition induced by famine was first reported to suppress symptoms of malaria during the Bengal famine of 1943 (Hendrickse 1967). Refeeding Somali nomad children with relief grain during the Sahelian famine of the mid-1970s precipitated previously asymptomatic malaria (Murray et al. 1978a). Cerebral malaria, which is often fatal, has been reported as more common in well-nourished West African children than in those with marasmus or kwashiorkor (Edington 1967, Hendrickse et al. 1971).

Adding iron to the diet of anemic patients precipitated malaria attacks in Tanzania (Byles and D'Sa 1970, Masawe et al. 1974) and Somalia (Murray et al. 1975, 1978b). Animal protein foods provide the bulk of the iron in the Vanatinai diet, and therefore, the food taboos prohibiting animal protein foods to young island children severely curtail their iron intake.

An all-milk or preponderantly milk diet has also been reported as suppressing symptoms of plasmodial infection in rodents, monkeys, and humans (Maegraith et al. 1952, Bray and Garnham 1953, Maegraith 1967). The Vanatinai food taboos ensure that island children consume an all-milk diet for the first six months of life, with a gradually increased supplementation of a largely breastmilk diet with vegetable foods, primarily starchy tubers, until they are weaned at about age three.

The age of greatest risk of death from malaria is virtually identical on Vanatinai with the age at which the taboo on consumption of animal protein foods is in effect. I therefore suggest that these food taboos constitute a cultural adaptation to an environment of endemic malaria, protecting young children in part against the disease and emphasizing the benefits of breastmilk for the child's health.

All of the other regions of the world in which similar food proscriptions are found, with the accompanying belief that the child would fall sick or die if fed the prohibited foods, are lowland tropical regions in which malaria is endemic. I further suggest that this overlap is no coincidence and that the food proscriptions in these other regions may also be cultural adaptations to an environment of endemic malaria which may benefit both the individual and the population as a whole. Cultural and behavioral adaptations to malaria have been noted in many parts of the world (e.g., May 1958, Brown 1981, Durham 1982), although an adaptive relationship between this type of food taboo and malaria has not previously been suggested by other authors.

## IMPLICATIONS FOR HEALTH POLICY AND FOR THE CROSS-CULTURAL STUDY OF CHILD TREATMENT

The hypothesis that food taboos and their probable consequence of mild to moderate child malnutrition may be a cultural adaptation which protects the child against death from malaria leads to obvious ethical and policy dilemmas. If such taboos are adaptive, should health workers refrain from intervening, even though child malnutrition may negatively affect the individual's physical and mental development and is synergistic with many other infectious diseases?

In the Vanatinai case, the period since World War II has led to increased contact with the outside world and probably a greater incidence of influenza, pneumonia, and other infectious diseases which are synergistic with the malnutrition which probably results from traditional food taboos.[4] Respiratory diseases are the leading cause of death in Papua New Guinea today. Deaths from bacterial pneumonia tend to follow as a complication of influenza, which sweeps the island three or four times a year. People in all age groups succumb. Thus food taboos which protect against malaria but increase risk of contracting or dying from a number of infectious diseases introduced by Europeans, to which the islanders have very low resistance, may be less adaptive today than they were in pre-colonial times. This may be the situation in other parts of the tropical world where such food proscriptions are found and which have had contact with European diseases in the last few hundred years.

Further study of the relationships among diet, nutritional status, malaria and other infectious diseases is urgently needed in areas where these food beliefs are traditional. If further research shows that in fact such food proscriptions protect against malaria, intervention might well still be indicated. Nutrition education campaigns could be combined with education concerning the risk of malaria for young children and suggestions as to how to reduce anopheline populations locally (e.g., in being vigilant about standing water, a common breeding site for some species) and how to keep children away from local anopheline habitats. This integrated approach combining nutrition and health education and health care has been emphasized recently as a successful and cost-effective means of improving public health and individual well-being (Taylor 1983, 1985).

In the Brazilian shanty-town situation described by Scheper-Hughes (1984, this volume), an extremely high risk of infant mortality is accompanied by a very dense population, a high birth rate, a short birth interval, and the expectation that many infants and young children will die. The parental strategy is to give birth to many children and to invest the greatest share of affection, nourishment and care in children who seem strong enough to survive in these conditions of poverty and disease.

Vanatinai is an island with a more moderate infant mortality rate where cultural and biological forces combine to produce a population of low density which is stable over time, a low birth rate and a long birth interval. The indigenous childcare strategy is to invest considerable amounts of parental care and attention in each infant who survives birth and, previously, the period at birth when infanticide was culturally permissible. Each Vanatinai child is therefore a wanted child, and its kin group has sufficient emotional and dietary resources to support it. According to local standards, the young infant receives more immediate food and attention than anyone else. "Food" in the Vanatinai language, *ghanika*, also means "yam," and children after six months of age are given as much *ghanika*, the staple yam and other starchy tubers, as they wish to eat.[5]

Traditional food taboos restrict the child's consumption of animal protein, but this category of food is withheld because it is locally believed to threaten the child's health and its life. The food taboos may in fact confer some protection against potentially lethal malaria, life-threatening diarrhea, and contaminated water, and they emphasize the benefit of maternal immunity for the child and protect it against the birth of a younger sibling while it is at a vulnerable age.

The Vanatinai demographic and cultural strategy of long birth intervals and intense parental investment in each child may be typical for food collecting and horticultural peoples with low populations where there are normally sufficient resources to maintain the population at or just above the replacement level (cf. Langness' 1981 discussion of child treatment in New Guinea and Konner's 1976 study of maternal care among the !Kung).

Infant mortality on Vanatinai is a threat to normal social relations in a subsistence society where cooperation among members is necessary for survival. Due to the personal causation theory of illness and death held by the islanders, most deaths or serious illnesses represent the destructive action of a neighbor who is practicing sorcery or witchcraft. More rarely, an infant death is attributed to taboo violation by its parents. Food taboos and post-partum sex taboos are often discussed but are rarely blamed in actual cases of death. Infant illness therefore has a social cost of creating fear and conflict among community members. Unlike in the Brazilian shanty-town, it is considered an abnormal and tragic situation.

The traditional Vanatinai food taboos must be studied as a part of a strategy of parental nurture which maximizes the survival chances of each viable infant according to indigenous theory and which emphasizes extra attention to the child's health needs. It is not a withdrawal of care, a withholding of nourishment or a form of child neglect. It is an adaptation to the recognized danger of infant mortality.

The food taboos-malaria hypothesis indicates the importance of caution in labeling traditional childcare practices as forms of child neglect, albeit "benign"or "unconscious". Researchers should at least take seriously the contention that these traditional practices such as food proscriptions are intended by a society's parents and adults to benefit the individual child. Child neglect as a culturally relative concept is a difficult issue for Western scientists. There are practices which are labeled by indigenous peoples in virtually every society as abusive or neglectful. The problem lies with practices which are normative to one population but which outside observers see as detrimental to the child's well-being even though the people themselves regard them as essential for the child's health or social well-being (Korbin 1981, Langness 1981). This chapter stresses the necessity of evaluating traditional childcare practices according to indigenous as well as Western standards of benefit and detriment before labeling them as neglectful and targeting them for intervention. Traditional practices often require careful study before their potential benefit to the individual or the population becomes obvious.

## NOTES

1. I conducted anthropological research in Papua New Guinea from November, 1977 to March, 1979 with a return visit in March and April of 1981. I became fluent in Vanatinai Ghalingaji, the unwritten language of Sudest Island. Data were collected through participant observation and informal interviews, supplemented by archival research. My research base during most of my stay was at Jelewaga Village, Sudest Island (Vanatinai), where I resided with a local family. I would like to give special thanks to Martin Peter, Nora Moses, Thomas Robutu, Jimmy, Daisy and Hina Martin and the people of Jelewaga, along with their neighbors on Vanatinai and nearby islands who shared their lives with me and offered me assistance, hospitality and friendship. Without their interest and moral support, none of my research would have been possible. I hope this research will benefit them and their children. I would also like to thank the late Dr. Colin Lewis, Milne Bay Provincial Health Officer from 1978–9, Dr. Festus Pawa, Milne Bay Provincial Health Officer from 1981 to present, and the staff of the Milne Bay Provincial Health Department for their assistance and their encouragement of this research. I wish to thank Nancy Scheper-Hughes for her helpful comments on an earlier draft of this chapter.

   Financial support for the 1977–9 research period was provided by the National Science Foundation and by the Chancellor's Patent Fund and the Department of Anthropology of the University of California, Berkeley. Transportation to Papua New Guinea in 1981 was subsidized by the Papua New Guinea Institute of Applied Social and Economic Research. Financial support during the period of library research and the writing of the first draft of this chapter was provided by the National Institutes of Health, National Institute of Child Health and Human Development through a Public Health Service Fellowship held at the School of Public Health, University of California, Berkeley. All of this financial support is gratefully acknowledged.

2. Diet on Vanatinai, although still based almost entirely upon subsistence, has changed significantly in the last few decades. As recently as forty years ago, the islanders relied to a greater degree upon the collection of wild vegetable foods and on sago making and less upon the cultivation of starchy tubers such as sweet potato and manioc. These two cultigens of New World origin were first brought to the island in the 1880s but were not grown in large quantities until after World War II. They are relatively easy to grow and do well on poor, sandy soil and in drought conditions. They may also be grown year-round, unlike yams, which are seasonal. This unplanned cultural change may have had a detrimental effect upon child and adult nutrition, as the earlier wild food-collecting diet was more varied and contained a wider range of micronutrients (see Lepowsky 1985 for a detailed discussion of this subject).

3. This survey was based upon data in Maternal and Child Health Clinic records. A majority of children in the Louisiade Archipelago are weighed once a year. In the Vanatinai and East Calvados region, the Mission of the Sacred Heart on Nimowa Island sends a boat to the coastal villages and sends word for children under five to be brought and weighed.

4. The initial period of widespread impact of European-introduced infectious diseases upon the

people of Vanatinai was probably in the mid-1880s. In 1885 71 men abducted and taken to labor on the Queensland sugar plantations were repatriated. Thirteen others were found by the Queensland government to have died on the plantations. The 1888 goldrush on the island briefly brought hundreds of Australian miners to the area as well as their contract laborers from other parts of former British New Guinea (Lepowsky 1981). Vanatinai people today say that Dobu Islanders brought in to labor on the goldfields taught their ancestors new and deadly sorcery spells. Dobu prowess in sorcery said to cause specific fatal conditions was made famous in anthropology with Reo Fortune's 1932 publication of *Sorcerers of Dobu*. Fortune reports that "measles (which kills natives), tuberculosis, influenza, dysentery, are recognized by the natives as being of introduced origin" and are attributed on Dobu to the malevolent action of a "devil" placed in local hot springs by Tauwau, the "mythological creator of the white race and of European artifacts" (1932: 136). It is possible that Vanatinai memories of new sorcery spells being introduced about 1888 by Dobu men reflect the realities of new killing diseases which first struck the local population during that period. The Vanatinai equivalent of Tauwau, named Alagh (or Ghalagh), is not held responsible for causing any category of illness or death. Vanatinai people explain a perceived rise in the amount of illness and death attributed to sorcery since the colonial suppression of warfare (a gradual process lasting from 1888 to 1942) by saying, "Before we killed with spears. Now we kill with sorcery." This belief may not only represent a cultural substitution of psychological for physical aggression but a rise in the incidence of serious illness and death from introduced infectious diseases over 100 years. However, despite these new introduced diseases, pre-colonial and colonial estimates and censuses of population on the island do not reveal any marked fluctuations since the 1880s (see Lepowsky 1981).

5. Similarly, the term "food" in Fiji "is used specifically for root and tree crop starches" (Pollock 1985: 195). *Ghanika moli* in the Vanatinai language means "true food" and refers to yams and other starchy tubers, plus sometimes bananas or pumpkin, boiled in coconut cream. This staple food is used to supplement the breastmilk diet of the child in gradually increasing amounts beginning at about six months of age (see Lepowsky 1985 for a more detailed discussion of indigenous concepts of food, historical changes in diet, and infant and child diet).

## REFERENCES

Beisel, William
  1982 Synergism and antagonism of parasitic diseases and malnutrition. Reviews of Infectious
       Diseases 4(4): 746–750.
Black, Robert H.
  1972 Malaria. *In* Peter Ryan (ed.), Encyclopaedia of Papua and New Guinea. Melbourne:
       Melbourne University Press, pp. 679–684.
Bolton, J.M.
  1972 Food taboos among the Orang Asli in West Malaysia: a potential nutritional hazard.
       American Journal of Clinical Nutrition 25: 789–799.
Bray, R.S. and P.C.C. Garnham
  1953 Effect of milk diet in P. cynomolgi infections in monkeys. British Medical Journal 1:
       1200–1202.
Brown, Peter J.
  1981 Cultural adaptations to endemic malaria in Sardinia. Medical Anthropology (Summer):
       313–339.
Burnet, Sir Macfarlane and David O. White
  1972 Natural History of Infectious Disease. (4th ed.) Cambridge: Cambridge University
       Press.

Byles, A.B. and A. D'Sa
   1970 Reduction of reaction due to iron dextran using chloroquin. British Medical Journal 3: 625–627.
Carlsson, B. et al.
   1980 The mechanism of immunity provided by breast-feeding. *In* S. Freier and A. Edelman (eds.), Human Milk: Its Biological and Social Value. Amsterdam: Excerpta Medica, pp. 122–126.
Carmichael, Ann G.
   1985 Infection, hidden hunger, and history. In Robert Rotberg and Theodore Rabb (eds.), Hunger and History: The Impact of Changing Food Production and Consumption Patterns on Society. Cambridge: Cambridge University Press.
Carroll, Vern (ed.)
   1970 Adoption in Eastern Oceania. Association for Social Anthropology in Oceania Monograph 1. Honolulu: University of Hawaii Press.
Cassidy, Claire
   1980 Benign neglect and toddler malnutrition. In Lawrence Greene and Francis Johnston (eds.), Social and Biological Predictors of Nutritional Status, Physical Growth, and Neurological Development. New York: Academic Press, pp. 109–139.
Durham, William
   1982 Interactions of genetic and cultural evolution: models and examples. Human Ecology 10(3): 289–323.
Eaton, J.W. et al.
   1976 Suppression of malaria infection by oxidant-sensitive host erythrocytes. Nature 264: 758.
Edington, G.M.
   1967 Pathology of malaria in West Africa. British Medical Journal 1: 715–718.
Ferro-Luzzi, A., N.G. Norgan and J.V. Durnin
   1978 The nutritional status of some New Guinean children as assessed by anthropometric, biochemical and other indices. Ecology of Food and Nutrition 7: 115–128.
Fortune, Reo F.
   1932 Sorcerers of Dobu: The Social Anthropology of the Dobu Islanders of the Western Pacific. Reprinted 1963. New York: E.P. Dutton.
Frisch, Rose
   1975 Critical weight, a critical body composition, menarche, and the maintenance of menstrual cycles. In E.S. Watts, F.E. Johnston, and G.W. Lasker (eds.), Biosocial Interrelations in Population Adaptation. The Hague: Mouton, pp. 319–347.
Frisch, Rose and J. McArthur
   1974 Menstrual cycles: fatness as a determinant of minimum weight for height necessary for their maintenance or onset. Science 185: 949–951.
Gerlach, L.
   1969 Socio-cultural factors affecting the diet of the Northeast Coastal Bantu. In L.R. Lynch (ed.), The Cross-Cultural Approach to Health Behavior. Rutherford, NJ: Fairleigh-Dickinson University Press, pp. 383–394.
Hamson, G.A., A.J. Boyce and C.M. Platt
   1975 Body composition changes during lactation in a New Guinea population. Annals of Human Biology 65: 341–349.
Hendrickse, R.G.
   1966 Some observations on the social background to malnutrition in tropical Africa. African Affairs 65: 341–349.
   1967 Interactions of nutrition and infection: experience in Nigeria. In G. Wolstonholme and M. O'Connor (eds.), Nutrition and Infection. CIBA Foundation study Group No. 31. Boston: Little, Brown.

Hendrickse, R.G. et al.
 1971 Malaria in early childhood. An investigation of five hundred seriously ill children in whom a clinical diagnosis was made on admission to the Children's Emergency Room at University College Hospital, Ibadan. Annals of Tropical Medicine and Parasitology 65: 1–20.
Jelliffe, Derrick
 1957 Social culture and nutrition: cultural blocks and protein malnutrition in early childhood in rural West Bengal. Pediatrics 20: 128–138.
Jelliffe, Derrick and E.F.P. Jelliffe
 1978 Human Milk in the Modern World: Psychosocial, Nutritional, and Economic Significance. Oxford: Oxford University Press.
Katz, M.
 1982 Discussion: malaria and malnutrition. Reviews of Infectious Diseases 4(4): 805.
Kolata, Gina
 1984 The search for a malaria vaccine. Science 226: 679–682.
Konner, M.J.
 1976 Maternal care, infant behavior and development among the Zhun/twa (!Kung) Bushmen. In Richard B. Lee and Irven DeVore (eds.), Kalahari Hunter-Gatherers. Cambridge: Harvard University Press.
Korbin, Jill (ed.)
 1981 Child Abuse and Neglect: Cross-Cultural Perspectives. Berkeley: University of California Press.
Langness, L.L.
 1981 Child abuse and cultural values: the case of New Guinea. In Jill Korbin (ed.), Child Abuse and Neglect: Cross-Cultural Perspectives. Berkeley: University of California Press, pp. 13–34.
Leach, Jerry and Edmund Leach (eds.)
 1983 The Kula: New Perspectives in Massim Exchange. Cambridge: Cambridge University Press.
Leonard, Dympna
 1980 Report on Food and Nutrition in Milne Bay Province. Milne Bay Development Study. Alotau, Papua New Guinea.
Lepowsky, Maria
 1979 A Preliminary Report on Cultural Factors Affecting Health and Nutrition: Sudest Island and the Louisiade Archipelago, Papua New Guinea. Report submitted to the Provincial Health Officer, Milne Bay Province. Mimeographed and distributed by the National Planning Office, Port Moresby, Papua New Guinea.
 1981 Fruit of the Motherland: Gender and Exchange on Vanatinai, Papua New Guinea. Ph.D. dissertation, Department of Anthropology, University of California, Berkeley.
 1983 Sudest Island and the Louisiade Archipelago in Massim exchange. In Jerry Leach and Edmund Leach (eds.), The Kula: New Perspectives in Massim Exchange. Cambridge: Cambridge University Press, pp. 467–501.
 1985 Food taboos, malaria and dietary change: infant feeding and cultural adaptation on a Papua New Guinea island. Ecology of Food and Nutrition 16(2): 105–126.
Lewis, Colin and David Henton
 1979 Nutrition Report: Child Nutrition in Milne Bay. Milne Bay Provincial Health Department, Alotau, Papua New Guinea.
Lewis, Gilbert
 1975 Knowledge of Illness in a Sepik Society: A Study of the Gnau, New Guinea. London: Athlone Press.
Maegraith, B.
 1967 Interaction of nutrition and infection. In G. Wolstonholm and M. O'Connor (eds.), Nutrition and Infection. CIBA Foundation Study Group No. 31. Boston: Little, Brown and Co., pp. 41–58.

Maegraith, B., T. Deegan and E.S. Jones
  1952 Suppression of malaria (P. berghei) by milk. British Medical Journal 2:1382–1384.
Malinowski, Bronislaw
  1922 Argonauts of the Western Pacific. London: Routledge and Kegan Paul.
  1935 Coral Gardens and Their Magic. (2 Vols.) London: George Allen and Unwin.
Masawe, A.J., J. Muindi and G. Swai
  1974 Infections in iron deficiency and other types of anemias in the tropics. The Lancet 11:
       314–317.
May, Jacques
  1958 The Ecology of Human Disease. New York: MD Publications.
Miller, Barbara
  1981 The Endangered Sex: Neglect of Female Children in Rural North India. Ithaca: Cornell
       University Press.
Molineaux, L. and G. Gramiccia
  1980 The Garki Project: Research on the Epidemiology and Control of Malaria in the Sudan
       Savanna of West Africa. Geneva: World Health Organization.
Murray, M.J. et al.
  1975  Refeeding, malaria and hyperferremia. The Lancet 1: 653–654.
  1978a Diet and cerebral malaria: the effect of famine and refeeding. American Journal of
        Clinical Nutrition 31: 1363–1366.
  1978b The adverse effect of iron repletion on the course of certain infections. British Medical
        Journal 3: 1113–1115.
Nardin, E.H. et al.
  1979 Antibodies to sporozoites: their frequent occurrence in individuals living in areas of
       hyperendemic malaria. Science 206 (November 2): 597–599.
National Planning Office
  1978 National Nutrition Survey. National Planning Office, Port Moresby, Papua New
       Guinea.
Norgan, N.G., A. Ferro-Luzzi and J.V. Durnin
  1974 The energy and nutrient intake of 204 New Guinean adults. Philosophical Transactions
       of the Royal Society of London, 268: 309–348.
Ogbeide, O.
  1974 Nutritional hazards of food taboos and preferences in Mid-West Nigeria. American
       Journal of Clinical Nutrition 27(2): 213–216.
Ogra, P., M. Fishaut and C. Theodore
  1980 Immunology of breast milk: maternal neonatal interactions. In S. Freier and A.
       Edelman (eds.), Human Milk: Its Biological and Social Value. Amsterdam: Excerpta
       Medica, pp. 115–120.
Parkinson, A.D.
  1974 Malaria in Papua New Guinea 1973. Papua New Guinea Medical Journal 17(1): 8–16.
Pasvol, G. et al.
  1976 Fetal haemoglobin and malaria. The Lancet, June 12, No. 7972: 1269–1271.
Pollock, Nancy
  1985 The concept of food in a Pacific society: a Fijian example. Ecology of Food and
       Nutrition 17: 195–203.
Scheper-Hughes, Nancy
  1984 Infant mortality and infant care: Cultural and economic constraints on nurturing in
       Northeast Brazil. Social Sciences and Medicine 19: 535–546.
Scrimshaw, Nevin S., C.E. Taylor and J.E. Gordon
  1968 Interactions of Nutrition and Infection. WHO Monograph No. 57. Geneva: World
       Health Organization.
Scrimshaw, Susan
  1975 Families to the city: a study of changing values, fertility, and socio-economic status

among urban in-migrants. In Moni Nag (ed.), Population and Social Organization. Paris: Mouton, pp. 309–328.

1978 Infant mortality and behavior in the regulation of family size. Population and Development Review 4(3): 383–403.

Sorenson, E. Richard
1976 The Edge of the Forest: Land, Childhood and Change in a New Guinea Protoagricultural Society. Washington, DC: Smithsonian Institution Press.

Spencer, Terence, Margaret Spencer and David Venters
1974 Malaria vectors in Papua New Guinea. Papua New Guinea Medical Journal 17(1): 22–30.

Stini, William
1979 Adaptive strategies in human populations under nutritional stress. In William Stini (ed.), Physiological and Morphological Adaptation and Evolution. New York: Mouton, pp. 387–403.

Targett, G.A.T.
1981 Malnutrition and immunity to protozoan parasites. In H. Isliker and B. Schürch (eds.), The Impact of Malnutrition on Immune Defense in Parasitic Infestation. Nestlé Foundation Publication, Series 2. Bern: Hans Huber, pp. 158–175.

Taylor, Carl E.
1983 Child and Maternal Health Services in Rural India: The Narangwal Experiment. Baltimore: Johns Hopkins University Press for World Bank.

1985 Synergy among mass infections, famines, and poverty. In R.I. Rotberg and Theodore K. Rabb (eds.), Hunger and History: The Impact of Changing Food Production and Consumption Patterns on Society. Cambridge: Cambridge University Press.

van der Hoeven, J.A.
1958 Taboos for pregnant women, lactating mothers and infants on the north coast of Netherlands New Guinea. Tropical and Geographical Medicine 10: 71–76.

Weinberg, Eugene
1978 Iron and infection. Microbiological Reviews 42: 45–66.

Wolff, R.J.
1965 Meanings of food. Tropical and Geographical Medicine 17: 45–51.

Wyler, David J.
1982 Malaria: host-pathogen biology. Reviews of Infectious Diseases 4(4): 785–797.

Wyon, John B. and John E. Gordon
1971 The Khanna Study: Population Problems in Rural Punjab. Cambridge: Harvard University Press.

# PART II

# INFANTICIDE: CULTURALLY SANCTIONED CHILD ABUSE

*LIMBO*

Fishermen at Ballyshannon
Netted an infant last night
Along with the salmon.
An illegitimate spawning,

A small one thrown back
To the waters. But I'm sure
As she stood in the shallows
Ducking him tenderly

Till the frozen knobs of her wrists
Were dead as the gravel,
He was a minnow with hooks
Tearing her open.

She waded in under
The sign of her cross.
He was hauled in with the fish.
Now limbo will be

A cold glitter of souls
Through some briny zone.
Even Christ's palms, unhealed,
Smart and cannot fish there.

Seamus Heaney, 1980

BARBARA D. MILLER

# FEMALE INFANTICIDE AND CHILD NEGLECT IN RURAL
# NORTH INDIA*

## INTRODUCTION

Sitting in the hospital canteen for lunch every day, I can see families bringing their children into the hospital. So far, after watching for five days, I have seen only boys being carried in for treatment, no girls (author's field notes, Ludhiana Christian Medical College, November 1983).

When the hospital was built, equal-sized wards for boys and girls were constructed. The boys' ward is always full but the girls' ward is underutilized (comment of a hospital administrator, Ludhiana Christian Medical College, November 1983).

In one village, I went into the house to examine a young girl and I found that she had an advanced case of tuberculosis. I asked the mother why she hadn't done something sooner about the girl's condition because now, at this stage, the treatment would be very expensive. The mother replied, "then let her die, I have another daughter." At the time, the two daughters sat nearby listening, one with tears streaming down her face (report by a public health physician, Ludhiana Christian Medical College, November 1983).

When a third, fourth, or fifth daughter is born to a family, no matter what its economic status, we increase our home visits because that child is at high risk (statement made by a public health physician, Ludhiana Christian Medical College, November 1983).

These quotations, taken from field notes made during a 1983 trip to Ludhiana, the Punjab, India, are indicative of the nature and degree of sex-selectivity in health care of children there. Ethnographic evidence gleaned from the work of other anthropologists corroborates that intrahousehold discrimination against girls is a fact of life in much of the northern plains region of India (Miller 1981: 83–106). The strong preference for sons compared to daughters is marked from the moment of birth. Celebration at the birth of a son, particularly a first son, has been documented repeatedly in the ethnographic literature (Lewis 1965: 49; Freed and Freed 1976: 123, 206; Jacobson 1970: 307–309; Madan 1965: 63; and Aggarwal 1971: 114). But when a daughter is born, the event goes unheralded and anthropologists have documented the unconcealed disappointment in families which already have a daughter or two (Luschinsky 1962: 82; Madan 1965: 77–78; Minturn and Hitchcock 1966: 101–102). The extreme disappointment of a mother who greatly desires a son, but bears a daughter instead, could affect her ability to breastfeed successfully; "bonding" certainly would not be automatically assured between the mother and the child; and the mother's disappointed in-laws would be far less supportive than if the newborn were a son (Miller, 1986).

A thorough review of the ethnographic literature provides diverse but strongly suggestive evidence of preferential feeding of boys in North Indian

95

*Nancy Scheper-Hughes (ed.), Child Survival, 95–112.*
© *1987 by D. Reidel Publishing Company.*

villages (Miller 1981: 93–94), as well as preferential allocation of medical care to boys. Sex ratios of admissions to northern hospitals are often two or more boys to every one girl. This imbalance is not due to more frequent illness of boys, rather to sex-selective parental investment patterns.

The practice of sex-selective child care in northern India confronts us with a particularly disturbing dilemma that involves the incongruity between Western values that insist on equal life chances for all, even in the face of our universal failure to achieve that goal, versus North Indian culture which places strong value on the survival of sons rather than daughters. Public health programs in North India operate under the guidance of the national goal of "equal health care for all by the year 2000" which was declared by many developing nations at the Alma Ata conference in 1978. Yet the families with whom they are concerned operate with a different set of goals less concerned with the survival of any one individual than with the survival of the family. In rural North India the economic survival of the family, for sociocultural reasons, is dependent on the reproduction of strong sons and the control of the number of daughters who are financial burdens in many ways.

This chapter examines a variety of data and information sources on the dimensions and social context of female infanticide and daughter neglect in rural North India, an area where gender preferences regarding offspring are particularly strong. I review what is known about outright female infanticide in earlier centuries and discuss the situation in North India today, examining the empirical evidence and current theoretical approaches to the understanding of son preference and daughter disfavor. The next section considers the role of a public health program in the Punjab. In conclusion I address the issue of humanist values concerning equal life chances for all versus North Indian patriarchal values promoting better life chances for boys than girls, and the challenge to anthropological research of finding an appropriate theoretical approach to the study of children's health and survival.

### INFANTICIDE: BACKGROUND

I consider infanticide to fall under the general category of child abuse and neglect which encompasses a range of behaviors. As I have written elsewhere:

... it is helpful to distinguish forms of neglect from those of abuse ... abuse is more "active" in the way it is inflicted; it is abuse when something is actually *done* to harm the child. In the case of neglect, harm comes to the child because something is *not done* which should have been. Thus, sexual molestation of a child is abusive, whereas depriving a child of adequate food and exercise is neglectful. One similarity between abuse and neglect is that both, if carried far enough, can be fatal (Miller 1981: 44–45).

Infanticide, most strictly defined, is the killing of a child under one year of age. Infanticide would be placed at one extreme of the continuum of effects of child abuse and neglect – it is fatal. At the opposite end of the continuum are forms of child abuse that result in delayed learning, slowed physical growth and development patterns, and disturbed social adjustment. Outright infanticide can be distinguished from indirect or "passive" infanticide (Harris 1977); in the former the means, such as a fatal beating, are direct and immediate, while in the latter, the means, such as sustained nutritional deprivation, are indirect.

Infanticide is further delineated with respect to the ages of the children involved. Most broadly defined, infanticide applies to the killing of children under the age of twelve months (deaths after that age would generally be classified as child *homicide*, although the definition and, hence, duration of childhood is culturally variable). *Neonaticide* usually pertains to the killing of a newborn up to twenty-four hours after birth and is sometimes given a separate analysis (Wilkey *et al.* 1982). The induced *abortion* of a fetus is sometimes categorized as a pre-natal form of infanticide that has been termed *"feticide"* in the literature.[1]

The discussion in this chapter encompasses both infanticide and child homicide, that is non-accidental deaths to minors from the time of birth up to the age of about fifteen or sixteen when they would become adults in the rural Indian context. For convenience, I will use the term infanticide to apply to the entire age range.

I have asserted (1981: 44) that where infanticide is systematically sex-selective, it will be selective against females rather than males. There are few cases of systematic male-selective infanticide in the literature that I reviewed. Some more recent work on the subject, however, has begun to reveal a variety of patterns. For example, a study conducted on several villages in a delta region of Japan using data from the Tokugawa era (1600–1868) reveals the existence of systematic infanticide which was sex-selective, but selective against males almost as frequently as females, depending on the particular household composition and dynamics (Skinner 1984).

Obviously all household strategies concerning the survival of offspring are not based solely on gender considerations, and it is doubtful that we can ever come close to a good estimation of just "how much" gender-based selective differential in the treatment of children exists, and how much of this is biased against females. Nevertheless, one part of the world where female-selective infanticide is particularly apparent is in North India, and across India's northwestern border through Pakistan (see Figure 1) to the Near East, and perhaps in a diminished form also in North Africa. Looking toward the East from India, it seems that Southeast Asia is largely free of the son preference/daughter disfavor syndrome, as opposed to China where one result of the one-child policy (see Potter, this volume) was the death of thousands of female infants.

## FEMALE INFANTICIDE IN PRE-TWENTIETH CENTURY INDIA

The British discovery of infanticide in India occurred in 1789 among a clan of Rajputs in the eastern part of Uttar Pradesh, a northern state.[2] All of the infanticide reported by British district officers and other observers was direct

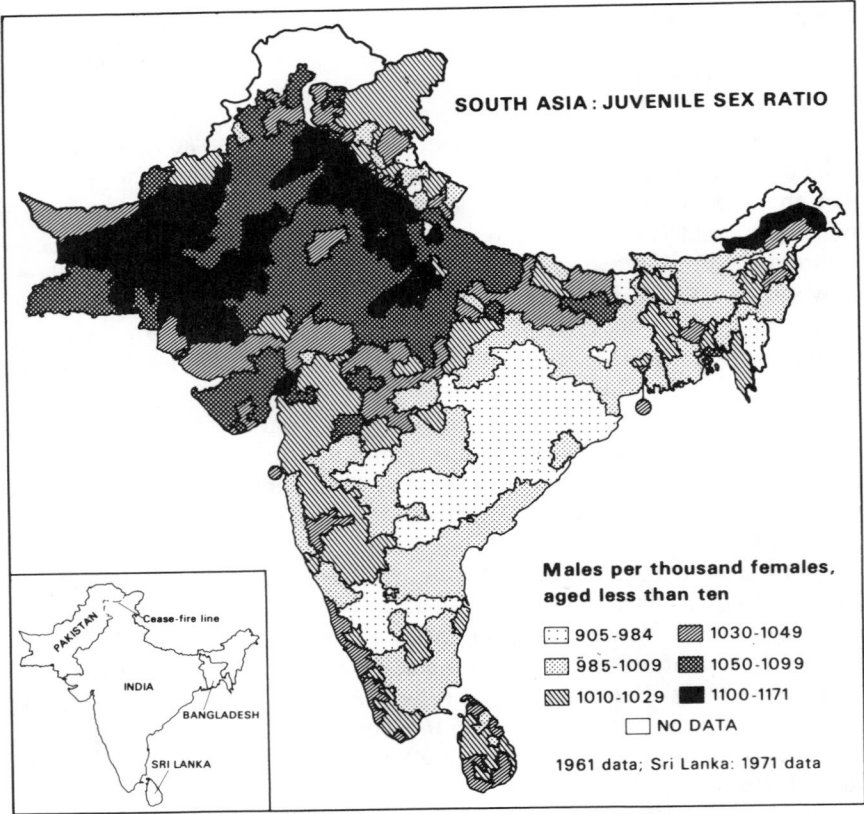

Fig. 1.   Juvenile sex ratios by district (urban and rural populations combined), India (1961), Pakistan (1961), Bangladesh (1961), and Sri Lanka (1971). Juveniles are children under ten years of age; sex ratio refers to the number of males per 1,000 females.

female infanticide. A lengthy quotation from a mid-nineteenth century description by a British magistrate in the Northwest Provinces of India demonstrates how open was the knowledge of the practice of female infanticide at that time:

There is at Mynpoorie an old fortress, which looks far over the valley of the Eesun river. This has been for centuries the stronghold of the Rajahs of Mynpoorie, Chohans whose ancient blood, descending from the great Pirthee Raj and the regal stem of Neem-rana, represents *la crème de la crème* of Rajpoot aristocracy. Here when a son, a nephew, a grandson, was born to the reigning chief, the event was announced to the neighboring city by the loud discharge of wall-pieces and matchlocks; but centuries had passed away, and no infant daughter had been known to smile within those walls.

In 1845, however, thanks to the vigilance of Mr. Unwin [the district collector], a little grand-daughter was preserved by the Rajah of that day. The fact was duly notified to the Government, and a letter of congratulations and a dress of honour were at once dispatched from head-quarters to the Rajah.

We have called this incident, the giving of a robe of honour to a man because he did not destroy his grand-daughter a *grotesque* one; but it is very far from being a ridiculous incident. When the people see that the highest authorities in the land take an interest in their social or domestic reforms, those reforms can give an impetus which no lesser influences can give them. The very next year after the investiture of the Rajah, the number of female infants preserved in the district was *trebled*! Fifty-seven had been saved in 1845; in 1846, one hundred and eighty were preserved; and the number has gone on steadily increasing ever since (Raikes 1852: 20–21).

A review of the secondary literature on female infanticide in British India reveals its practice mainly in the Northwest, and among upper castes and tribes. Not all groups practiced female infanticide, but there are grim reports that a few entire villages in the northwestern plains had never raised one daughter.[3] On the basis of juvenile (under ten years of age) sex ratios for districts in the Northwest Provinces, 1871, I have estimated crudely that for nineteenth-century Northwest India it would not be unreasonable to assume that one-fourth of the population preserved only half the daughters born to them, while the other three-fourths of the population had balanced sex ratios among their offspring (Miller 1981: 62). This assumption yields a juvenile sex ratio of 118 (males per 100 females) in the model population, which is comparable to current juvenile sex ratios in several districts of northwestern India and Pakistan (Miller 1981, 1984). It seems clear that female infanticide in British India was widespread in the Northwest rather than of limited occurrence.

The British investigated the extent and causes of female infanticide, and in 1870 passed a law against its practice. Other policy measures, based on their assessment of the causes of the practice, included subsidizing the dowries of daughters that were "preserved" by prominent families, and organizing conferences in order to enlighten local leaders and their followers about the need to prevent infanticide (Cave Browne 1857).

There are two areas of ignorance about the wider context of the historic practice of female infanticide in India. First, we know little about the apparent and gradual transition from direct to indirect infanticide. It appears that either deep-seated social change and/or British policy against the practice of female infanticide succeeded in bringing about the near-end of direct female infanticide by the beginning of this century. In the twentieth century we hear little about female infanticide in census reports, district gazetteers, or anthropological descriptions of rural life. What is needed is a careful tracing of the situation from roughly 1870 when the practice was outlawed to the present time in order to plot the dynamics of change from outright to indirect infanticide. Second, we need to know much more about the sociocultural determinants of female infanticide in British India. The British pointed to two causal factors – "pride and purse." The pride of upper castes and tribes is said to have pushed them to murder female infants rather than give them away as tribute to a more dominant group, or even as brides which is viewed as demeaning in rural North India today. By "purse" is meant dowry, and most groups that practiced infanticide did have the custom of giving large dowries with daughters.[4] But there is some contradictory evidence. In the undivided Punjab, it has been documented for the early twentieth century that dowry was not widely given among the rural Jats, a caste which nonetheless exhibited very high sex ratios (i.e., males over females) among its juvenile population. In fact, the Jats, a landed peasant caste, often secured brides through brideprice, which should have provided an economic incentive for parents to preserve daughters (Darling 1929; see also the discussion in Miller 1984). Further exploration of archival materials for the nineteenth century would help illuminate this matter.

### FEMALE INFANTICIDE AND NEGLECT: THE CURRENT CONTEXT

It is beyond doubt that systematic indirect female infanticide exists today in North India. It is possible that outright infanticide of neonates is also practiced, though nearly impossible to document due to the extreme privacy of the birth event and the great ease with which a neonate's life may be terminated.[5] This section of the paper is concerned with indirect female infanticide, which is accomplished by nutritional and health-care deprivation of children, and which results in higher mortality rates of daughters than sons.[6]

There is a strong preference for sons in rural North India and there are several strong sociocultural reasons for this preference. Sons are economic assets: they are needed for farming, and for income through remittances if they leave the village. Sons play important roles in local power struggles over rights to land and water. Sons stay with the family after their marriage and thus maintain the parents in their old age; daughters marry out and cannot contribute to the maintenance of their natal households. Sons bring in dowries with their brides; daughters drain family wealth with their required dowries and the constant flow of gifts to their family of marriage after the wedding. Sons, among Hindus, are also needed to perform rituals which protect the family after the death of the father; daughters cannot perform such rituals.

Elsewhere I have argued that extreme son preference is more prevalent in North India than in the South and East, and that it is more prevalent among upper castes and classes than lower castes and classes (Miller 1981). By extension, daughter neglect would follow the same pattern. Some of the key research questions include: how extensive is daughter disfavor in different regions and among various social strata in India? How serious are its consequences in terms of mortality and in health status of the survivors (not to mention more difficult to diagnose conditions such as emotional and cognitive development)? Are these patterns changing through time? At this point, scattered studies help illuminate some aspects of these questions, but there is no study that addresses them all systematically either for one locale or for India as a whole.

First, let us consider the question of the extent of the practice in India. In a recent publication, Lipton (1983) suggests that fatal discrimination against daughters in India is a very localized, and thus minor, problem. But my all-India analysis (1981), using juvenile sex ratios as a surrogate measure of child mortality, shows that while the most afflicted area encompasses only two or three states of India, there are seriously unbalanced sex ratios among children in one-third of India's 326 rural districts, an area spanning the entire northwestern plains.[7] Simmons *et al.* (1982) provide results from survey data on 2064 couples in the Kanpur region of Uttar Pradesh (a state in northern India) which reveal that reported infant and child mortality rates for girls aged one month up to three years of age are much higher than the rates for boys. This finding is similar to, though less astonishing than, Cowan and Dhanoa's (1983) report that in a large sub-population carefully monitored in Ludhiana district, the Punjab, 85 percent of all deaths to children aged 7–36 months were female. Another dependable database that has been carefully analyzed by Behrman (1984) and Behrman and Deolalikar (1985) concerns an area of India where juvenile sex ratios are not notably unbalanced, south-central India in the area between Andhra Pradesh and Maharashtra. The authors have found that there is a noticeable nutrient bias in favor of boys in the intrahousehold allocation of food. This unequal distribution has a seasonal dimension: in the lean season boys are more favored over girls in the distribution of food in the family, while in the surplus season distribution appears quite equal.

Class/caste variations in juvenile sex ratios are also important. Simmons *et al.* (1982) unfortunately do not present findings on class or caste patterns. They mention that education of the parents is a positive influence on child survival in the first year of life, less so in the second and third. If parental education can be used as a crude indicator of class status, then it would seem that survival for both boys and girls would be more assured in better-off families. Demographic data from the Ludhiana area of Punjab state have been analyzed for class differences by Cowan and Dhanoa (1983). Among upper class, landed families (termed "privileged" by Cowan and Dhanoa), there is a large disparity between survival rates for male and female children and also in the nutritional status of those surviving (Table I). These disparities are mirrored, though less severe, in the lower class, landless population. Cowan and Dhanoa found that birth order strongly affects the survival and status of daughters. Second-born and third-born daughters are classified by health care personnel as "high risk" infants, as are high birth order children of both sexes born to very large families, regardless of socioeconomic status. The extent of fatal daughter disfavor in this relatively affluent state of India is severe, and it contributes to Punjab's having infant (up to one year of age) mortality rates higher that those of poorer states where daughter discrimination is less severe (Miller 1985).

Caldwell's data on a cluster of villages in Karnataka (southern-central

TABLE I

Prevalence of 2nd/3rd degree malnutrition in 911 children in second and third year of life,
Ludhiana, the Punjab

| | Number | Sex ratio[a] | With 2nd/3rd degree malnutrition[b] | Ratio of male to female malnourished |
|---|---|---|---|---|
| Privileged Males | 231 | 111.0 | 2 | 1:6.5 |
| Privileged Females | 208 | | 13 | |
| Under-Privileged Males | 244 | 102.5 | 11 | 1:2.6 |
| Under-Privileged Females | 228 | | 29 | |
| TOTAL | 911 | 106.5 | 55 | 1:3.2 |

[a] Sex ratio refers to the number of males per hundred females.
[b] The numbers in this column were read from a graph and may be off by a small margin.
*Source*: Cowan and Dhanoa (1983: 352).

India), with a total population of more than 5000, revealed "surprisingly small" differences in infant and child mortality by economic status, father's occupation and religion (1983: 197). (This area of the country is characterized by balanced juvenile sex ratios at the district level.) The authors do not mention whether there are any sex differentials in child survival and health. Infant mortality rates are, however, much lower in households with an educated mother than those where the mother has little education. Girls tend to receive less food than boys, and family variables are mentioned as being involved in this matter.

Another report from a region with balanced juvenile sex ratios, a two-village study in West Bengal reported on by Sen and Sengupta (1983), produced some provocative findings. The authors did not look at mortality but rather at levels of undernourishment in children below five years of age according to caste and land ownership status of the household. Results were surprising: the village with a more vigorous land redistribution program had a greater nutritional sex bias, even among children in families who had benefited from the redistribution. In the second village, children in poor families had higher nutritional standards and a lower male-female differential than their counterparts in the first village.

Rosenzweig and Schultz (1982) used a sub-sample of rural households in India, presumably nationwide, and found that boys have significantly higher survival rates relative to girls in landless rather than in landed households. Horowitz and Keshwar report that survey data from a Punjab village (northern India) demonstrate more pronounced son preference among the proper-tied peasant castes, although the phenomenon is "nearly" as strong among agricultural laborers (1982: 12); they do not provide health or survival statistics, but use data on stated preferences of parents.

The above review indicates that, while we do not possess an ideal picture of the extent and nature of daughter disfavor, there is evidence that its practice does exist widely in India and does tend to exhibit class/caste patterns – though the exact nature of these is in dispute. We know very little about the question of change through time since few good sources of longitudinal data exist, and those that do exist have not been examined for sex disparity information as yet.

## SEX-SELECTIVE ABORTION

Several years ago a Jain woman in her sixth month of pregnancy came to Ludhiana Christian Medical Hospital for an amniocentesis test. The results of the test showed that genetic defects such as Down's syndrome or spina bifida were not present in the fetus. The test indicated that the fetus was female. The woman requested an abortion and was refused. She went to a clinic in Amritsar, another major city in the Punjab, and had the abortion done (report by a physician, Ludhiana, November 1983).

This anecdote was told to me at Ludhiana Christian Medical College as an explanation why Ludhiana CMC no longer performs amniocentesis. There were so many requests for abortion of female fetuses following amniocentesis that the hospital made a policy decision not to provide such services.[8] Today a person with intent to abort a female fetus in Ludhiana must take the train about 90 miles to Amritsar where the service is available. An especially poignant aspect of the anecdote is the information that the woman was a Jain. Jainism supports nonviolence toward all life forms. Orthodox Jains sometimes wear cloths over their mouths so as not to swallow a fly, and Jains do not plow the earth for fear of inadvertently cutting in half a worm. But the Jain woman in the anecdote was willing to abort a female fetus in the sixth month of gestation, so strong was the cultural disfavor toward the birth of daughters.

At this time I do not have access to data on the number of female fetuses aborted each year in India, nor to data on the social characteristics of those people who seek to abort their female fetuses. Nonetheless, several considerations are important: how can we estimate the extent of the practice? What are the social and economic characteristics of those families seeking to abort female fetuses? What are the demographic characteristics of the families seeking sex-selective abortion? There are some clues.

In 1980 an article published in *Social Science and Medicine* provided some evidence of the extent of the phenomenon based on clinic records in a large city of western India (Ramanamma and Bambawale 1980). In one hospital, from June 1976 to June 1977, 700 individuals sought prenatal sex determination. Of these fetuses, 250 were determined to be male and 450 were female.[9] While all of the male fetuses were kept to term, fully 430 of the 450 female fetuses were terminated. This figure is even more disturbing in light of the fact that western India is characterized by a less extreme son preference than the Northwest.

There is an eager market in India for sex-selective abortion, although the cost of the service may make it prohibitive for the poorest villagers. A report in *Manushi* (1982) states that the service is available in Chandigarh, the Punjab, for only 500 rupees.[10] Another report mentions that the charge was 600 rupees at a clinic in Amritsar, the Punjab (*Washington Post* 1982). A recent visitor to Ahmedabad, Gujarat, reports a charge of only 50 rupees in a clinic there (Everett 1984). Whether the charge is 50 rupees or 500 rupees, the cost is minor compared to the benefits reaped from the possibility of having a son conceived at the next pregnancy, or compared to the money that would have been needed to provide a dowry for the girl were she to survive.

## DETERMINANTS OF SON PREFERENCE AND DAUGHTER DISFAVOR

Why does son preference exist, and why does it often exist in tandem with the practices of sex-selective abortion, female infanticide, and female neglect? Anthropologists have proposed "explanations" for the practice of female infanticide in simple societies, but less work has been done for complex civilizations. Recent problems in China, provoked by the one-child policy, have attracted attention to the subject, but little scholarly thinking, with few exceptions (see Wasserstrom 1984, and Potter, this volume). A range of hypothesized causal factors has been suggested to account for female infanticide in the past few years. They can be divided into ecologic/economic determinants, social structural determinants and sociobiological determinants.

From the broadest population ecology perspective, Harris (1977) proposes that female infanticide, and by extension sex-selective abortion, will most likely occur when a society has reached a crisis level in its population/ resources ratio, or right after that crisis when the society has moved into a more intensive stage of resource exploitation. Thus, female offspring are a necessarily expendable portion of the population in relation to resources. This theory has explanatory power for some cases, but we might bear in mind that infanticide is only one of many possible strategies for ameliorating a high population/ resources ratio. Other options include migration, and the reduction of natural population growth through delayed marriage, abstinence, abortion, and other forms of birth control both traditional and modern.

My interpretation, based on the case of North India, gives more emphasis to economic demand factors. I have hypothesized that labor requirements for males versus females (themselves ecologically, agriculturally and culturally defined) are key in determining households' desires regarding number and sex of offspring (Miller 1981, 1984). Although I take the sexual division of labor as primary, I view it as creating a secondary and very powerful determinant in the domestic marriage economy. In the case of India, the contrast between dowry marriages and bridewealth marriages illustrates the "mirroring" of the sexual division of labor in marriage costs: generally where few females are employed in the agricultural sector, large dowries prevail, but where female labor is in high demand, smaller dowries or even bridewealth are the main form of marriage transfers.

Other more orthodox economic approaches stress rational decision-making on the part of the family based on perceived "market opportunities" of offspring (Rosenzweig and Schultz 1982) or intrafamily resource allocation systems (Simmons *et al.* 1982). Sen and Sengupta propose that land distribution patterns are an important determinant of sex differentials in children's nutritional status (1983).

The major exponents of a social structural theory are Dyson and Moore (1983). They identify the patriarchal nature of North Indian society as the basis for the neglect of daughters and other manifestations of low female status. They do not seek to explain why society in North India is strongly patriarchal – that is simply a given.

Dickemann, who studied female infanticide cross-culturally and particularly in stratified societies such as traditional northern India and China, provides a sociobiological interpretation for female infanticide (1979, 1984). Her early observation of the connection between hypergynous marriage systems and female infanticide was a particularly important contribution (1979). Dickemann views sex ratio manipulation among offspring as one reproductive strategy that will, under alternate resource conditions, result in maximum reproductive success for the family. She has recently stated that:

Like other acts of reproductive management, infanticide-pedicide seems to be best understood at present, in all species, as one parameter of interindividual and interfamilial competition for the proportional increase in genes in the next generation . . . (1984: 436).

In terms of the explanatory power of evolutionary models with respect to the cause of violent mistreatment of human offspring, however, Hrdy and Hausfater (1984: xxxi) agree with Lenington (1981) that "only a portion of such cases" will be thus explained.

## PUBLIC HEALTH AND PATRIARCHY

Ten years ago when I began my research on fatal neglect of daughters in rural India the problem was not widely accepted by scholars in the West or in India as a serious one.[11] Today the practice of fatal daughter disfavor is more widely recognized by scholars as a serious social issue. Current concern in India about the growing recourse to sex-selective abortion, using information on sex of the fetus derived from amniocentesis, adds a new and important dimension to problems of female survival and the ethics of abortion (Ramanamma and Bambawale 1980; Kumar 1983).

Operating within such a patriarchal system, could any health care program seeking to provide equal health care for all have any success? There is controversy concerning the impact of health care programs in alleviating sex differences in child survival in patriarchal cultures, particularly North India.

Some writers suggest that a simple increase in health care services will improve the situation for girls (Minturn 1984). Others have found evidence that increased services will be diverted to priority children, most often boys, and that only secondarily will low priority children, most often girls, benefit.[12] Finally, the introduction of new medical technologies – such as amniocentesis – can be manipulated to advance patriarchal priorities (Miller 1986).

*Focus on the Punjab*

The Punjab, India's wealthiest state, is located in the northwestern plains region adjacent to Pakistan. Its economy is agricultural with wheat the major food crop, but there is a well-developed industrial sector also. Within the Punjab, Ludhiana district is usually recognized as the most "developed" district. Ludhiana district also stands out because it houses one of the best medical colleges and community health programs in India, Ludhiana Christian Medical College. Ludhiana, and the Punjab district, are squarely in the area in northwestern India where juvenile sex ratios are the most masculine and excess female child mortality the greatest (Miller 1985).

Since the early 1970s, Ludhiana CMC has been monitoring the reproductive and health status of the surrounding population – first as a pilot project in three rural locations and one urban location, and later in the entire block of Sahnewal (an administrative subdivision of the district), with a population of about 85 000. The monitoring is part of a decentralized, comprehensive basic health care program that focuses on the welfare of mothers and children and includes both health care delivery at village centers and home-based educational programs. For each of the nearly 14 000 families in Sahnewal block, the CMC Ludhiana program maintains family folders containing information on all family members and their health status. Mortalities are carefully recorded in each folder and also in Master Registers kept in 49 village centers throughout the block. Some analysis of these data has been performed (Cowan and Dhanoa 1983) which provides startling figures on sex differentials of mortality for children aged 7–36 months in which female deaths constituted 85 percent of the total (1983: 341).

Cowan and Dhanoa note that one important result of their intensive home-based visiting approach in the rural Punjab is a reduction in the percentage of female child deaths (1983: 354). There is no doubt that their approach can be effective for saving the lives of high-risk children, though it requires great effort and entails much surveillance of private life. Two questions arise from this finding: a related result of increased survival for girls is an increase in the percentage of malnourished girls – girls' lives have been saved, but the quality of those lives may not be at all equal to that of males. Would even more intensive home visiting help alleviate this problem? Furthermore, some would argue that the death of unwanted children might be preferable to their extended mistreatment and suffering (Kumar 1983; and see the discussion in Cassidy, this volume).

We have not estimated the unit health care costs by sex and priority of the child, but the cost of saving the life of a low priority female child must far outweigh the cost of saving and improving the life of a high priority male. It is not unthinkable that the time will arrive when, with fiscal stringency the watchword of the day, the cost of intensive health care and survival monitoring for girls becomes a barrier to programs such as the one at Ludhiana CMC. Two arguments can be developed to counter policies which would limit special efforts to equalize life chances between boys and girls. First, one might look to the broader social costs of a society in which the sex ratio is seriously unbalanced. It cannot be proven that unbalanced sex ratios invariably lead to social disturbances, but there is much cross-cultural evidence to support this (Divale and Harris 1976). A balanced sex ratio does not guarantee social tranquility, but it could minimize some sources of social tension. Second, in a strongly son-preferential culture, women bear many children in the attempt to produce several sons. The pattern of selective care which promotes son survival to the detriment of daughter survival is built on "over-reproduction" and much child wastage. Mothers bear a physical burden in this system. The Ludhiana program seeks to keep children alive and wanted, and to promote family planning after a certain number and sex composition of children have been born in a household; this goal should reduce the physical burden on mothers created by extended childbearing.

## HUMANISTIC VALUES, PATRIARCHAL VALUES AND ANTHROPOLOGY

This chapter discusses an extreme form of sex-selective child care, one which is not universally found throughout the world though it is not limited to rural North India. [Strong preference for sons which results in life-endangering deprivation of daughters is "culturally" acceptable in much of rural North India with its patriarchal foundation.] It is not acceptable from a Western humanistic or altruistic perspective (see Cassidy, this volume) nor from that of an emergent, international feminist "world view." But, how can anthropological research, with its commitment to nonethnocentric reporting of cultural behavior, contribute to an amelioration of the "worldview conflicts" that create inappropriate public health programs targeted at high-risk children, that sometimes only prolong the suffering of these disvalued ones?

As Cassidy (this volume) hints in her conclusion, perhaps positivistic anthropology and Western altruism can work together. First, let me hasten to soften the hard edges of the "conflict" in world views that Cassidy has constructed: there is no such thing as purely objective and nonethnocentric anthropological research and there is, increasingly, less and less culturally uninformed altruism being foisted on the Third World. All anthropologists, as Schneider so clearly states (1984), have their own unavoidable, culturally-influenced presuppositions and biases through which they choose subjects for research and through which they analyze their data. The best an anthropologist can do is state the nature of his/her presuppositions at the outset: mine, influenced by my white, middle class, American upbringing, are based on the precept that human life, its duration and quality, is something to which all persons should have equal access, although I am fully aware of the fact that scarcity (real or culturally defined) results in priorities about the quality of life that certain groups will receive. Thus I define female infanticide and skewed sex ratios as a social "problem." As an applied anthropologist I believe that socio-behavioral data can provide the key to successful public programs which seek to ameliorate the "problem."

My experience, though too brief, in working with Dr. Betty Cowan and Dr. Jasbir Dhanoa (two "altruists") in Ludhiana convinced me that there is hope for a realistic solution to the conflict between altruism and, in this case, extreme patriarchy, in the sensitive applications of social science knowledge and research. The public health program at Ludhiana is perhaps never going to dilute the force of Indian patriarchy, but knowledge about the patriarchal culture can help promote more effective health care. For instance, the Ludhiana hospital built equal-sized wards for boys and girls, on the Western model. But families bring their boys in for health care in much greater numbers than their girls; the girls' ward is relatively empty while the boys' ward is overflowing. Health care practitioners thus realized the need for very decentralized health care rather than only hospital-based services, including frequent home visiting, if health care was to reach girls.

Anthropologists can provide important information to health care intervenors which will allow those intervenors to be more effective in delivering their services. The most important issue in the Ludhiana area still to be resolved is the impact of class and caste stratification on female survival. Health care practitioners see daughter disfavor largely as a result of poverty. My own research would question poverty as the principal determinant in Ludhiana because there is a marked disparity in survival of boys and girls in the propertied class as well as in the unpropertied class. Although the larger picture is unclear because of lack of data across North India, it is obvious that policy implications differ greatly depending on class/caste dimensions of village life. If health care programs are to be targeted to "high-risk" groups, anthropologists can help by providing data on the nature of these groups and the potential implications of intervention in their lives.

## NOTES

* Much of my recent research on this subject has been supported by grants from the Wenner-Gren Foundation for Anthropological Research. I am grateful for the Foundation's support which enabled me to visit two hospitals in India during November 1983 in order to learn about their community health programs: Ludhiana Christian Medical College in the Punjab and Vellore Christian Medical College in Tamil Nadu. While in India, I received help from many people, but I especially want to thank Dr. Betty Cowan, Principal of Ludhiana CMC, and Dr. P.S. Sundar Rao, Chief of the Biostatics Department at Vellore CMC. An earlier version of this chapter was presented at a seminar sponsored by the Department of Anthropology and the Asian

Studies Program at the University of Pittsburgh in March 1985, and I am grateful for the comments I received from those who attended. Finally, I must thank The Metropolitan Studies Program, The Maxwell School, Syracuse University, for support of my work.

1. A discussion of abortion and infanticide from a Western philosophical view is provided in Tooley (1983); compare his presentation with Potter's description of the Chinese view (this volume).

2. We know very little about the practice of female infanticide in India before the British era. The discussion that follows is extracted in large part from Miller (1981: 49–67).

3. Critics are quick to point out that without daughters, villages will not "survive." But in the case of North India, marriage is village exogamous, particularly for Hindus; that is, brides must come from a village other than the groom's. Villages without daughters would "survive" because they would bring in daughters-in-law. More anecdotally, the Community Health Program at Ludhiana CMC was started by a woman physician who was the third daughter of the Grewal lineage to be preserved; even without daughters, the Grewal lineage has "survived" for centuries.

4. Another effect, largely urban and upper-class, of the dowry system in North India is the murder of young wives by their in-laws in order to procure a second bride with her dowry (Sharma 1983).

5. Knowledgeable physicians who have worked with the community health care program in the rural areas surrounding Ludhiana, the Punjab, know that there is a preponderance of female neonatal deaths as compared to those of males. They are averse to labelling this as due to infanticide since an autopsy may well not reveal an intentional death as opposed to a stillbirth or an unintentional death. The physicians do know that neonatal deaths constitute a serious problem, and one that is the hardest for them to deal with due to the secrecy surrounding births in rural India.

6. A detailed discussion of the dynamics of son preference in India can be found in Miller (1981), and a comparison between Pakistan and Bangladesh in Miller (1984).

7. This pattern in Northwest India extends over the Indian border into Pakistan (see Fig. 1).

8. The central government of India has banned prenatal sex determination tests in government hospitals throughout the country for the same reason.

9. The preponderance of females in the sample is probably due to sheer accident.

10. In 1984–85, one dollar equalled approximately twelve rupees.

11. There are some notable exceptions to this generalization (Bardhan 1974; Chandrasekhar 1972; Dandekar 1975; Visaria 1961), although none of these scholars emphasized the major role of sex-differential survival of children in creating the preponderance of males over females.

12. Srilatha (1983) reports that in a large study area in Tamil Nadu, South India, infant and child mortality rates have declined significantly in the last ten years, but the decline was dramatic for boys and only slight for girls. The implication is that improved health services may be differentially allocated to boys and girls in this area of India.

## REFERENCES

Aggarwal, Partap C.
    1971 Caste, Religion and Power. An Indian Case Study. New Delhi: Shri Ram Centre for Industrial Relations.
Bardhan, Pranab K.
    1974 'On Life and Death Questions.' Economic and Political Weekly 10(32–34): 1293–1303.
Behrman, Jere R.
    1984 'Intrahousehold Allocation of Nutrients in Rural India: Are Boys Favored? Do Parents Exhibit Inequality Aversion?' Unpublished manuscript, University of Pennsylvania, Department of Economics. (Revised 1985.)

Behrman, Jere R. and Anil B. Deolalikar.
  1985 'How Do Food and Product Prices Affect Nutrient Intakes, Health and Labor Force
      Behavior for Different Family Numbers in Rural India?' Paper presented at the 1985
      Meetings of the Population Association of America, Boston.
Caldwell, J.C., P.H. Reddy, and Pat Caldwell.
  1983 'The Social Component of Mortality Decline: An Investigation in South India Employ-
      ing Alternative Methodologies.' Population Studies 37: 185–205.
Cave Browne, John.
  1857 Indian Infanticide: Its Origin, Progress, and Suppression. London: W.H. Allen.
Chandrasekhar, S.
  1972 Infant Mortality, Population Growth and Family Planning in India. Chapel Hill, NC:
      University of North Carolina Press.
Cowan, Betty and Jasbir Dhanoa.
  1983 'The Prevention of Toddler Malnutrition by Home-based Nutrition Education.' In
      Nutrition in the Community: A Critical Look at Nutrition Policy, Planning, and
      Programmes. D.S. McLaren (ed.), pp. 339–356. New York/London: John Wiley and
      Sons.
Dandekar, Kumudini.
  1975 'Why Has the Proportion of Women in India's Population Been Declining?' Economic
      and Political Weekly 10(42): 1663–1667.
Darling, Malcolm Lyall.
  1929 Rusticus Loquitur or the Old Light and the New in the Punjab Village. London: Oxford
      University Press.
Dickemann, Mildred.
  1979 'Female Infanticide, Reproductive Strategies, and Social Stratification: A Preliminary
      Model.' In Evolutionary Biology and Human Social Behavior: An Anthropological
      Perspective. N.A. Chagnon and W. Irons (eds.), pp. 321–367. North Scituate, MA:
      Duxbury Press.
  1984 'Concepts and Classification in the Study of Human Infanticide: Sectional Introduction
      and Some Cautionary Notes' In Infanticide: Comparative and Evolutionary Perspec-
      tives. Glenn Hausfater and Sarah Blaffer Hrdy (eds.), pp. 427–439. New York: Aldine
      Publishing Company.
Divale, William and Marvin Harris.
  1976 'Population, Warfare, and the Male Supremacist Complex.' American Anthropologist
      78: 521–538.
Dyson, Tim and Mick Moore.
  1983 'Gender Relations, Female Autonomy and Demographic Behavior: Regional Contrasts
      within India.' Population and Development Review 9(1): 35–60.
Everett, Jana.
  1984 Personal communication. (Dr. Everett is a political scientist at the University of
      Colorado, Denver.)
Freed, Stanley A. and Ruth S. Freed.
  1976 Shanti Nagar: The Effects of Urbanization in a Village in North India: 1. Social
      Organization. Anthropological Papers of the American Museum of Natural History.
      Vol. 53: Part 1. New York: The American Museum of Natural History.
Harris, Marvin.
  1977 Cannibals and Kings: The Origins of Cultures. New York: Random House.
Horowitz, B. and Madhu Keshwar.
  1982 'Family Life – The Unequal Deal.' Manushi 11: 2–18.
Hrdy, Sarah Blaffer and Glenn Hausfater.
  1984 'Comparative and Evolutionary Perspectives on Infanticide: Introduction and Over-
      view' In Infanticide: Comparative and Evolutionary Perspectives. Glenn Hausfater and
      Sarah Blaffer Hrdy (eds.), pp. xii–xxxv. Aldine Publishing Company.

Jacobson, Doranne.
1970 'Hidden Faces: Hindu and Muslim Purdah in a Central Indian Village.' Unpublished doctoral dissertation, Columbia University.
Kumar, Dharma.
1983 'Male Utopias or Nightmares?' Economic and Political Weekly January 15: 61–64.
Lenington, S.
1981 'Child Abuse: The Limits of Sociobiology.' Ethnology and Sociobiology 2: 17–29.
Lewis, Oscar.
1965 Village Life in Northern India: Studies in a Delhi Village. New York: Random House.
Lipton, Michael.
1983 Demography and Poverty. World Bank Staff Working Papers, Number 623. Washington, DC: The World Bank.
Luschinsky, Mildred S.
1962 'The Life of Women in a Village of North India: A Study of Role and Status.' Unpublished doctoral dissertation, Cornell University.
Madan, T.N.
1965 Family and Kinship: A Study of the Pandits of Rural Kashmir. New York: Asia Publishing House.
Manushi.
1982 'A New Form of Female Infanticide.' 12: 21.
Miller, Barbara D.
1981 The Endangered Sex: Neglect of Female Children in Rural North India. Ithaca, NY: Cornell University Press.
1984 'Daughter Neglect, Women's Work and Marriage: Pakistan and Bangladesh Compared.' Medical Anthropology 8(2): 109–126.
1985 'The Unwanted Girls: A Study of Infant Mortality Rates' Manushi 29: 18–20.
1986 'Prenatal and Postnatal Sex-Selection in India: The Patriarchal Context, Ethical Questions and Public Policy.' Working Paper No. 107 on Women in International Development (East Lansing, MI: Office of Women in International Development, Michigan State University).
Minturn, Leigh.
1984 'Changes in the Differential Treatment of Rajput Girls in Khalapur: 1955–1975.' Medical Anthropology 8(2): 127–132.
Minturn, Leigh and John T. Hitchcock.
1966 The Rajputs of Khalapur, India. Six Cultures Series, Volume III. New York: John Wiley and Sons.
Raikes, Charles.
1852 Notes on the North-Western Provinces of India. London: Chapman and Hall.
Ramanamma, A. and Usha Bambawale.
1980 'The Mania for Sons: An Analysis of Social Values in South Asia.' Social Science and Medicine 14B: 107–110.
Rosenzweig, Mark R. and T. Paul Schultz.
1982 'Market Opportunities, Genetic Endowments, and Intrafamily Resource Distribution: Child Survival in Rural India.' American Economic Review 72(4): 803–815.
Schneider, David M.
1984 A Critique of the Study of Kinship. Ann Arbor, MI: The University of Michigan Press.
Sen, Amartya and Sunil Sengupta.
1983 'Malnutrition of Children and the Rural Sex Bias.' Economic and Political Weekly Annual Number, May: 855–864.
Sharma, Ursula.
1983 'Dowry in North India: Its Consequences for Women.' In Women and Property, Women as Property. Renee Hirschon (ed.), pp. 62–74. London: Croom Helm.

Simmons, George B., Celeste Smucker, Stan Bernstein, and Eric Jensen.
   1982 'Post Neo-Natal Mortality in Rural India: Implications of an Economic Model.' Demo-
       graphy 19(3): 371–389.
Skinner, G. William.
   1984 'Infanticide as Family Planning in Tokugawa Japan.' Paper prepared for the Stanford-
       Berkeley Colloquium in Historical Demography, San Francisco.
Srilatha, K.V.
   1983 Personal communication. (Dr. Srilatha is an epidemiologist, Senior Training and
       Research Officer, Rural Unit for Health and Social Assistance, Vellore Christian
       Medical College, Tamil Nadu, India).
Tooley, Michael.
   1983 Abortion and Infanticide. Oxford: Oxford University Press.
Visaria, Pravin M.
   1961 The Sex Ratio of the Population of India. Census of India 1961. Vol. 1. Monograph No.
       10. New Delhi: Office of the Registrar General.
Washington Post. August 25.
   1982 'Birth Test Said to Help Indians Abort Females.'
Wasserstrom, Jeffery.
   1984 'Resistance to the One-Child Family.' Modern China 10(3): 345–374.
Wilkey, Ian, John Pearn, Gwynneth Petrie, and James Nixon.
   1982 'Neonaticide, Infanticide and Child Homicide.' Medicine, Science and the Law 22(1):
       31–34.

DOROTHY S. MULL AND J. DENNIS MULL

# INFANTICIDE AMONG THE TARAHUMARA OF THE MEXICAN SIERRA MADRE

It is axiomatic to anthropology that human behavior must be understood within the context of the culture in which it occurs. For example, the extreme fear of lightning among the Tarahumara, noted as early as the 17th century (González Rodríguez 1982: 178, 196) and today expressed in their baptismal ceremonies (Mull 1985), at first glance seems irrational – a "primitive" fear. It becomes more understandable, however, once it is realized that (a) lightning bolts are common in the region, causing considerable destruction and death, and (b) lightning, like certain other celestial phenomena such as a haze-covered sun, is interpreted by the Tarahumara as a sign of serious cosmic disruption. So too the existence of culturally-sanctioned infanticide may seem incomprehensible unless we understand the internal and external constraints at work to produce it.

For the Tarahumara, these constraints include the harsh environmental conditions in which they must eke out an existence, the consequent high value placed on ability to work, and the fact that the two-parent nuclear family is the basic unit in which children can be effectively nurtured. Other factors allowing the maintenance of infanticidal behavior are the characteristic independence and reserve of the Tarahumara people, their reliance on traditional rather than modern forms of health care, and the continued isolation of the region from the mestizo Mexican legal system. In order to convey some understanding of these constraints, any discussion of Tarahumara infanticide must begin with a brief description of the people and their milieu.

## THE PEOPLE AND THEIR CULTURE

The Tarahumara are a Uto-Aztec-speaking indigenous people occupying the vast, remote reaches of the Sierra Madre Occidental in the Mexican state of Chihuahua. Approximately 50 000 in number, they are – except for the Navajo – the largest indigenous American group north of Mexico City. They are famous for their marathon foot races, which can last for several days. The Tarahumara first became known to outsiders when Jesuit missionaries reached the Sierra in 1607, but despite repeated contact since that time, they have maintained much of their traditional culture. According to the Mexican census of 1980, for example, 28% of the Sierra Tarahumara speak no Spanish at all.

A major reason for this maintenance of cultural integrity is their geographic isolation. Living in an area the size of three New England states, the Tarahumara populate a rugged terrain characterized by formidable granite

113

*Nancy Scheper-Hughes (ed.), Child Survival, 113–132.*
© *1987 by D. Reidel Publishing Company.*

peaks, dense pine forests, and precipitous canyons. In the midst of the region is the famous Barranca del Cobre (Copper Canyon), approximately as deep as the Grand Canyon but broader and more branched. Scattered throughout the Tarahumara territory, isolated nuclear or extended families typically live several miles from their nearest neighbors. The relatively small quantity of grassy terrain and arable land would seem to be partly responsible for this settlement pattern.

The material culture and social organization of the Tarahumara has been well described in several excellent anthropological studies beginning with that of Lumholtz in 1902. Among the more outstanding subsequent work is that of Bennett and Zingg (1935), Pennington (1963 and 1983), Kennedy (1978), and Merrill (1978 and 1983). These and other observers describe a milieu in which the Tarahumara live primarily as subsistence farmers outside the cash economy, growing corn and beans and herding goats and sheep. Most live in log houses with dirt floors and no running water or electricity, and a minority who lack even the scant resources needed to build such modest dwellings live in caves. Others own houses but occupy caves for part of the year, usually while working in outlying fields or while living in the warm, low-lying barrancas during the winter months. When the rains fail and the corn is meager or stunted, Tarahumara men may be forced to hire themselves out as laborers in mestizo-managed enterprises such as sawmills located at some distance from their homes.

In a society in which life is difficult and resources scant, those people who can work hardest are regarded as the best marriage partners (Bennett and Zingg 1935: 225, de Velasco Rivero 1983: 83). Physical strength is highly valued in children as well, since 8- to 10-year-olds must often assume heavy responsibilities (herding, care of younger siblings, etc.) to ensure the economic survival of the family as a whole. Adult labor tends to be sex-differentiated, with women grinding corn, cooking, carrying water, weaving, and making pottery while men build houses, gather firewood, plow fields, plant crops, and hoe corn (Kennedy 1978: 72). Infants whose fathers are absent from the household are severely disadvantaged, since the mother, performing not only her own traditional tasks but also heavy labor normally done by men, may be unable to provide adequate nurturance.

Although the extended family may step in to help in such situations, ordinarily the Tarahumara are strikingly independent of each other (including their own kin), wary of the outside world, and noted for their reserve, a quality highly valued in the culture (Lumholtz 1902: 259–261, Passin 1942, Fried 1969, Burgess 1981). The extreme shyness of the women was noted by the Jesuits shortly after the first Spanish contact was made (González Rodríguez 1982: 159). Even today, young women tending their goats will turn their faces away and sometimes flee when a stranger approaches. Not only shyness but also a historically-justified fear of rape by mestizo loggers and other outsiders motivates this behavior. Such outsiders are widely – and apparently correctly

– believed to transmit gonorrhea (Tarahumara *bikarí*)[1] to the Tarahumara people.

The limited diet, often inadequate shelter, and pervasive lack of sanitation in the region pose other threats to health. During the rainy season, overflowing rivers mix with fecal matter and gastroenteritis is rampant. In the winter cold, pneumonia is a major killer. As one might expect, tuberculosis is common in all seasons and infant mortality is extremely high (Mull and Mull 1983). A further obstacle to health is that although the majority of their diseases are curable, most Tarahumara remain aloof from the small, often poorly-equipped clinics dotting the region, preferring to rely on traditional healing methods instead (Anzures y Bolaños 1978: 66).

Tarahumara curing ceremonies typically involve dancing, chanting, ritual drinking of homemade corn beer (Spanish *tesgüino*, Tarahumara *batári*), dreaming by a shamanistic curer (Tarahumara *owirúame*), and animal sacrifice.[2] In addition, nearly 300 different medicinal herbs are used (Bye 1976). Belief in witchcraft is strong, and many illnesses are attributed to fright sickness (Tarahumara *maharí*) or to anger directed at the victim by individuals or personified entities such as the peyote plant. Natural disasters such as drought or hail are often blamed on God's "annoyance" or his "illness." Preventive as well as curative rites are performed. Some of these, such as the Tarahumara baptismal ceremony to protect the infant against lightning bolts and other hazards, are normally concealed from outsiders.

The Tarahumara abandon their reserved and reticent manner chiefly during fiestas known as *tesgüinadas*. Here, Tarahumara families meet and socialize, and work such as planting, weeding, and blanket-weaving is combined with drinking of *tesgüino* until a state of inebriation is reached. Most acts of violence between adults, as well as instances of sexual dalliance, occur during these drinking parties (Lumholtz 1902: 351–352, Kennedy 1978). Sometimes the violence comes to the attention of Mexican authorities, who take the offender to jail, but more often the government does not become involved and indigenous laws are the means of social control. Elected tribal leaders adjudicate disputes and allocate punishments following the patterns first described by Lumholtz (1902) and Bennett and Zingg (1935).

In some cases, violence appears to be culturally accepted, or at least tolerated. Kennedy, for example, reports (1978: 199–200) that after a slaying at a *tesgüinada*, the killer was ostracized for a short time but was soon reabsorbed in the community. Although several people said he would be excluded from heaven after death, most excused his behavior on the grounds that he was drunk at the time of the murder and therefore could not help himself. (Mexican authorities had initially been called in, but after the murderer escaped from custody, the police were apparently deterred by the inaccessibility of the region and did not bother to pursue the matter further.)

Reliable informants also told us of three cases during the 1980s in which individuals believed to be evildoers were killed without the knowledge or involvement of Mexican officials. One man, who was said to have beaten many women, was tied hand and foot by fellow Tarahumara and put in a cave that was then walled off with rocks; his skeleton was seen there in 1983 by a member of a Catholic religious order. In another case, a famous, politically powerful shaman (*owirúame*) was knifed in his sleep, reportedly because he was thought to have become a witch (*sukurúame*) who put hexes on people instead of curing them. In a third incident, which took place in an area so remote that many inhabitants have never seen a car, a woman murdered a female witch by driving a stake into her back, and then buried her.[3] The Tarahumara spoke guardedly of these killings, but sanctioned them as necessary for the good of the community as a whole.

### TARAHUMARA INFANTICIDE: THE CASE OF CECILIA

The possible existence of culturally-sanctioned infanticide, as well as homicide, among the Tarahumara first came to our attention when one of us (JDM) was serving as a volunteer physician at a hospital in the Tarahumara region in 1982. A 12-month-old child had been admitted to the same hospital five months earlier with severe diarrhea, and intravenous fluid had been given via a vein in her foot. Tragically, a rare iatrogenic mishap had allowed medications and salt solutions to leak into the tissues. The result was massive necrosis that had necessitated amputation of half the toddler's foot.

Subsequent problems with infection and pain had kept the child in the hospital for months following the amputation, where she became a favorite of the doctors and nurses. Meanwhile, however, her mother gradually stopped coming to see her. By the time we became familiar with the case, the mother's visits had changed from lengthy interactions to very cursory affairs – often only a few minutes spent at the hospital while she was in town on other business. In her conversations with us, the mother expressed a restrained but deeply felt anger toward the medical staff, remarking that her daughter was not "like that" (i.e. lacking half her foot) before she entered the hospital. Except for the amputation the child was in good health and was almost ready to be discharged.

Shortly after returning to the United States, we learned that a messenger had been sent to find the mother and to ask her to take the child home, which she agreed to do. Initially all seemed well, but a few weeks later, Tarahumara patients from the same area reported to hospital staff that the child had "failed" and died several days after she returned home. The doctors and nurses were shocked and appalled. Many expressed the belief that the child had died of "neglect" as a result of the mother's ignorance, laziness, and lack of concern, as evidenced by the decreasing frequency of her visits. The mother was not seen again in the town.

On returning to the Sierra in the summer of 1983, we dicussed the case with several Tarahumara informants. One said immediately, "Oh, her family killed her – probably by hitting her. Or they gave her a poisoned drink." Another agreed, adding, "Well, after all, with only half a foot she'd never be able to walk right, or work hard. She might never find a husband." Still another said that the sight of her mutilated foot might have caused fright sickness – Spanish *susto*, Tarahumara *maharí* – in beholders. (Belief in fright sickness, a potentially fatal illness involving soul loss, is very strong among the Tarahumara as among many other Latin American groups. The Tarahumara say that it can result from viewing unattractive physical abnormalities as well as from undergoing frightening experiences such as falls and assaults. Thus, burn victims may be abandoned in hospitals if they are severely disfigured; health workers told of many such cases, and in 1983 we observed one ourselves.)

We next asked several health care providers in the Tarahumara region whether they had ever treated or nurtured a child over a long period of time only to have it die at home soon after discharge. Most had had such an experience. For example, a nurse who was acting essentially as a physician in a remote hospital recounted the frustrating case of a baby born with a cleft lip and palate. She had rescued the baby from near starvation and had arranged for corrective surgery. As she described it, neither the lip nor the palate could be closed completely, but both were enough improved to allow her to spoon-feed the baby by placing liquids far back in its mouth. Finally, after the infant was thriving, she summoned the parents and taught them her feeding method. The baby was discharged but died less than a month later.

Afterwards, neighbors reported that the parents had largely ignored the baby and that it had died as a result of not being fed. The same nurse recalled that the family had not shown much enthusiasm for using such a time-consuming feeding method, and she expressed both grief for the baby's death and disgust with the parents' "ignorance" and "laziness." As Cecilia's doctors had done, she attributed the unexpected infant death to parental incompetence.

But the comments of our Tarahumara informants, as reported above, suggest that a conscious decision to eliminate a deformed baby may have been involved. In addition, a well-known Mexican physician who has worked extensively with the Tarahumara told us that he had never seen a case of cleft lip during his years in the Sierra. (Worldwide, it is estimated that one case occurs in every 800 births.) He said that children with such deformities were eliminated because they were thought to cause life-threatening fright sickness. Indeed, many Tarahumara classify anomalous births of this kind with other rare occurrences such as meteor showers as portending the end of the world. We decided to search the literature for additional cases that might shed light on the matter.

## PUBLISHED REFERENCES TO TARAHUMARA INFANTICIDE

Given the extreme sensitivity of the subject, it is not surprising that published allusions to Tarahumara infanticide are few and brief. The entire literature on the topic can be reproduced in a few short paragraphs. Nevertheless, the five scholars who have alluded to the practice since the turn of the century – Lumholtz (1902), Bennett (1935), Gajdusek (1953), Fried (1969), and de Velasco Rivero (1983) – have impeccable credentials and are respected observers of the Tarahumara.

The famed Norwegian naturalist and world traveler Carl Lumholtz was the first to study the Tarahumara in a systematic fashion. He writes (1902: 243), "I have been told that in some rare instances a Tarahumare [sic] woman will sit on her child right after its birth to crush it, in order to save herself the trouble of bringing it up. . . . [Still,] crimes of this kind are exceedingly rare." He states further (1902: 417–418) that "a few instances are known in which women have left their half-caste [i.e. fathered by non-Tarahumara] babies in the woods to perish, and such children are often given away to be adopted by the Mexicans."

Wendell Bennett, then chair of the anthropology department at Yale, contributed the section on social organization in a classic volume on the Tarahumara. He asserts (1935: 348) that Tarahumara infanticide is "uncommon, although unmarried girls may let their children fall on the rocks or choke them. This is to avoid social disgrace." He cites the following anecdote (1935: 229): "Maricela became pregnant and, when cross-examined, finally admitted that her brother was the guilty party. Considerable scandal arose. . . . The girl killed the baby by letting it fall on the rocks. Not long afterward, she was properly married."

D. Carleton Gajdusek, the physician and Nobel laureate perhaps best known for his studies of *kuru* in New Guinea, relates another incident (1953: 38):

Albinism occurs occasionally among pure-blooded Indians. Near Guachochi we learned of an albino Tarahumara boy who lived with a mestizo family. His father, suspecting a Caucasian intruder into the Sierra, had refused to keep the child and had thereafter kept his wife under close supervision. The birth of an albino girl the following year finally convinced him of his wife's innocence. This second child was dropped over a cliff, we were told. No other example of infanticide was encountered.

Sixteen years later, Jacob Fried, a distinguished anthropologist who wrote the chapter on the Tarahumara for the *Handbook of Middle American Indians*, states straightforwardly (1969: 868) that "infanticide is practiced for a variety of reasons, psychological as well as economic."

Finally, Pedro de Velasco Rivero, the Jesuit author of a book on Tarahumara religious beliefs and rituals, quotes one of his informants, a woman from Tewerichi in the northeast part of the Tarahumara zone, as saying (1983: 71) that

algunas mujeres no quieren tener otro hijo, y . . . cuando ya están a punto de dar a luz se salen de
la casa sin que las vea el marido y se van lejos a tener su niño. Una vez nacido lo "paran" dentro
de algún encino hueco, o lo dejan en la arena y se vuelven a su casa. Ella supo de una mujer que
hizo esto y, cuando el marido volvió a su casa notó que ya había dado a luz y le preguntó dónde
estaba el niño, ella respondió que lo había dejado en la arena. El marido fue a recogerlo y lo
encontró casi muerto porque "había comido mucha tierra".

(some women do not want to have another child, and . . . when they are at the point of giving
birth they leave the house without their husband seeing them and go far away to have their child.
Once the child is born, they "stand it up" in some hollow oak tree, or they leave it on the ground
and return to their house. She knew of a woman who did this, and when the husband came home
he noticed that she had already given birth and asked her where the child was. She replied that
she had left it on the ground. The husband went to get it and found it almost dead because it had
"eaten a lot of earth.")

De Velasco Rivero goes on to state his opinion (1983: 71) that

a pesar de estos relatos, no parece que realmente estas prácticas sean comunes. Tanto más
cuanto que el índice de mortalidad es de por sí muy elevado y que en esta sociedad los niños
representan una verdadera ayuda, tanto en la casa como en ciertas labores como el pastoreo,
desde muy temprana edad.

(in spite of these tales, it does not really appear that these practices are common, especially since
the infant mortality rate is in itself very high and since in this society, children represent a real
economic advantage from a very early age, both in the house and in certain tasks like herding.)

These, then, are the published scholarly references to Tarahumara infanticide – all apparently based on the comments of one or at most several
informants. In addition, it is perhaps noteworthy that in the late 17th century,
a Jesuit priest remarked on the small number of Tarahumara with birth
defects (González Rodríguez 1982: 184), which suggests that such individuals
might have been disposed of as infants or young children.

Thus our investigation led us to conclude that infanticidal behavior might
occur among the Tarahumara under the following circumstances: (1) situations in which *any* birth is unwelcome because the mother has no male
support (the father being absent or inappropriate, as in incest) or already has
"too many" children; (2) situations in which the infant is defective or sickly or
is perceived as such (e.g. albinism). The infanticidal methods attributed to the
Tarahumara in the literature include throwing or allowing the infant to fall
from the edge of a cliff, sealing it up in a hollow tree, abandoning it on a
hillside, and rolling on the infant to suffocate it. In addition, our experience
with Cecilia and the cleft palate case reported by the hospital nurse suggested
that defective or sickly children might sometimes be disposed of by severe
neglect (i.e. starvation) or in rare instances by more direct and aggressive
means, such as a blow to the head or a poisoned drink. However, the
evidence to date has been anecdotal; no survey of knowledge of these
practices had ever been undertaken.

THE PRESENT STUDY

*Method*

Since we were engaged in a study of Tarahumara obstetric beliefs and practices (Mull and Mull 1984) and were collecting information on that subject from Tarahumara women, we decided to add to the study an inquiry into infanticide. During the summer of 1983 and 1984, one author (DSM) questioned 20 Tarahumara women from different parts of the Sierra on their knowledge of infanticidal practices. The interview sites were the town of Creel (population 5000) and the village of Norogachi, much smaller than Creel and separated from it by 100 km of rough dirt road. Sampling was opportunistic: those women were questioned who had time to talk while they were in town to go to church, to seek medical care, or to buy provisions such as salt and coffee.

Most women ($N = 13$) were interviewed in Spanish, but those who spoke no Spanish, or so little that they could not express themselves easily in the language, were interviewed in Tarahumara by a bilingual Tarahumara woman acting as an interpreter. The questions were formulated with the information supplied by the literature and by our previous informants in mind. They were incorporated into the obstetrics survey instrument, a structured interview, in as natural a way as possible. For example, a question about possible causes of birth defects was followed by a question about what should be done if a child were born with cleft lip. Because of the sensitive nature of the topic, not every woman was asked every question; therefore it is likely that actual knowledge of infanticidal practices was greater than the results indicate.

*Results*

Results from the obstetrics portion of the questionnaire have been presented elsewhere (Mull and Mull 1984). Table I summarizes the demographic characteristics of the 20 women interviewed. Though all but two lived within four hours' walk – for a Tarahumara – of the interview sites, their homes were distributed over a wide area. One woman had lived in a cave as a child and one migrated to a cave in the barrancas every winter to avoid the cold at higher altitudes.

As noted above, seven spoke no Spanish or so little that a Tarahumara-Spanish interpreter was used. One of those who spoke Spanish could also read and write. Sixteen women said that they were married, but it should be noted that "married" often means for these women that they are living in a stable union with a man; only a minority of Tarahumara are legally married. All of the women interviewed were nominally Catholic. In other words, like the vast majority of the Tarahumara (Kennedy 1978: 2, de Velasco Rivero 1983: 72, Merrill 1983: 295), they had received a Catholic baptism and had

TABLE I
Demographic profile of informants ($N = 20$).

| Residence | Near Creel | 12 |
|---|---|---|
| | Near Norogachi | 6 |
| | Other | 2 |
| Age | 16 – 80 years | |
| | Mean = 38.5, median = 37.5 | |
| Language | Much Spanish | 10 |
| | Little Spanish | 6 |
| | No Spanish | 4 |
| Marital status | "Married" | 16 |
| | Widowed | 2 |
| | Single or separated | 2 |

TABLE II
Reproductive history of informants age 40 or older ($N = 10$).

| | |
|---|---|
| Number of pregnancies | 10.9 per woman |
| Number of live births | 9.1 per woman |
| Number of children who had died before age 5 | 4.3 per woman (47.3% of the live births) |
| Age of these 43 children at death | |
| Less than 6 months | 6 |
| 6 months to less than 1 year | 11 |
| 1 year to less than 2 years | 15 |
| 2 years to less than 3 years | 7 |
| 3 years to less than 4 years | 2 |
| 4 years to less than 5 years | 2 |

accepted certain beliefs and practices of the Catholic Church, most notably those resembling their own indigenous traditions.

Table II presents the reproductive histories of the 10 women interviewed who were 40 years of age or older and whose families were therefore essentially complete. It shows an extremely high infant mortality rate (47.3% of the live births) and a clustering of these 43 infant deaths in the "6 months to 2 years" age range, a pattern that is consistent with the dangers associated with weaning. (The youngest infant who was reported to have died was two weeks old.) The major stated causes of the 43 deaths were gastroenteritis, pneumonia, and measles. Fright sickness and bewitchment were also mentioned. No mother said or even hinted that infanticide or maternal neglect was implicated in any of these deaths.

With respect to knowledge of infanticidal behavior, Table III shows that 95% of the 20 women questioned knew of at least one case of infanticide when the mother "had no husband" (i.e. lacked male support) or had "too

TABLE III

Tarahumara infanticidal practices known to informants ($N = 20$).

| | Number knowing of at least one case of infanticide, by category |
|---|---|
| *Reason for infanticide* | |
| Mother with "no husband" (no male support) | 19 (95%) |
| Mother with "too many" children | 19 (95%) |
| Infant "damaged" (defective) | 11 (55%) |
| Infant sickly | 2 (10%) |
| *Method used* | |
| Throw infant or allow it to fall from cliff | 12 (60%) |
| Deny food to infant* | 11 (55%) |
| Seal infant up in hollow tree | 9 (45%) |
| Abandon infant on hillside | 3 (15%) |
| Roll on infant to suffocate it, then bury it | 3 (15%) |
| Give poisoned drink to infant* | 2 (10%) |
| Bury infant alive immediately after birth | 1 (5%) |

* Method used only if the infant was "damaged" or sickly.

many" children. 55% knew of at least one case associated with a "damaged" (i.e. defective) infant, and 10% knew of at least one case in which a sickly infant had been killed.[4] (All of the women knew of infanticide having occurred under at least one of these circumstances.) In almost all instances, the infant was said to have been killed *by the mother*, making her decision autonomously and acting alone, immediately after it was born. The cultural preference for unattended birth (Mull and Mull 1984), although apparently motivated principally by female modesty, would facilitate this practice. (Other family members were said to sometimes become involved in unusual cases, such as that of Cecilia, in which immediate infanticide was delayed.)

The methods allegedly used to dispose of an unwanted infant were essentially the same ones described in the literature and by our previous informants. For healthy but supernumerary babies, these methods were, in order of frequency: (1) throwing or allowing the infant to fall from the edge of a cliff; (2) placing the infant in a hollow tree in a standing position and sealing the hole with stones (recalling the way in which the man was sealed up in the cave); (3) abandoning the infant on a hillside; (4) rolling on the infant to suffocate it and then burying it; and (5) burying the infant alive immediately after birth. (In addition, two women stated that babies were sometimes given away.) Defective or sickly infants, such as those born with cleft lip, were reportedly sometimes allowed to die by neglect (i.e. they were not fed), or, rarely, they were killed by more aggressive means such as a poisoned drink. Killing with blows, however, was not mentioned.

Other information obtained during the questioning was also of considerable interest. For example, two women volunteered that they themselves had close relatives (an aunt and a daughter-in-law) who had committed infanticide. The aunt "had no husband" and had put her baby in a hollow tree; the daughter-in-law had stopped feeding an 8-month-old whom she perceived as sickly. (While we were conducting the study, this same daughter-in-law attempted to give away another of her children, a 7-year-old girl who had suffered from frequent illnesses.) Although this woman was disapproved of by the community, informants said that infanticide carried out immediately after birth was not strongly condemned, especially if the baby had physical defects. Further, we were told that if a woman had decided to kill an unwanted child, she preferred to do so immediately after birth in order to avoid "knowing" the infant.

Two other informants said that older people in the community – usually female – frequently cautioned young women not to kill their babies if no birth defects were present. One said that her own father had warned her against this, stating that God would punish her for it after she died. When she tried to enter heaven, God would bar her way, asking, "And where are all those babies you killed?" – a casual but telling allusion to multiple killings by one woman. The other informant reported that "the old women say" that if babies who have no defect are killed, God will send the mother back to earth to search endlessly, like the Llorona of Spanish folklore, for the murdered infants.[5] (She went on to say that she knew many women who had done it anyway.)

In an effort to determine how widespread the practice of killing defective infants might be, we asked each informant whether she had a "damaged" infant in her own family who was still alive. Three said yes. One had a niece who had been born blind, one had a grandchild with a "short arm and leg," and one had a daughter who was still unable to speak at age 7. (It might perhaps be noted that in only one of these cases would the defect have been apparent at birth.) Though all 20 women knew what cleft lip was, describing it as being born "without a nose," none knew of any living child with this condition.[6]

## Discussion

Obviously, the frequency of infanticide among the Tarahumara cannot be determined from a small exploratory study such as this one, which must of course be regarded as preliminary and provisional. The possibility that some informants were simply repeating village hearsay rather than recounting first-hand observations cannot be ruled out. Because of the sensitivity of the subject, it was not possible to elicit precise numbers of cases or, except in the two instances mentioned above, the names of infanticidal mothers. Nevertheless, it seems clear that the practice of killing an infant when a woman has no male support or "too many" children is not rare, since 19 of our 20 informants (95%) claimed to know of such events. A health worker in the Tarahumara region told us that she personally knew two women who had committed infanticide in the 1980s under these circumstances.

An uninitiated observer might wonder why contraception or feticide (induced abortion) is not practiced instead in such cases, since infanticide is a relatively inefficient, physiologically wasteful form of reproductive management, depleting the mother's body and exposing her to childbirth-associated risks. The fact is that, at least in the more remote parts of the Tarahumara region, contraceptive and abortive methods that are both effective and harmless to the woman seem to be unknown. Only two ways of inducing abortion were mentioned to us, and both were said to be unreliable: the drinking of three liters of red oak-bark tea per day for three days (*Quercus chihuahuensis*; Tarahumara *rohá sitákame*; Spanish *encino colorado*)[7] and the drinking of massive quantities of wormseed-plant tea (*Chenopodium ambrosioides*; Tarahumara *pasóte, basóta*; Spanish *epazote*). The latter herb is also used to aid expulsion of the placenta after birth.

Although Tarahumara contraceptive and abortive methods have not yet been studied in any systematic way, Bennett reports (1935: 348) that "contraceptive measures are unknown. Abortion is considered ugly and rarely practiced. The woman accomplishes this by herself through a violent massaging of the abdomen when well advanced in pregnancy. Another method is to fill a heavy olla [clay pot] with water and to place it upon the abdomen." Writing almost half a century later, de Velasco Rivero (1983: 71) comments that

no parece haber ni prácticas anticonceptivas ni prácticas abortivas. Lolita [the author's informant] afirma que no hay hierbas para no tener hijos; sin embargo, dijo que cuando una mujer no quiere tener hijos va con el owirúame quien tiene poder para hacer que no los tenga.[8] [*Author's note*: Sin embargo la carencia de medios anticonceptivos se confirma por la pregunta de Chabela de Tewerichi a una de las religiosas respecto a qué cosa tomaban para no tener hijos, pues ella no quería tener más.] Dijo también que hay una planta – una variedad de pino[9] – que les dan a las mujeres para que "salga al niño", pero que se la dan cuando están ya para dar a luz.

(neither contraceptive nor abortive practices seem to exist. Lolita [the author's informant] declares that there are no herbs to prevent having children; nevertheless, she said that when a woman does not want to have children she goes to an *owirúame* who has the power to make her not have them.[8] [*Author's note*: However, the lack of contraceptive methods is confirmed by the fact that Chabela from Tewerichi questioned one of the nuns regarding what they were taking to avoid having children, since she did not want to have any more.] She also said that there is a plant – a variety of pine[9] – that they give to women to make the child "come out," but that they give it when the women are already at the point of giving birth.)

Thus – though the evidence is sketchy at best and obviously merits further investigation – it appears that contraception and induced abortion are not re? possibilities for many Tarahumara women, and that infanticide may in effect be their only choice when a pregnancy is unwanted. Under such circumstances, it would not be surprising if infanticide occurred fairly freque

The situation with regard to defective children is somewhat less clearcut than it is with regard to supernumerary ones. As noted above, three of our informants had such children in their own families and the children were still living. Further, Lumholtz reports (1902: 236–237) that in the course of his travels among the Tarahumara he saw eight cases of cleft lip, a man with only stumps for arms, and a boy with clubfoot; and crippled Tarahumara are occasionally seen today in the Sierra. It may be that those babies with the worst deformities – cleft palates so severe as to prevent nursing, for example – are allowed to die while those with lesser defects survive. This would be consistent with the fact that the three defects present in our informants' families were not ones that would preclude successful breast-feeding.

The phrase "allowed to die" is used advisedly in the preceding paragraph, for several informants made a verbal distinction between actively "killing" a child and passively "letting it die" by denial of food or abandonment in the wild. Thus, one woman responded in the negative when asked whether children with cleft lip were "killed," but then said, "Sometimes they can't eat with cleft lip," and, after a moment's pause, added, "And sometimes they don't give them anything to eat." A preference for passive rather than violent infanticidal methods is suggested by the data reported in Table III and has been described in other societies (Scrimshaw 1984: 443).

The Tarahumara practice of delaying their indigenous name-giving cere-mony for a period of three days to one year after birth (Mull 1985) may also have the effect of deferring "human" status and allowing the avoidance of murder as it is culturally defined (murderers are believed to be excluded from heaven after death). Our research indicates that all but the most acculturated Tarahumara regard this ceremony as of crucial importance in confirming the infant's identity both as a person and as a Tarahumara. In fact, the Tarahumara word for 'to have a name,' *rewérama*, can also be used to mean 'to be, to exist.'[10]

Despite the apparent tolerance of at least some types of infanticide within their own culture, the Tarahumara exhibit considerable discomfort and evasiveness when discussing such practices. All know that both the Catholic Church and Mexican law forbid murder, and although the Mexican legal system has little impact on their culture, Catholic teachings do have an influence on many, especially since church personnel operate schools in the region. The widely-known pro-life convictions of the Catholic missionaries scattered throughout the Sierra have undoubtedly contributed to continued concealment of the existence of infanticide. Many informants were willing to discuss it only after looking furtively about to be certain that no church personnel were nearby. In a few instances they even insisted on getting away from all buildings and going out into the open spaces where no one could possibly overhear the conversation.

Because of such understandable sensitivities and fears, it is difficult to ascertain the prevalence of Tarahumara infanticide. In addition, the flexibility and adaptability of the people, together with their varying degrees of acculturation and economic resources, make generalizations extremely hazardous. Thus, we found several instances in which mothers of twins were making every effort to keep both infants alive, just as we found instances in which children with handicaps were being nurtured. Similarly, it is by no means true that most Tarahumara mothers who lack male support commit infanticide; we ourselves met many such women who had come, with their babies, to sell handicrafts in areas frequented by tourists, and informants told us of many more. It appears that mothers are likely to resort to infanticide only when the child has a severe birth defect or when circumstances conspire to make their life situations extremely stressful. Nevertheless, in view of the universal knowledge of the practice among our informants, it seems indisputable that infanticide is a part of Tarahumara culture, now as in the past.

## CLINICAL IMPLICATIONS

Recent work on infanticide brought together in Hausfater and Hrdy (1984) suggests that an array of conscious and unconscious forces may contribute to the practice. Some of these are as yet poorly understood. For example, some forms of delayed infanticide, such as death induced by child abuse in our own society, are difficult to comprehend, yet we know that they occur. What is certain is that infanticide seems to be motivated by powerful human needs, including the survival instinct itself. If we contemplate the strength of these needs, we are likely to conclude that traditional explanations for infant mortality, however compelling, should be re-examined.

In the case of the Tarahumara, for example, detailed histories of 150 families taken between 1983 and 1985 by one author (JDM) revealed childhood mortality rates at approximately 50% from birth to age 5. (This figure is supported by the observations of three other contemporary investigators [Kennedy 1978: 164, Murray 1981: 208, de Velasco Rivero 1983: 71] and by the present survey.) Approximately 40% of the living children under age 5 in these 150 families showed poor growth and insufficient weight gain. Such growth failures, which are known to predispose to high mortality, are clearly related to inadequate food intake. Originally, we regarded this as the unfortunate result of crop failure and economic privation, and as a misfortune that affected all members of the family more or less equally. In the light of some recent work on infanticide and differential feeding practices, however (McKee 1984: 96–97, Scrimshaw 1984: 444, 448), we decided to re-examine the eating patterns of the Tarahumara nuclear family.

We found that in most families, there were no fixed mealtimes as we know them. Food was simply cooked and put out so that those who wished could help themselves. Mothers were frequently unaware of what their children actually ate, and in what quantity. In such a setting, adults and older children are in a position to acquire more food than are smaller children, so that what at first appears to be merely permissive child-rearing can actually amount to selective neglect. Reliable observers told us that on occasion, food donations from the United States that had been targeted for flagrantly malnourished children had been eaten by adults instead. Could it be that such behaviors are culturally designed to favor adults and older children who have already demonstrated their value to the family unit and their ability to survive?

Such questions are difficult to ask, and even more difficult to answer, but recent studies suggest that explanations of this kind should not be rejected out of hand. One wonders whether, as has been suggested by Scheper-Hughes (1984 and this volume), mother-infant bonding may under some social conditions be delayed until the child has survived to age 3 or even later. Certainly the Tarahumara practice, cited above, of delaying name-giving for up to a year after birth suggests that they have a cautious attitude toward child survival. Infants who have not been named are regarded as "the Devil's children" and are not buried with those who have been baptized; two Tarahumara legends (Mares Trías 1975: 33, 37) describe how such infants were placed on a river bank to attract a serpent identified with the Devil. The deferral of breast-feeding until the colostrum has been replaced by milk, common among the Tarahumara as among other indigenous groups, may also serve to discourage the formation of mother-child bonds until the period of highest infant mortality has passed.

The recent view of infanticide as a widespread and perhaps universal human behavior (Scrimshaw 1984) comes at a fortuitous time for those who have been studying medical decision-making by patients, e.g. the choice of a folk healer or folk remedy instead of a physician. Investigators have attempted to identify the factors determining such choices, but after some initial insights, the field has virtually come to a halt. Although entities such as access (distance to health care facilities, cost, etc.), perceived seriousness of the illness, and folk belief models have been shown to be important (e.g. Young and Garro 1982), the decision-making models that have been proposed suffer from significant gaps and limited predictive power. In a society such as that of the Tarahumara, for example, seemingly irrational and harmful decisions not to seek a doctor are often made. The perplexing nature of such health care choices may be resolved if we take into consideration the existence of conscious or unconscious infanticidal intent. The following case is cited as an example.

### The Case of Victor

In 1983, a 15-month-old child with diarrhea and dehydration was seen by one author (JDM) during a program to teach home-based oral rehydration therapy to Tarahumara parents. The teaching was done in a makeshift clinic located about 5 km from the nearest town. The child's mother and father, who lived near the clinic, were taught that diarrhea causes dehydration, that dehydration in turn causes cessation of tears and urine, and that this often fatal condition can be effectively treated with an orally-administered solution of sugar, salt, and water. After being shown how to make up the solution, the parents administered it to the child under supervision. They were given a spoon for measuring the sugar and salt, which they said they had at home, and a container to mix it in. Finally, they were asked to bring the child back the next day for re-evaluation of his condition.

The parents did not appear the next day, however; and not knowing where they lived among the numerous caves and canyons dotting the area, we were at a loss to find them. We returned to town without having re-examined the child. Some time later, we learned from neighbors that he had died 48 hours after being seen at the clinic, and that his parents had not given him the sugar and salt solution, although the solution could have saved his life.

Our original conclusion, echoing traditional anthropological theory about health care choices (summarized in Kroeger 1983), was that the parents had not administered the solution because it was not perceived as medicine. In other words, we assumed that – since access to the clinic was not a problem – our medical advice was not heeded because of a dominant folk belief model or a preference for folk remedies (Mull 1984:487). Now, in the light of current thinking about infanticide, we question this conclusion. Could it be that not taking medical advice, not giving the prescribed solution, and not returning to see the physician were less the result of an erroneous decision or a preference for folk medicine than of a parental decision to accept the child's death?

The answer to such a question has extremely important implications for international health care initiatives. Oral rehydration therapy, for example, was unsuccessfully recommended in the case recounted above, yet it is the centerpiece of the current, widely-hailed World Health Organization effort to bring health to all by the year 2000. Millions of dollars of U.S. Agency for International Development money, training programs around the world, dozens of publications, and an international conference on the subject have all canonized oral rehydration therapy (ORT) as the cheapest and most effective way to save the lives of the nearly five million children who die each year from diarrhea and dehydration.

That ORT saves lives has been proved beyond dispute, but whether people are motivated or *can* be motivated to use it is not yet known. Experiences such as the one cited above suggest that this initially promising form of therapy may face more obstacles than simply a set of ethnomedical models in conflict with biomedical ones. Without intending to minimize the importance of such obstacles, but to add perspective, we suggest that other powerful social and psychological forces may prevent ORT programs from ever becoming an unqualified success, at least in some cultures.

Health workers attempting to implement such programs need to understand the "logic" of noncompliance as a survival strategy in the larger social context within which parenting takes place. For example, a mother who chooses not to invest time and energy in an infant who has no paternal support or is unlikely to survive to adulthood can often improve not only her own prospects but those of other children she may have. One wonders whether the Tarahumara, whose indulgent affection for their children has been justly praised by observers from Lumholtz on (1902: 273–275), could afford to be quite so nurturant if every child survived infancy.

A question that awaits resolution is whether the impulse toward infanticide can be modified through betterment of social and economic conditions. There is some evidence that it is affected by the worsening of such conditions. Medical volunteers combatting the East African famine in 1984 and 1985 reported that traditional family ties, normally strong in that region, were so eroded that it was not uncommon to see well-fed parents with hungry children.[11] Certainly the relationship between a child and his or her parents does not occur in a vacuum but in a dynamic and changing context affected by such matters as the economic welfare of the family unit and the parents' stress level.

Thus, infanticidal practices might be more common in societies such as that of the Tarahumara where corrective surgery for birth defects is not easily obtained and where supernumerary children may threaten the well-being of the family unit in an ecology of scarcity. If so, it would follow that improved health care, family planning programs, and other forms of social and economic support might diminish the forces that would contribute to a mother's wish to destroy her own child. Although a dispassionate perspective is hard to achieve with a topic such as infanticide, it seems clear that only further study from such a perspective is likely to illuminate this crucial issue.

## NOTES

1. Tarahumara words have been transcribed in the orthography described and used by Pennington (1983: 276n.).
2. Bennett (1935: 288) reports that infant sacrifice was practiced in the past.
3. Lumholtz (1902: 325) and de Velasco Rivero (1983: 424n.) also mention occurrences of this kind.
4. Although the women were not questioned specifically about the birth of twins, one informant volunteered that if a woman had twins and her breast milk was inadequate to feed both, one of the twins – usually the female if they were of different sexes – might be given away so that the other would survive. (Health workers in the Tarahumara region confirmed that babies had been given away, or given to them to care for, in such situations.) This same informant added that she herself had had twins and had had plenty of milk for both. When asked whether one of a pair of twins might be killed rather than given away, she said that she had heard rumors of such events but did not know of any specific cases.
5. This may be related to the Tarahumara belief that after death, a person must find, gather up, and present to God all items that were once part of his or her body, e.g. fingernail parings, hair, and even (according to Burgess 1981: 13) spoken words. One's umbilical cord stump and the placentas of one's children, if any, must also be presented (Mull and Mull 1984), for, as one informant put it, "That is your flesh." If dead babies are indeed classified with items of

this nature, this may indicate that they are not considered bona fide "people" who once had an independent existence.

6. When questioned about the possible causes of deformities such as cleft lip and clubfoot, all but one informant mentioned eclipse of the moon and 9 informants (45%) mentioned eclipse of the sun as well. One said that two of her grandchildren had been born "dark" – supposedly "burned" by the sun – after their mother was exposed to a solar eclipse. The underlying belief is that the eclipsed moon or sun is annoyed and "eats" part of the fetus (or sometimes, in the case of the sun, burns it) in revenge. The notion that a pregnant woman who looks at a lunar or solar eclipse risks giving birth to a baby with cleft lip was recorded among the Aztecs by Sahagún before 1569 (Book V, Chapter XIX, Section 2; reprinted in Sahagún 1956: II:34), and thus probably antedates the Conquest. Fear of lunar eclipse as a cause of birth defects is widespread in present-day Mexico and in many other areas of Latin America (Kelly 1965: 116). Though we are not aware that attribution of fetal deformity to solar eclipse has been documented elsewhere in modern times, the sun is of course extremely important for many indigenous groups. Today the Tarahumara commonly identify it with God.

7. Pennington (1963: 180) states that the bark of *rohá* (*Quercus chihuahuensis*) is used by the Tarahumara to make "a medicinal tea taken by women during pregnancy" and that this tea is also believed to cure heart ailments. In Mexico, red-colored remedies such as pieces of red cloth or crosses drawn on the skin with lipstick are often placed over the heart to "strengthen the blood" of people with heart disease, and it is possible that the Tarahumara see some such magical connection between a reddish tea and the blood of an induced abortion.

8. Tarahumara informants said that the shaman dreams of the woman's uterus "closing up" to accomplish this, but that the ritual is not always successful in preventing conception.

9. This is undoubtedly *Cupressus arizonica* (Tarahumara *wa'á*, Spanish *táscate*), a type of evergreen whose needles are made into a tea to stimulate labor, according to our informants. (Slow birth is greatly feared by Tarahumara women.) The branches of this tree are also used in ceremonial cures, including cleansings and sweat baths.

10. An infant who has not undergone the indigenous baptismal ceremony not only cannot enter heaven but attracts lightning bolts that threaten the entire community. Informants told of a curing ritual performed in 1985 around a stand of trees that had been repeatedly struck by lightning, supposedly because an unbaptized new born had been left there to die by his mother. This potential danger to others may help to explain why such infants are normally disposed of in places remote from dwellings and tilled fields.

11. *The New York Times*, February 10, 1985.

## REFERENCES

Anzures y Bolaños, María del Carmen
    1978 La Relación Médico-Paciente en la Sierra Tarahumara. *In* Estudios sobre Etnobotánica y Antropología Médica. Vol. 3. Carlos Viesca Treviño (ed.), pp. 59–71. México, DF: Instituto Mexicano para el Estudio de las Plantas Medicinales.
Bennett, Wendell C., and Robert M. Zingg
    1935 The Tarahumara: An Indian Tribe of Northern Mexico. Reprinted 1976. Glorieta, NM: The Rio Grande Press, Inc.
Burgess, Don
    1981 Tarahumara Folklore: A Study in Cultural Secrecy. Southwest Folklore 5: 11–22.
Bye, Robert A., Jr.
    1976 Ethnoecology of the Tarahumara of Chihuahua, Mexico. Ph.D. dissertation, Department of Biology, Harvard University.
de Velasco Rivero, Pedro
    1983 Danzar o Morir: Religión y Resistencia a la Dominación en la Cultura Tarahumar. México, DF: Centro de Reflexión Teológica.

Fried, Jacob
   1969 The Tarahumara. *In* Handbook of Middle American Indians. Robert Wauchope (ed.), Vol. 8, Ethnology, part 2. Evon Z. Vogt (ed.), pp. 846–870. Austin: University of Texas Press.
Gajdusek, D. Carleton
   1953 The Sierra Tarahumara. The Geographical Review 43: 15–38.
González Rodríguez, Luis
   1982 Tarahumara: La Sierra y el Hombre. México, DF: Fondo de Cultura Económica.
Hausfater, Glenn, and Sarah Blaffer Hrdy
   1984 Infanticide: Comparative and Evolutionary Perspectives. New York: Aldine Publishing Company.
Kelly, Isabel
   1965 Folk Practices in North Mexico. Austin: University of Texas Press.
Kennedy, John G.
   1978 Tarahumara of the Sierra Madre: Beer, Ecology, and Social Organization. Arlington Heights, Illinois: AHM Publishing Corporation.
Kroeger, Axel
   1983 Anthropological and Socio-Medical Health Care Research in Developing Countries. Social Science and Medicine 17: 147–161.
Lumholtz, Carl
   1902 Unknown Mexico, Vol. 1. Reprinted 1973. Glorieta, NM: The Rio Grande Press, Inc.
McKee, Lauris
   1984 Sex Differentials in Survivorship and the Customary Treatment of Infants and Children. Medical Anthropology 8: 91–108.
Mares Trías, Albino
   1975 Jena Ra'icha Ralámuli Alué 'Ya Muchígame Chiquime Níliga: Aquí Relata la Gente de Antes Lo Que Pasaba en su Tiempo. México, DF: Instituto Lingüístico de Verano.
Merrill, William L.
   1978 Thinking and Drinking: A Rarámuri Interpretation. *In* The Nature and Status of Ethnobotany. Richard I. Ford (ed.), University of Michigan Museum of Anthropology Anthropological Paper 67, pp. 101–117. Ann Arbor: University of Michigan.
   1983 Tarahumara Social Organization, Political Organization, and Religion. *In* Handbook of North American Indians. William C. Sturtevant (ed.), Vol. 10, Southwest. Alfonso Ortiz (ed.), pp. 290–305. Washington, DC: Smithsonian Institution.
Mull, Dorothy S.
   1985 Consejos Contra el Rayo: A Tarahumara Baptismal Rite. Paper presented at the California Folklore Society Annual Meetings, Irvine, CA, April 20.
Mull, Dorothy S., and J. Dennis Mull
   1983 Algodoncillo: White Sign of Danger. Medical Anthropology Quarterly 14(4): 4–13.
   1984 Tarahumara Obstetrics. Paper presented at the American Anthropological Association Annual Meetings, Denver, November 17.
Mull, J. Dennis
   1984 Oral Rehydration Therapy: An Oasis of Hope in the Developing World. The Journal of Family Practice 18: 485–487.
Murray, William Breen
   1981 The Relevance of Anthropology in Medical Education: A Mexican Case Study. Ph.D. dissertation, Department of Anthropology, McGill University.
Passin, Herbert
   1942 Tarahumara Prevarication: A Problem in Field Method. American Anthropologist 44: 235–247
Pennington, Campbell W.
   1963 The Tarahumar of Mexico: Their Environment and Material Culture. Salt Lake City: University of Utah Press.

    1983 Tarahumara. *In* Handbook of North American Indians. William C. Sturtevant (ed.),
         Vol. 10, Southwest. Alfonso Ortiz, ed., pp. 276–289. Washington, DC: Smithsonian
         Institution.
Sahagún, Bernardino de
    1569 Historia General de las Cosas de Nueva Espana. Reprinted 1956. México, DF:
         Editorial Porrua. 4 vols.
Scheper-Hughes, Nancy
    1984   Infant Mortality and Infant Care: Cultural and Economic Constraints on Nurturing in
         Northeast Brazil. Social Science and Medicine 19: 535–546.
Scrimshaw, Susan C.M.
    1984 Infanticide in Human Populations: Societal and Individual Concerns. *In* Infanticide:
         Comparative and Evolutionary Perspectives. Glenn Hausfater and Sarah Blaffer Hrdy
         (eds.), pp. 439–462. New York: Aldine Publishing Company.
Young, James Clay, and Linda Young Garro
    1982 Variation in the Choice of Treatment in Two Mexican Communities. Social Science and
         Medicine 16: 1453–1465.

# PART III

# SOCIAL TRAUMA: THE EFFECTS OF POVERTY, SOCIAL DISRUPTION, AND CATASTROPHE ON CHILD TREATMENT

I have been assured by a very knowing American of my acquaintance in London, that a young healthy child well-nursed is at a year old a most delicious, nourishing and wholesome food, whether stewed, roasted, baked or boiled, and I make no doubt that it will equally serve in a fricasee or a ragout.

Jonathan Swift's "Modest Proposal for Preventing the Children of Ireland from being a Burden to their Parents or Country" during a period of wide-spread famine, 1729

LUCILE F. NEWMAN

# FITNESS AND SURVIVAL

## INTRODUCTION

The birth weight of an infant is the single most important determinant of his or her chances of survival. Because birth weight is influenced by the age, health, nutritional and social status of the mother, the proportion of preterm infants serves as an indicator of the health status of the communities into which they are born. Key factors contributing to low birth weight are low socioeconomic status, mother's very young age, multiple pregnancies, many children, and close birth spacing (Zuckerman *et al*, 1984; Garn *et al.* 1977).

While more and smaller infants are saved each year through the technological interventions of neonatal intensive care, attention must be paid to the social circumstances into which these children go. What is the meaning for a family of a traumatic beginning to their child's life? What social factors contribute to situations of risk? What is the relation of survival of very low birth weight infants to the evolutionary concept of "fitness"?

This chapter is an exploration of vulnerability and resilience in children who have been born prematurely, and in which is identified a high risk high risk spiral, referring to high risk mothers with high risk infants. The potential vulnerability of infants in these circumstances to physical, social or environmental insult is central to the following analysis. We will begin with the concept of fitness, then a description of the effects of premature birth as revealed through the Social and Sensory Environment Studies Project, to be followed by discussions of the high risk subset, and finally, the vulnerable child.

## THE CONCEPT OF FITNESS

The separate development of theory and research methods in physical and social anthropology has resulted in a divergence of these human studies into separate fields reflecting differing definitions and differing research questions based on the now outmoded nature-nurture controversy. There is a trend, however, among a number of theorists to reintegrate these fields through the conceptual integration of biological and social factors in human development. For example, Dubos consistently stressed the flexibility of the human organism in relation to environments in his designation of the "continually evolving phenotype" (1965).

The construct of "biosocial adaptation" suggests biological adaptations with culture as the adaptive mechanism (Cohen 1968: 5). Johnston has noted as an aspect of what he has termed "microevolution" of human populations, plasticity of genetic expression, or phenotype in response to environmental

135

*Nancy Scheper-Hughes (ed.), Child Survival, 135–143.*
© *1987 by D. Reidel Publishing Company.*

differences (1973: 125). Recently Chisholm has developed an evolutionary perspective based on an ontological view of natural selection (1983: 24). Oyama stresses the need to recognize both genetic and environmental contributions to phenotypic variation since nature does not inhere in genes, but emerges in processes; "it is on these processes and their phenotypic outcomes that natural selection operates" (1982: 101). While fitness, in the simplest evolutionary sense, refers to survival to reproductive capacity, Dobzhansky (1968: 115) preferred to describe fitness as differential persistence of genotype or genetic systems, a relative term. Johnston (1973) includes non-selective adaptation, the phenotypic changes resulting from plasticity or variableness within the genotype as aspects of fitness.

It is our view that through plasticity, or individual-environment adaptations within the genotype, human variability derives in some part from variations in the process of development (Lerner 1984; Hinde and Bateson 1984). Implications of these formulations for biobehavioral research include not only a reintegration of organic and environmental forces, but an alignment of them with developmental process and with social situation (Kagan 1984).

In American medical parlance, the concept of *risk* is a statement of statistical probability. Epidemiological studies isolate prevalent "risk factors" from existing cases that then become defining characteristics of a population perceived as "at risk." The fine tuning of the concept of risk and its implications provides an opportunity for investigation of ranges of human behavior – in statistical terms an exploration of the standard deviation. Risk may be seen as those factors potentially compromising fitness of populations. It is necessary then to define as exactly as possible the risk factors experienced by particular populations.

### PREMATURE BIRTH: THE SOCIAL AND SENSORY ENVIRONMENT STUDIES

The Social and Sensory Environment Study of Low Birthweight Infants, focusing on the individual premature infant in the controlled environment of an incubator, derives from a conceptual framework stressing the mutual processes of maturation and adaptation, in an effort to identify the nature of the reciprocity of the infant organism and the incubator environment. The methods of the studies have been ethological, using observation according to identified behavioral categories in conjunction with tape recording of environmental sound and infant vocalization and observers' notes of motor behavior. The original question of these studies was "What is the life experience of the preterm infant in intensive care?" And what factors in this early experience might have any known relationship to later functioning?

The hypothesis was that in the last two months of external development in the very specific environment of the incubator, maturation would take place in a different context and therefore in a different progression than for those who were developing *in utero*. While many persons born prematurely develop consistently with species-typical developmental systems, certain regularities in deviations from the norms of human development have been observed in the lives of some who begin as premature infants. These may be classified as post birth (immediate survival, irritability, distorted forms of parental interaction); early childhood (delayed speech, hyperactive behavior); or at school age (attentional deficit disorders, dyslexia, reading disabilities, and the like). Whether the deficits are interactional, in language, or in social functioning, they can result in a child whose ability to cope with his or her environment is compromised. If the environment itself is a difficult one, the outcome may be a vulnerable child in a high risk situation.

## THE STUDIES

The Social and Sensory Environment Studies of Low Birth Weight infants, carried out from 1978 to the present, are descriptive of the social life and sensory experience of prematurely born infants (Newman 1980, 1981, 1982). They are studies of first contact of a social nature for this special population. The infant's development proceeds in the particular environment of neonatal intensive care – itself an artifact of scientific medicine. In an evolutionary sense neonatal intensive care may be said to create a cultural construction of fitness, that may be termed "medical selection," a differential persistence deriving from the medically defined requirement to survive.

Very low birth weight refers to infants born at 1500 grams or less. They constituted 1.15% of all live births in 1979 (McCormick 1985: 83).

In 1979, in the city of Providence, there were 156 infants born at very low birthweight, (between 900 and 1500 grams) at the Women and Infants Hospital. Of these, 52 did not survive the neonatal period. Of the 104 survivors, 14 were the result of twin births and 14 mothers were age 19 or under.

The numbers are not large, but certain findings already stand out.

1. The prematurity rate for women 19 and under was 8.3% as compared with 4.7% for women 20 and over in this population.
2. Nine of the teenaged mothers were single. Of the other two, no teenaged parent partnerships (whether marriage or stable relationship) has been able to withstand a preterm birth.
3. Among the Social and Sensory Environment study infants, only half of the infants in intensive care were visited by parents. Lack of parent visiting in the Special Care Nursery was found to be predictive for the study group of lack of commitment to follow-up care. Those visiting least at that time were later lost to follow-up completely.

A review of hospital records of the 1979 cohort of infants born at 900–1500 grams was undertaken to investigate patterns of risk. The question in this study was – what factors lead to differences between potential risk and realized risk? Our objective was to determine the nature of vulnerability when examined from different perspectives.

## THE HIGH RISK HIGH RISK SPIRAL

Of the 1979 cohort, there was a small subset of particular concern that was "off the charts" in terms of reproductive failure. We took a closer look at these families.

There were eleven in this category out of the total population of 90 mothers of surviving very low birthweight infants. The numbers here, however, represent only the more immediately visible and surface manifestations of more profound human costs. The eleven high risk women identified in the 1979 cohort had had 37 pregnancies (plus six elective abortions) totaling 43 conceptions. They had 24 living children of which 14 had been premature. They had suffered five spontaneous abortions and eight post birth child deaths.

The records of each of the High Risk mothers was compared with those of the three next Special Care Nursery patient parents file (three records were incomplete and the comparison group is 30). Table I presents the data profile of the two groups. The High Risk group is younger – many of them having first birth under age 17. The comparison group is older and have more living children. All are mothers of preterm infants and about equal numbers in both groups have had previous pregnancy loss or premature deliveries.

By the time these individuals were identified as in trouble, they were lost to follow-up or had already experienced child death and were no longer under the care of the clinical service that had identified them. They constituted a population of high risk mothers of high risk infants. Teenage mothers tend to have often been themselves products of teenage pregnancy (Zuckerman et al, 1985), and can be seen to represent a continuing generational effect that results for some in a high risk high risk spiral.

TABLE I
Descriptive data high risk and comparison group 1979 cohort

|  | High Risk | Comparison Group |
|---|---|---|
|  | (N = 11) | (N = 30) |
| Mean Age | 18.09 | 23.86 |
| Mean Age at First Birth | 17 | 21.63 |
| Married or Stable |  |  |
|    Relationship | 2 (18%) | 24 (80%) |
| Single | 9 (82%) | 6 (20%) |
| Some Prenatal Care | 6 | 28 |
| No Prenatal Care | 5 | 2 |

TABLE II
Qualitative psychosocial risk scale

|  | High Risk | Comparison |
|---|---|---|
|  | (N = 11) | (N = 30) |
| 1. Maternal age at first pregnancy under 17. | 9 (82%) | 3 (10%) |
| 2. Multigravida, high parity | 3 (27%) | 4 (13%) |
| 3. Pregnancies spaced by one year or less. | 1 (9%) | 2 (7%) |
| 4. Late, little or no prenatal care. | 5 (45%) | 2 (7%) |
| 5. Prior pregnancy wastage/Prior preterm birth. | 3 (27%) | 9 (30%) |
| 6. Single (separated, divorced, never married) | 9 (82%) | 4 (13%) |
| 7. Father not identified. | 5 (45%) | 3 (10%) |
| 8. Socially isolated, with poor support system. | 2 (18%) | – |
| 9. SES Stress (precarious financial situation). | 4 (36%) | – |

The picture these cases present is of social isolation, early first pregnancy, history of reproductive loss, no involvement (beyond the minimum of delivery) with health or social services, and no consistent effective contraception. This population appears to be made up of individuals suffering a lack of social support and alienation from the institutions of modern society. We reviewed the records to determine what were their defining common characteristics and we developed a Qualitative Psychosocial Risk scale to see if it would be possible to identify those at risk for reproductive distress on their admission to the hospital. It is the basis for Table II.

Other investigators have combined quantitative with qualitative methods of research with comparable findings. Margaret Boone (1982), analyzing combined data from an inner-city Black population in Washington, D.C. all of whom had low educational levels and who were mostly young and unmarried, found that the standard criteria of age, education and marital status or even drug abuse and sexually transmitted disease did not necessarily correlate with their poor pregnancy outcome. That is, factors related to low birth weight in this group are not identical to those in the general low S.E.S. population. In her study she found that – in addition to alcoholism, smoking, low maternal weight at delivery, hypertension history, ineffective contraception, closely spaced pregnancies, and no prenatal care, there were additional stressors including isolation factors such as migrant status, violence from abusive partners or others, and a poor support system.

Hunter, Kilstrom, Kraybill and Loda, (1978) in North Carolina, in a prospective study of child abuse had noted, as have others, a high incidence of child abuse of children born prematurely, and developed a psychological assessment scale predictive of child abuse.

In our study, in a predominately white population, the mothers so defined seem, as a group, to be characterized also by a mistrust of social institutions, both educational and medical, as reflected in a tendency to drop out of school (in a society where social class is measured by educational achievement), and by poor use of medical care even when its was available, encouraged, and free.

Premature delivery is only one reproductive expression of this group of women at social disadvantage. Another one concerns high risk pregnancy wastage – high unspaced parity, fetal death, spontaneous and induced abortion, child death. In addition, for this population, these maternal factors would be expected to dominate neonatal and early childhood life experience to the degree that they would constitute a major aspect of the child's environment. Although small in absolute numbers, this group accounts for a large amount of pregnancy loss, social dysfunction, and developmental deficit, thereby accounting also for a proportionately high degree of human cost as well as economic cost to society.

## THE VULNERABLE CHILD

Retrospective studies suggest the increased risks to children who are already at a disadvantage (Wise et al. 1985).

McCormick, in a review of the 'Contribution of Low Birth Weight to Childhood Morbidity' (1985) points out that the effect of birth weight on post neonatal mortality is modified by socioeconomic factors. "The risk of developmental delay is not independent of factors that act to increase the risk of low birth weight. Thus, low birth weight infants of disadvantaged mothers are more likely to fail in school (Ramey et al. 1978), or to have lower IQs than infants of similar weight in more advantaged families" (Hardy et al. 1979, Escalona 1982).

Rutter refers to these characteristics of disadvantage as "environmental hazard." As he writes, in the best of circumstances, the hazards seem non existent, "but there seems to be an interactive effect so that the effects of low birth weight are greatest in deprived social circumstances " (1982: 100). He attributes this phenomenon to lowered adaptability resulting from the biological handicap, thereby increasing vulnerability to environmental hazard. Some of these hazards are social, some accidental, and some related directly to circumstances of birth.

The incidence of prematurity in the general population of Rhode Island has changed over the period from 1979–1984 from 7.1% to 6.1%. In a study of the more than 600 victims of certified child abuse in the state over that same period, the incidence of prematurity in the backgrounds of child abuse victims was 23.6%, comparable to that found in North Carolina (Hunter et al. 1978), and other urban areas.

Many studies have demonstrated child death and child abuse to be high among children born at low birthweight, handicapped children, and children who are perceived as slow (McCormick 1985). Scrimshaw's cross-cultural review of infanticide includes child death of high parity children and those of close birth spacing, and suggests these as unconscious parental strategies for providing optimum survival opportunity for the strongest children in situations with no other form of effective fertility regulation (1984: 460).

Our own studies are demonstrating, in minute but consistent ways, that the commitment of a parent to an infant is expressed in multiple ways, but that for pre-term infants the issues of parental investment is especially complex. It includes such indicators as having sought prenatal and follow-up care for the infants, and parent involvement from the beginning in their child's hospital care (Newman 1983).

While a preterm birth is not easy for anyone, there is great variation in outcome, and in functional abilities for infants born at low birth weight that is not relatable only to ethnicity, socioeconomic status or marital status or to the social or biological factors that characterize those at risk for low birth-weight itself, but rather to adult commitment to the child. We have found, for example, that parent commitment as demonstrated by visiting in the hospital in the first few weeks of life is associated with an earlier and more consistent weight gain (Newman 1982). In our current study of vocalization, visiting is associated with more vocalization in week four by a factor of two (Newman, 1986). Many parents, however, perceiving a potentially dying child, begin a distancing process of coping, and do not participate in their infant's hospital care (Newman, 1980).

In the best of circumstances these early differences "wash out," and the infants are not distinguishable at later ages from their full term peers. In difficult circumstances, an extended loss of weight, delayed speech, a lack of follow-up for ameliorative care, and a demonstrated lack of parent commitment may increase the category of risk realized. In these cases a vulnerable child may not survive to reproductive age. This raises the question of a tension between "medical selection" and the realities of life at what Escalona has termed "double hazard." In this sense survival against odds may not correspond with fitness, and may only postpone death (Buehler et al. 1985).

In summary, neonatal intensive care is a product of scientific medicine's research orientation and aggressive intervention on behalf of human survival. While there is of course, expressed concern for longterm outcome, medical action is directed toward immediate survival, rather than long term wellness. The family system, often vulnerable and facing extremely difficult situations is left to cope with the long term. Certainly, some infants with potential risk fare well. Parents in the High Risk High Risk group, that is, those mothers with high pregnancy loss and children with developmental disabilities face the realized risk and all the suffering that entails.

More integration of intensive individual and epidemiological study is necessary before this configuration of factors can be conclusively demonstrated as causally related. They do, however, provide a continuing research direction, and an example of an evolutionary framework for the definition of fitness.

## NOTES

The research reported here has been supported by the Rhode Island Chapter of the March of Dimes, the Department of Pediatrics of Women and Infants Hospital, and Biomedical Research Support Grants from Brown University. Grateful acknowledgement for support and encouragement is made to Dr. William Oh, Pediatrician-in-Chief and to Dr. Richard Cowett, Director of the Special Care Nursery. For imaginative research assistance, I am indebted to Sarah Aronson, Gwyn Cattell, and Lise Johnson.

The term "High Risk High Risk Spiral" to describe the continuing dynamics of high risk mothers with high risk infants, was derived in conversation with Dr. Beatrix Hamburg, Adolescent Psychiatrist. It reflects her concern with the disadvantage, stressful environment and long term outcomes of both mother and infant in these circumstances.

## REFERENCES

Audy, J. Ralph
    1980 Man the Lonely Animal *in* The Anatomy of Loneliness edited by Joseph Hartog, J.Ralph Audy, and Yehudi A. Cohen. New York: International Universities Press.
Buehler, James W., Carol J.R. Hogue, and Susan M. Zaro
    1985 Postponing or Preventing Deaths? Trends in Infant Survival, Georgia, 1974 through 1981. JAMA 253 (24): 3564–3567.
Boone, Margaret S.
    1982 A Socio-medical study of infant mortality among disadvantaged Blacks, Human Organization 41 (3): 227–236.
Center for Disease Control
    1984 Morbidity and Mortality Weekly Report 33 (31, 32), CDC, Atlanta, Georgia.
Chisholm, James S.
    1983 Navajo Infancy. An Ethological Study of Child Development New York: Aldine.
Cohen, Yehudi A.
    1968 Man in Adaptation: the Biosocial Background.
Dobzhansky, Theodosius
    1968 Adaptedness and Fitness, pp. 109–118 *in* Population, Biology and Evolution edited by Richard C. Lewontin. Syracuse, New York: Syracuse University Press.
Garn, Stanley M., Helen A. Shaw, and Kinne D. McCabe
    1977 Effects of Socioeconomic status and race on weight–defined and gestational prematurity in the United States. *In* D.W. Reed and F.J. Stanley (eds.) The Epidemiology of Prematurity, pp. 127–143. Baltimore–Munich: Urban and Schwarzenberg.
Escalona, S.D.
    1982 Babies at Double Hazard: Early Development of Infants at Biologic Risk. Pediatrics 70: 670–676.
Hardy, J.M.B., J.S. Drage, and E.C. Jackson
    1979 The First Year of Life: The Collaborative Perinatal Study of the National Institute of Neorological and Communicative Disorders and Stroke. Baltimore: The Johns Hopkins University Press.
Hinde, Robert A. and Patrick Bateson
    1984 Discontinuities versus continuities in behavioral development and the neglect of process, International Journal of Behavioral Development, 7: 129–143.
Hunter, R.S., N. Kilstrom, E.N. Loda and F. Kraybill
    1978 Antecedents of child abuse and neglect in premature infants: a prospective study in a newborn intensive care unit. Pediatrics 61: 629–635.
Johnston, Francis E.
    1973 Microevolution of Human Populations. Englewood Cliffs, New Jersey: Prentice Hall.

Kagan, Jerome
1984 The Nature of the Child. New York: Basic Books.
Lerner, Richard M.
1984 On the Nature of Human Plasticity. Cambridge: Cambridge University Press.
McCormick, M.C., S. Shapiro, B. Starfield
1982 Factors Associated with Maternal Opinion of Infant Development Clues to the Vulnerable Child? Pediatrics 69: 537–543.
McCormick, M.C.
1985 The Conribution of Low Birthweight to Infant Mortality and Childhood Morbidity. New England Journal of Medicine 312 (2): 82–90.
Newman, L.F.
1980 Parents' Perceptions of Their Low Birth Weight Infants, Pediatrician 9: 182–190.
Newman, L.F.
1981 Social and Sensory Environment of Low Birth Weight Infants in a Special Care Nursery: An anthropological investigation. Journal of Nervous and Mental Disease 169 (7).
Newman, L.F.
1982 The Special Care Nursery: An Anthropological Study in Birth, Interaction and Attachment edited by M.H. Klaus and M.O. Robertson. Johnson and Johnson Baby Products Company.
Newman, L.F.
1982 Teenage Parents, Preterm Infants. Paper presented at International Congress of Adolescent Psychiatry and Psychology. Dublin, Ireland. July, 1982.
Newman, L.F.
1983 Preterm infants, their parents, and the neonatal intensive care nursery. In Gynecology and Obstetrics edited by J.J. Sciarra. Vol. 6, Chaper 80, pp. 1–6. Philadelphia: Harper and Row.
Newman, L.F.
1986 Premature Infant Behavior: An Ethological Study in a Special Care Nursery. Human Organization 45(4): 327–333.
Oyama, S.
1982 A reformulation of the idea of maturation. In Perspectives in Ethology, Vol. 5 Ontogeny, edited by P.P.G. Bateson and P.H. Klopfer. New York: Plenum.
Ramey, C.T., D.J. Stedman, A. Borders-Patterson, W. Mengel
1978 Predicting school failure from information available at birth. Am J Ment Defic 82: 525–34.
Rutter, M. (ed)
1983 Developmental Neuropsychiatry. New York, London: The Guilford Press.
Scrimshaw, Susan C.M.
1984 Infanticide in Human Populations: Societal and Individual Concerns in Infanticide edited by Glenn Hausfaber and Sarah Blaffer Hrdy. New York: Aldine.
Wise, Paul H., Milton Kotelchuck, Mark L. Wilson, and Mark Mills
1985 Racial and Socioeconomic Disparities in Childhood Mortality in Boston. New England Journal of Medicine, 313 (6): 360–366.
Zuckerman, Barry S., Deborah K. Walker, Deborah A. Frank, Cynthia Chase, and Beatrix Hamburg
1984 Adolescent Pregnancy: Biobehavioral Determinants of Outcome. Pediatrics 105: 857–863.

LIZABETH HAUSWALD

# EXTERNAL PRESSURE/INTERNAL CHANGE: CHILD NEGLECT ON THE NAVAJO RESERVATION

> Difficulties multiply during periods of rapid social and cultural change, for then the old customary relationships and ways of doing things no longer are appropriate and yet are not replaced . . . And everywhere under new conditions parents are unprepared how to care for their children and the old support system, the back-up system for poor parenting, has broken down. (Mead 1978)

## INTRODUCTION

On the Navajo Reservation today, family maladjustment is characterized by marital discord, weak support networks, breaks in affiliation and interaction between family members and kinsmen, alcohol abuse and child neglect. The existence of such families is not unique to the Navajo Reservation, but the context within which child abuse and neglect occurs is culturally specific.

The recent history of the Navajos is one in which language, religion, and childrearing practices have all been disrupted to a greater or lesser degree. The Navajo Reservation continues to be assaulted with economic, educational, religious, and social alternatives, many of them in direct conflict with traditional lifestyles and values. The maintenance of stable childrearing patterns in this rapidly changing and stressful social context is often impossible.

The external pressure of changes brought about through Anglo education and wage labor and the loss of the cultural heritage of religion and language has created internal pressure in families. As the primary socializing unit, the family must mediate between the old ways and the new, retaining enough of traditions to provide continuity between generations, to ensure enculturating children into meaningful adult roles and to prepare them for satisfying interpersonal relationships. When social pressure disrupts the internal workings of the family to an extent that creative adaptation is impossible, the psychological adjustment of individuals dependent on that family system is threatened. In problem families, successive generations of inconsistent and weak parenting lead to maladjustment in children and eventual neglect and abuse in childrearing.

This paper proposes that the patterns of child neglect and abuse seen on the Navajo Reservation today are the result of social pressures and economic change that have eroded the values and lifestyle necessary to sustain traditional Navajo childrearing. In the absence of social and moral support, and in the face of disparaged self-identity and unclear social roles, parents falter in

145

*Nancy Scheper-Hughes (ed.), Child Survival, 145–164.*
© *1987 by D. Reidel Publishing Company.*

the difficult task of caring for and socializing their children. The chapter starts with a social/historical overview of the disruptions that have affected Navajo families in the last 100 years. In abusive and neglectful families, the breakdown of traditional childrearing patterns often can be traced back two or more generations to social situations outside the family's control. The generational cycle of abuse and neglect is culturally unique in the ways in which the social and cultural environment impact on individual families. The incidence of abuse and neglect today, the attitudes that shape "characteristic" patterns, and how cultural ideals and norms constrain successful intervention will be discussed.

I collected data on childrearing and on child abuse and neglect during fieldwork in the Ft.Defiance and Chinle agencies of the Navajo Reservation between June 1981 and September 1984. Interviews on childrearing and family life were conducted with mothers in 110 normal and problem families in these two agencies, and with Navajos and Anglos employed in social welfare, nursing, the police department, community health, alcohol rehabilitation, legal and court positions, and other jobs related to child protective services in the Chinle agency. I focus on child neglect more than physical abuse because approximately 90% of the child protective services cases reported to this agency involve neglect, and because neglect is more likely to be misinterpreted, overlooked, or tacitly accepted than abuse [see Scheper-Hughes and Stein, this volume]. In 1985, when I returned briefly to the Reservation to conduct training workshops on assessment and early intervention for child abuse and neglect, I found a new growing awareness of, and concern with, sexual abuse.

### The Incidence of Child Neglect and Abuse Cases on the Navajo Reservation

The only statistical study to date on child abuse and neglect on the Navajo reservation was conducted in 1977 by Roger White. Unfortunately, the absence of accurate records in child protective services agencies makes the collection of statistics very difficult. By the author's own estimation, the data "suffered from incompatible and imprecise definition," in the reporting of cases within as well as between agencies (White 1977: 2). Most problematic is the inability to distinguish new cases (never before reported) from those children and their siblings previously identified as at-risk. White found a rate of 13.5 validated cases per year per 1000 children under the age of 9. With an estimated 40 000 children on the Reservation in the 0–8 year group, White's rate would mean that at least 540 children per year are at risk. In 1984 I found accurate statistics no easier to come by, but White's figures are somewhat lower than estimates I received in 1985 from the Navajo Tribe Division of Social Welfare (DSW). Four agency offices (Tuba City, Chinle, Ft.Defiance, and Eastern) gave average rates of two to three verified reports per week. The Shiprock agency has a rate of reporting almost twice as high, but whether this difference is due to more actual cases or to a greater willingness to report child maltreatment in this more acculturated area of the Reservation is unclear. This comes to a total of 12–18 cases per week, or roughly 600–900 cases per year. These statistics reflect the total number of verified incidences of abuse or neglect but may include more than one report for a given family.

The ratio of neglect to abuse in White's study of 370 cases was 6 : 1. Severe harm to the child was assessed in 25 percent of the neglect and 19.6 percent of the abuse cases. Twenty-three percent of the children were hospitalized and over 50 percent were placed in foster care. All agencies encountering suspected cases of child abuse or neglect are supposed to file a report with the DSW.

Social workers in the Chinle Agency, where I did my research, reported a very low incidence of physical abuse cases. One administrator stated that in 1982 her case load of 80 included only one physical abuse case. By 1985, about 10–15 percent of all reported cases involved physical or sexual abuse. Virtually all physical abuse cases are initially referred from the Indian Health Service hospital, while reports of neglect originate from many sources, including police, school personnel, alcohol rehabilitation counselors, and individuals. Previously most sexual abuse was reported by hospital personnel, however in 1985 the number of reports of sexual abuse coming directly from the community had increased dramatically. In 1985, the Chinle office reported that new sexual abuse reports were occurring at a rate of close to 1 per week, a 5–10 fold increase from the preceding year.

## THE SOCIAL AND HISTORICAL CONTEXT OF NAVAJO ABUSE AND NEGLECT

### Background: The Navajo Nation Today

The Navajo Nation occupies 25 000 square miles of high, semi-arid plateau land in Northeastern Arizona, Northwestern New Mexico, and Southern Utah. This is the largest reservation in the United States. The territory is expansive, but more than half is classified as desert and another 40 percent is steppe, semi-arid land used only for grazing. The average population density for rural areas is 6 persons per square mile. The traditional economy was based on herding and small scale agriculture. Residence was matrilocal, with extended families living in camps of clustered housing that were often separated by several miles from adjacent camps. Today, approximately one-third of the reservation population is clustered in agency-towns and near coal and uranium mines where employment is available (Goodman 1982). Most residences in these more densely populated areas are single family, neolocal houses.

Very few Navajos can live on the traditional economic resources of herding, weaving, and farming without some kind of supplemental cash income.

Only a minority of all adult Navajos have permits to raise sheep, and those families with herds usually do not have enough livestock to support a large extended family. Many families live well below poverty level, with an increasing income gap between those who have high-paying, full-time jobs with the federal or tribal governments or at the mines and those who eke out a living from the combined resources of family members, including social security, welfare, food stamps, part-time employment, weaving, jewelry making, and herding. Estimates of unemployment on the Reservation range from thirty to seventy percent. It is common for men to seek part-time or temporary employment away from home, but in rural areas it is likely that many men in an extended family will be unemployed at any given time (Navajo Times Newspaper 1982). In 1980, the Navajo tribe reported the average per capita income on the Reservation to be $2300, including federal and state income received from Aid to Families with Dependent Children, General Assistance, and Aid to the Disabled.

The Navajo population is young – in 1978 the median age was 16.4 years as compared with a median of 29 years for the United States' population as a whole. The fertility rate among Navajos is very high, with an average of 4.6 children per woman as compared to an average of 1.8 children per woman in the U.S. population as whole. Though neonatal mortality rates are similar to the overall U.S. rate, the Navajo post-neonatal rate is two and one-half times higher (Broudy and May 1983). The factors that contribute to a high mortality risk for Navajo children include environmental health problems related to sanitation and isolation from medical services. Most rural homes are without electricity and indoor plumbing, and many are dependent on hauled water. However, many children are at-risk for social rather than medical or environmental reasons. Lack of parental guidance, patterns of heavy drinking, and weak social roles for young adults all place young Navajos at risk for injury or death associated with alcohol use and abuse.

## Navajo Childrearing Traditions

The prototype for kinship and the strongest bond in Navajo society is the mother-child relationship. This close relationship embodies the ideal of all kinship relationships. In myths, the Navajo woman is depicted as protective and nurturing, strong and dependable. The presumption of continuity and reciprocity between family members is basic to the everyday life of Navajos who follow the traditional religious and kinship systems. To cut a child off from this is to cut his lifeline to security and to participation in the culture.

Navajo "camps", residential enclaves made up of a group of houses of related kinsmen, allowed for indulgent care of young children by aunts and grandmothers as well as by mother and father. Childrearing and socialization patterns were supported by economic, residential, kinship, and religious systems. One older male informant described traditional childrearing as follows:

The method of discipline is mainly by word of mouth and example reinforced by words of love . . . words that give the feeling of worth. Fear is sometimes used as an influence to control the child. An example being that 'so and so will cut off your ears.' Sometimes discipline is severe, but when the manner in how it is carried out is considered one cannot help but see it is out of concern and love that the child is disciplined.

This is a story told by a former councilman: 'I was told to get an axe and go down to the water pond, chop a hole in the ice and jump in. I did as I was told because my father had a horsewhip. After jumping into the water I got out and ran for the hogan. I thought I would turn into an icicle but I kept on running because my father was right behind me. Many mean thoughts went through my mind, and I felt that my father could not love me. When I opened the door I fell upon the sheep skin my father had spread near the fireplace. Then my father wrapped me in blankets, sat down beside me, put his hand upon my forehead and said, 'son, you may think I am just a mean old man to treat you like this. But I did it because I love you. I did it so you will be able to endure all kinds of hardships.'

Ideally, the parents' role was as teacher and protector. Discipline took place when it was necessary to strengthen or to protect rather than to punish the child. Children learned at a young age how to do simple household tasks, how to care for younger siblings, and how to herd sheep. Under the supervision of adults, age and sex appropriate tasks were frequently assigned to children, and idleness and laziness were scorned. Yet there was indulgence of the child, with attempts made to fulfill "childish" demands and a reluctance to say no to a strongly made request. Enforcement of discipline came in areas that were essential for safety and well-being, such as following religious taboos and learning self-discipline and endurance in physical tasks. The expectation that children should learn to endure hardship, as exemplified in the above example should not be confused with physical punishment used for disciplinary reasons. Many times I heard an elder informant make a statement like this:

You should not hit a child because the hitting is endless . . . 'You don't do this, my baby,' that is the way my father talked to me . . . This way my children were aware of the rights and wrongs at a very young age. If you hit them you can damage their thinking, their brains, and they won't listen to you.

In traditional families, "fostering" of children does take place. Usually the receiving adult will be the mother's mother or the mother's sister. In Navajo kinship, "mother" and "mother's sister" are both addressed as "shima", and mother's mother is "shimasani". The role of mother and grandmother is often the same; grandmothers in Navajo culture are ideal as mothers. Free from many constraints of heavy chores and tasks such as shopping, grandmothers are typically even more indulgent in their care of children than parents. Grandparents are most often the people who teach the children the traditional myths and who instill in them a sense of respect for and involvement with the traditional ways. It is not unusual for the mother to 'give' her first born child to her mother, particularly if her mother has no children remaining at home. The receiving parent in these cases becomes the mother and is addressed "shima" by the child (Shomaker 1984).

## THE IMPACT OF SOCIAL CHANGE

### Economics

Forced economic change, subsequent shifts in patterns of residence from extended nuclear to nuclear family households, boarding school education, and loss of the Navajo language and religion all threaten the integrity of the Navajo family. Changes in domestic group structure and in kinship interaction and ties weaken the strength of the family and make the socialization of children through teaching cultural values and history and by example of parental behavior more difficult.

Families in which child abuse and child neglect occur show the impact of one or more generations of disruption in family life. Historically, the sources of disruption are many, with some events impinging on particular families more than others. Forced reduction of livestock in the 1930s reduced by 50% the total number of sheep on the Reservation and dramatically changed the economic livelihood and social status of many families. Before the livestock cuts, most families were self sufficient, but following them, supplemental income from wage labor and/or welfare became essential for many. Since the thirties the Reservation economy has become increasingly dependent on wage labor. This has resulted in a shift to neolocal residence near employment centers on the Reservation and to an increase in periodic migration as well as some permanent relocation to urban areas beyond the Reservation (Callaway 1977; Chisholm 1981). Adult children are neither geographically as close nor economically as dependent on their parents as in the traditional economy. Although a great deal of visiting still takes place between most parents and their adult children, grandparents play a less central role in rearing and teaching their grandchildren than they did in previous generations.

### Education

The presence of classroom education has also affected change. The Navajo Treaty of 1868 which returned the Navajos to their native lands included a promise by the Navajos to educate the children, and one by General William T. Sherman to furnish a classroom and a teacher for every thirty children between the ages of six and sixteen. The dispersed population on the Reservation (an average of less than 5 people per square mile) made local schools a logistically difficult alternative. Furthermore, it was believed that children were better off away from the influence of their families. However, the experience of Navajos at boarding schools both on and off the Reservation has largely been negative. From the 1880s until after World War II it was generally assumed that a primary task of the boarding school was to purge the Indian child of his or her heritage and replace traditional language, religion and culture with that of White Americans. The task of educating Navajos was approached in a harsh and often brutal militaristic environment. Children worked four or more hours a day at manual labor, were marched to and from classrooms and dormitories, were severely punished for the use of the Navajo language, were required to adopt a Christian religion, and often were not free to visit home. The shock of being removed from the security and warmth of a loving family and being placed in an impersonal and alien environment would have been difficult at best. The added insults and punishment for being themselves, that is to say Navajo, made the adjustment to boarding school particularly negative and humiliating (Bergman 1967).

Boarding school placement still continues today, with children as young as 6 years old being sent away to school. Although these schools are less punitive than in the past, the adult to child ratio is approximately 1 to 50 after classroom hours. The individual attention and informal interaction commonplace in families is virtually unknown in these institutionalized environments. If the lessons learned in the traditional Navajo family are disrupted by residential change, they are virtually annihilated by boarding school placement. In this environment, the child may give up seeking attention and withdraw from adults, looking only to age peers for comfort and stimulation. Time spent at home may be inadequate to compensate for the months away. Summer is a time of much activity and travel for traditional Navajo families. Unlike the winter months during which group games and story telling take place, families are often divided between residences and sheep camps, and may travel frequently to help with and participate in squaw dances and other ceremonials.

The impact of boarding school on children is perhaps seen most clearly when they become parents themselves, for they have internalized a negative self-image and are insecure in their parental roles (Metcalf 1975). They have not had the experience of family life that would allow them to raise their children as their own parents were raised; they have not internalized patterns of kinship affiliation and religious belief that their parents took for granted. They may live a "traditional" lifestyle, but they do not teach the traditions to their children. Feeling that the Navajo Way is disadvantageous in the "modern" world, they do not teach the Navajo language or religion to their children and are at a loss as to how to teach or discipline their children; so, although they now have the alternative of using public day schools, they frequently send their own children to Bureau of Indian Affairs (BIA) boarding schools or Mormon Placement foster homes, a common pattern in neglectful and abusive families.

*Religion*

The traditional religion, taught as an integral part of everyday family life, prescribed appropriate behavior for both parent and child. Within the fabric of traditional family and religious life lay the implicit answers to essential questions such as "Who am I?" and "How should I relate to others?" Those aspects of childrearing that were previously most clear cut were prescribed and sanctioned in a particular ecological and religious environment. Child-rearing in a secular environment, without moral guidelines, creates problems of both a moral and interpersonal nature. Why are rules established, how should they be reinforced, when does a parent know better than the child? Present day parenting in unstable families is often indulgent without bound-aries, or strict without reason. In non-problem families, continuity in religious affiliation and childrearing values is maintained even when families "modern-ize", by joining the Native American Church or converting to Christian faiths, or working at wage labor jobs.

## The Generational Cycle of Child Abuse and Neglect

Strong reinforcement of kinship roles, social values, and family relationships provide a positive self-image and supportive social network for children. In problem families, social changes such as those mentioned above, have re-sulted in problems in childrearing that are exacerbated in successive genera-tions. Child abuse and neglect are the most extreme symptoms of failures in nurturance that can often be traced back two, three, or four generations to disruptions in traditional childrearing and socialization patterns.

The following illustration (Figure 1) of 'The Generational Cycle of Navajo Child Abuse and Neglect' depicts the multigenerational character of abuse and neglect. External pressure generated by social and cultural changes results in internal changes in the family. In problem families, these changes lead to family instability and to increasingly pathological parenting patterns. Alcohol is often blamed as the root cause of child abuse and neglect, but breakdown in cultural traditions associated with rapid change in family interaction and childrearing actually precede the use of alcohol in many neglectful families.

In the cycle of external pressure and change internal to the family, alcohol becomes a substitute for cohesive and satisfying kinship relationships that have been lost. The perpetuation of culturally and socially disruptive patterns such as decline in the use of the Navajo language, disrespect for the religious and cultural traditions, loss of work opportunity, degradation of fathers and fathers' roles, increase in neolocal residence, and forced relocation off of traditional land, all contribute to the continued weakening of the family as the primary socializing agent and exacerbate parents' problems in establishing values and setting boundaries for their children.

Families of abused and neglected children are characterized by high rates of unemployment, divorce and alcohol abuse. When the pattern of disruption and alienation goes back one or more generations, though the mother's

GENERATIONAL CYCLE OF ABUSE AND NEGLECT

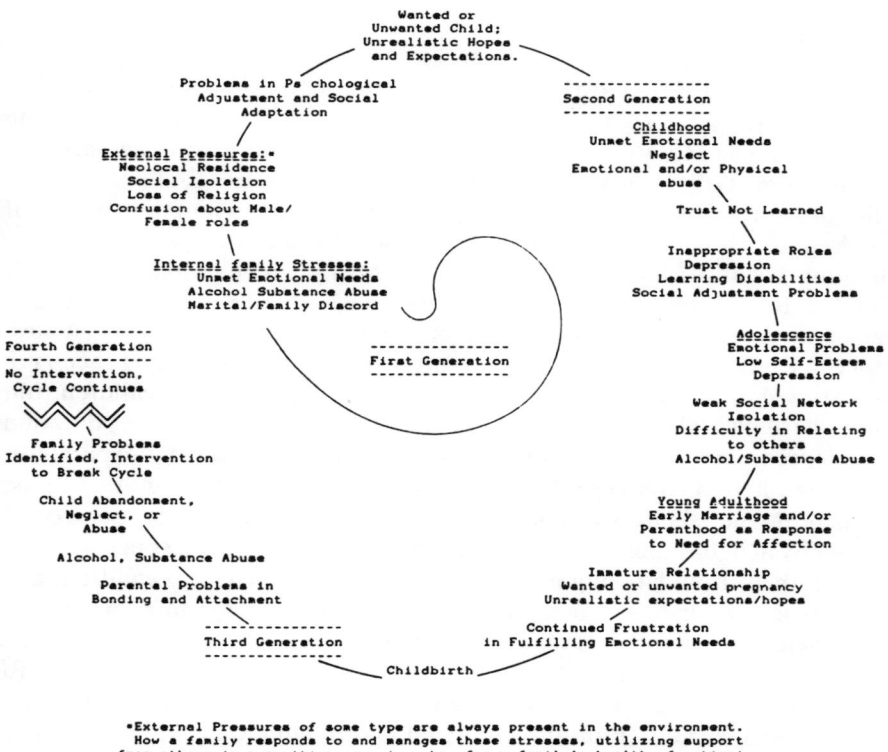

Fig. 1. Generational cycle of abuse and neglect

parents may be physically present, they are neither emotionally nor economically supportive of the young mother. Neglectful and abusive parents from an emotionally unstable family have a negative self-image and are frustrated by adult roles. When faced with emotional demands and responsibilities, they fail to respond to the needs of their children. Cultural childrearing norms are misinterpreted to provide an excuse for parental neglect and/or abuse of children.

## THE CULTURAL CONTEXT OF CHILD NEGLECT AND ABUSE

### Navajo Views of Neglect

Much traditional childrearing was characterized by passive strategies rather than by active interference in child's behavior. Ignoring a child or turning ones back on an activity communicates disapproval. There were few surprises or unknown dangers in the confines of the family camp. Children learned rules of interpersonal behavior and tasks by watching and imitating adults. If children were left, they were not totally alone, as some adult would be within shouting distance, and children could go to a relative's house for food. Children learned to cook, to do housework, to weave, to herd, etc. at a young age, and many other adulthood responsibilities were assumed in "adolescence." Tasks were learned gradually through experience. Herding sheep is a primary cultural example of the responsibility given to young children, but even "herding" takes different forms. The distance from the home, duration of time, presence of other children or adults, amount of previous experience, size of the herd all are considerations. For with herding, as with other tasks, the parent will balance the ability of the individual child against the need of the family in determining how much the child will do. Watching grazing sheep to keep them from straying is the task most often assigned to children, and this is much easier than moving the herd from one location to another.

Problems that occur in child rearing are the reverse of the positive virtues and prescriptions in the culture. In Navajo culture, proscriptions against adults directly saying "no" or forbidding certain behavior result in tolerance and respect for children on the one hand and in emotional withdrawal as a means of control on the other. A mother who is frustrated at her child's behavior will withdraw affection and attention as a means of communicating her displeasure. Taken in the extreme, this normative practice can turn into a failure to guide, teach, and care for the child.

Today as in the past, children are perceived as capable of responsibility, work, and decision-making at a young age. This cultural norm is reflected in the frequent use of siblings as caretakers and the inclusion of children in family decision making. However, in parenting today, rules must be established that pertain to the child outside the immediate control of the parent, either when the child is in school or when the parent is away from the geographically isolated nuclear family home.

The cultural traditions of sibling caretaking and of giving young children responsibilities is misinterpreted and misused by neglectful parents. In more benign cases, this may mean not adequately supervising activities in which a youngster may get injured or ignoring an infant's cries. Families who neglect their children often are reported by IHS physicians for failing to treat injuries and illnesses. In more serious circumstances, neglectful parents will leave infants and toddlers alone for several hours or will leave a preadolescent child alone for days without adequate food, clothing and heat, to care for several siblings.

Neglectful parents will sometimes try to excuse their behavior as being consistent with Navajo traditions of "trusting" their children. However, this "trust" becomes neglect when the actual capacity of the oldest child to care for the younger siblings is not assessed, and when the needs of the parent are the only consideration.

In my 1984 interviews with 30 Navajo mothers, no one condoned leaving young children alone for extended periods of time with siblings under 13 years of age, and leaving children alone overnight without adult supervision was not approved of. Yet in neglect cases, children as young as 5 years will be left for prolonged periods with younger siblings, and the parents will justify their behavior in terms of Navajo childrearing traditions.

Perhaps the most widespread problem is the young mother who forgets about her infant while she is away drinking. In these situations, the infant or young child will be found by police or reported abandoned in a pick-up truck, at a squaw dance, or in the home. Parents are most likely to "ditch" their children if they have weak kin networks. Even if a woman lives near her mother, their relationship may be poor if this is a family that has had problems for several generations.

In other neglectful families, children may be left with an unwilling or incapable grandmother. If the grandmother is either physically unfit to care for young children or emotionally disinterested, she may abuse or neglect the children herself. The cultural myth that grandmothers are the ideal mothers does not take into account multigenerational problems.

Children will be "abandoned" by their parents for days or weeks, and the relatives they are left with sometimes feel trapped and report the parents to the DSW. Typically these parents are shamed into taking custody of their children, with further neglect often being the consequence. In these situations, forcing the children on their unwilling parents is not a good solution. Alternatives include finding a stable home with family or clan relatives in which a foster placement can be made until the parents are stable, or considering adoption if the situation continues for more than a couple of years. However, the Navajo idealization of the mother-child relationship greatly inhibits such responses.

*Navajo Views of Physical Abuse*

The idea of harming a child through violence inflicted to the body is shunned in traditional teachings not only because of the danger to the child but because of the negative spiritual impact on the whole family. It is believed that if one hurts a human or an animal, it [the action] comes back to hurt the perpetrator. There are also repercussions in the relationship to the child, who becomes alienated so that when s/he leaves home s/he will often never return. If treated this way, children will not take care of their parents in their old age.

The general prohibition against hurting others does not inhibit violence between adults in Navajo society today. Heavy drinking is often associated with violence between men who are drinking together and between husbands and wives when they drink together or when a drunken husband returns home. However, even when violence occurs between spouses in the home, children generally are not physically accosted. Blatant physical abuse is neither excused nor overlooked when it is observed by someone in the extended family or by someone outside the family, but is seen as a danger to the child.

Yet, child abuse cases involving hitting or more severe whipping as corporeal punishment are ambiguous. As discussed earlier, traditional Navajo childrearing was strict and required children to perform physically difficult and sometimes unpleasant tasks to build stamina and courage and to protect children against vulnerability to physical hardship and other difficulties they might face later in life. Today Navajo parents who use corporeal punishment defend the practice as traditional, "strict", childrearing, taking the example of their parents or grandparents. However, this actually confounds strictness and control over the behavior of children with physical punishment, the latter a non-traditional approach. In the context of traditional teachings, self-control over the body and the emotions, and the maintenance of harmony between oneself and the natural and supernatural world are linked. Teaching a child to be self-disciplined is not equivalent to punishing a child who misbehaves.

A Navajo legend tells of a mother who severely punished her child. Finally the child ran away, and when she came looking for him, he hid under the ground, and became a prairie dog and never returned to his family. Though many traditional sanctions existed against assaulting children, some incidences of physical abuse invariably occurred against which the legend served as a warning.

In the past, boarding schools introduced many Navajos to corporeal punishment as an appropriate means of control over children. Many early boarding school programmes were run by ex-military men, and regulation and physical punishment for the transgression of rules were commonplace. Students attending these institutions were taught to disrespect the traditional teachings, were often away from home for ten months out of the year, ar  he primary models for adult-child relationships became those learned in boarding school.

Today, Navajos who use corporeal punishment are in the minority, but it is not uncommon. As with the mainstream culture, the reason for punishment and the manner in which punishment is administered is crucial in determining if the parent is abusing or disciplining the child. Social workers and judges who themselves come from a diversity of acculturated and bicultural backgrounds often have a difficult time evaluating the severity and intention of punishment in individual cases. Nonetheless, child battering cases are rare, and discussions as to the appropriate intervention in such cases are quite open.

Physical abuse tends to occur in two rather different contexts. The first is among older Navajos caring for their grandchildren. These grandparents attended boarding schools but subsequently returned to live "traditional" adult lives. They misinterpret the strict religious taboos and prescriptions of earlier generations regarding child behavior as equivalent to the harsh physical discipline they experienced in boarding school. These individuals do not utilize religious moral or behavioral guidelines in their childrearing, but depend on physical control more than instruction to keep children in line. Older grandparents in this situation often have difficulty taking care of their energetic grandchildren and some may resent that the parents are not doing this job themselves.

The second context is physical assault by young Navajo parents which seems to be very similar in character to other cases of child abuse found in the mainstream American culture. Though these parents face the economic stress of rural life, they are not embedded in either Navajo or Anglo social and cultural systems, and are emotionally alienated and socially isolated. They have little or no contact with traditional religion and ceremonial systems, they probably do not speak Navajo, and they may have been raised in an urban area of the reservation in an isolated nuclear family, out of contact with other relatives. Child abuse in these families is the product of the loss of culture and the loss of those positive reinforcements and negative sanctions that previously inhibited the incidence of abuse.

### Sexual Abuse

Sexual abuse is the most difficult pattern to typify for the Navajo. Though both hospital and social welfare professionals view sexual abuse as a grave problem, the number of reported cases is still relatively small, and an understanding of the circumstances in which these cases take place is poor. Misinterpretation of cultural traditions by contemporary perpetrators is common, often serving as a rationalization for sexual assault. For example, a Navajo girl who has had a 'kinaalda' puberty ceremony is, by traditional definition, a woman available for marriage. In traditional times, she would not be available as a sexual partner before marriage, but the current warping of her status as "a woman" sometimes serves as an excuse for sexual aggression by adult men. Secondly, traditional marriage patterns included preference for sister-in-law's sister, and step-daughters (as second wives). Assault against these girls is justified in terms of their appropriateness as sexual partners although, once again, the tradition was with respect to marriage, and not promiscuity with children. Again, in these situations, the cultural tradition becomes an excuse masking underlying psycho-social problems similar to those found in incestuous relationships in other cultures.

### INTERVENTION: PROBLEMS AND STRATEGIES

*Health and Social Services*

Starting in 1978 with the passage of the Indian Child Welfare Act (Public Law 95–608) the Navajo Tribe Division of Social Welfare (DSW) has been fully responsible for custody, placement, and litigation regarding child neglect and abuse cases on the Reservation. All suspected cases of child abuse and child neglect are referred to the DSW. The Navajo Tribe receives funds that previously supported the Bureau of Indian Affairs Social Services program and receives additional funds for community-based social services workers. Virtually all of the Tribal social workers are Navajos. They often have no training except that received on the job.

Official rules and regulations and funding decisions are made at the central DSW office in Window Rock, but day to day procedures are independently handled by each of the five agency offices. Child protective services is one of the duties of the Special Services Unit in each agency. In the Chinle agency this unit consists of 7 workers and a unit supervisor serving a population of approximately 25000. These workers are also responsible for the placement of juveniles in boarding schools or foster homes, and for the supervision of social welfare and social security funds for minors. The average caseload is 95 cases, about half of them related to child protective services. Being Navajo, the DSW social workers are familiar with the language and the culture of their clients, but most of them have little or no training in child abuse and neglect or in counseling. The cultural backgrounds of the Navajo social workers range from very traditional to very acculturated with respect to education, religion, and values orientation.

Child abuse and neglect cases that result in litigation are usually brought before the Navajo Tribal Courts. Felony cases cannot be tried under the jurisdiction of the Navajo Tribe, so there are limits as to the charges that can be made against the perpetrators in these cases. Felony charges associated with physical or sexual abuse must be investigated by the FBI and tried in federal courts. Incidences that take place off the Reservation in border towns such as Gallup and Farmington sometimes are under the jurisdiction of the

State (Arizona, New Mexico, or Utah) department of social welfare. However, under the Indian Child Welfare Act, the Navajo Tribe Division of Social Welfare must be involved in any case requiring the removal of children from the parental home for more than 3 days. Cooperation between Tribal and Federal agencies on the Reservation and Tribal and State agencies in border towns such as Gallup and Farmington varies from office to office, but cases that are not clearly in one jurisdiction or another often remain in limbo for extended periods of time.

The United States Government Department of Public Health provides free medical services to Native Americans through Indian Health Service (IHS) hospitals and clinics. The initial reporting of child abuse cases is often through IHS physicians who have seen the child in the emergency room or in pediatrics for treatment. IHS physicians are Anglos who are either career employees or recent graduates who have to do two years of service to pay back for medical school financial assistance. Some of the nurses and most of the auxiliary staff are Navajo. In contrast to DSW employees, hospital nurses and social workers are highly educated. Though some of the IHS staff are Navajo, they tend to agree with their Anglo colleagues in negatively assessing the Tribal social workers and judges.

Other individuals and agencies involved with Navajo families at risk for, or identified as, abusive or neglectful include Tribal alcohol rehabilitation counselors, Tribal community health workers, IHS field health nurses, public school counselors, Bureau of Indian Affairs (BIA) boarding school counselors, early childhood education and child care teachers, Tribal police, BIA police, Tribal court judges and probation officers, prosecutors for the Tribal court, IHS mental health services workers, IHS physicians and religious personnel (Christian church clergy, Native American Church roadmen, and traditional Navajo Way healers) who act as counselors or who perform traditional ceremonies to help troubled families. The official responsibility for cases lies with the DSW, but other agencies will report suspected cases and, sometimes, do investigate cases.

Each IHS hospital has a Child Advocacy Committee (CAC) composed of individuals from all of the agencies involved in the child protective services and from all of the hospital personnel who might be involved in a hospital case. Ideally this broad representation should allow for coordination and cooperation between agencies, but in reality misunderstandings and feelings of manipulation are more common than is positive communication.

### Problems in Intervention

Though a complex and seemingly thorough system of reporting and intervening in child abuse and neglect cases exists, effective action to either rehabilitate the family or to place a child permanently is rare. The reasons for this can only be explained by looking back at the cultural and historical backdrop of abuse and neglect.

In the initial reporting and investigation of a case, the DSW administrators often prefer to have the original reporting agency do a preliminary investigation because the DSW has neither the manpower nor the travel funds to visit every family suspected of abuse or neglect. However, once the Tribal police, BIA police or IHS conduct the investigation, further communication with the DSW is poor. The BIA and IHS are staffed by Anglos and by "modern" Navajos who see the DSW as unprofessional because its workers often lack formal training and because of a history of refusing to terminate Navajo parents' parental rights and to permanently place children in foster homes. There is distrust on both sides, the BIA and IHS assume that the DSW workers are incompetent and the DSW workers assume that there are cultural issues that are not adequately respected by BIA and IHS personnel. This failure in interagency communication exacerbates the problem however, because the DSW personnel are rendered helpless in intervention if they have inadequate data on the family.

The DSW social workers often show tremendous resistence in child neglect cases with respect to acknowledging the potential seriousness of the situation. The mother-child relationship tends to be idealized as does the belief in kinship interdependency throughout the life cycle. When a mother claims that she loves her children and will reform and take care of them, she will generally be given the benefit of the doubt by DSW workers, whether it is the first or the twentieth time she has made such a claim.

The following case exemplifies some of the symptoms exhibited by neglectful families. Both the mother and father were heavy drinkers. They were recently divorced with wife battering implicated in the separation. The four children, 2, 4, 7, and 10 years of age were in the mother's custody. The father was employed but did not pay child support and claimed he had no responsibility for the children. Relatives reported that the children were frequently left alone when the mother went out to drink. Though the mother's sister was willing to take the children, the mother would not voluntarily give them to her.

During one five month period, the mother was reported twice by the family for leaving the children alone for extended periods of time, the mother was arrested for drunk driving with the children in the vehicle, IHS reported the family for medical neglect when the ten year old took herself to the hospital following a 3 week bout with strep throat, and the public school reported that the school-aged children were underfed.

Each report was treated as a discreet incident. The children who were left alone were placed in temporary custody until the mother was located, the mother was informed that she should provide medical care, the mother was told about a free breakfast program for the children, and family finances and the lack of financial support by the father were seen as the focus of the families problems. In this case, alcohol rehabilitation was not mandated; when it is, a child may be placed with relatives for 1–2 months while the mother dries out, but he/she will be returned to the mother as soon as she returns from the rehabilitation program.

The family is not viewed from a systems perspective. In this family, the willingness of the father to abandon his children, the unwillingness of the mother to trust her sister with the care of the children, repeated incidences of nutritional and medical neglect in addition to abandonment, all indicate underlying and chronic bonding and attachment problems that are not simply symptoms of binge drinking.

One dimension of the failure to see deviant patterns or to treat the long-term problem of raising healthy children is the kind of cultural myopia discussed here. Excuses are found for the mother's actions, and the mother convinces the social worker that she will reform, or that this was an atypical incident due to circumstances beyond her control, or that her husband is to blame because he is not paying child support. The Navajo social worker wants to believe that the mother is a victim of circumstance and that she will be a good mother if only. . . . To remove the children and place them in long-term or permanent foster care is to blame the victim. There is a fear that long term placement will only contribute to the further dissolution of the family, and there is no assessment of the potential benefit to the child of being placed in a secure and stable environment. The handling of this case is typical of neglect cases that are carried in the active DSW case files for five, ten, and fifteen years without resolution. This problem represents the reverse side of the one discussed by Hughes (this volume); both analyses concern different dimensions of cultural misunderstanding.

The pattern that is emerging in cases of sexual abuse is similar. There is a tendency to excuse the perpetrator's actions as due to a cultural "misunderstanding" as described above, or to accept the defense that the victim had given her consent. There is much more uneasiness about sexual abuse than there is about neglect, but there is still tremendous reluctance to removing a child from the parent's home. If the perpetrator can be convinced to leave voluntarily, every one is greatly relieved, but people are slow to press criminal charges. When criminal charges are made, the BIA must conduct its own investigation because all felony cases are handled in federal rather than tribal courts. In these cases, coordination between agencies is often inadequate.

The children most likely to be placed in foster care institutions and non-related families are those who have been physically abused. Though there is some cultural debate about the appropriateness of physical punishment, severe abuse is recognized as life-threatening and quick action is taken. However, according to IHS physicians who report abuse to the DSW and who testify in court hearings if the child is to be removed from the home, the DSW rarely presses for termination of parental rights, but will eventually return the child to the home if there is any indication that the situation has improved. There are cases in which a mother voluntarily places her children in a long-term foster care arrangement with relatives, but in my two years experience with the DSW, only when a mother had abandoned her children for many months were parental rights legally terminated. Among both social workers and judges there is recognition of these problems in the abstract, but continued inaction in actual cases.

More successful intervention strategies must take into account the organizational and cultural problems in the present child protective services system.

## CONCLUSION

In approaching Navajo social workers, judges, prosecutors, counselors, and administrators, it is essential to be knowledgeable about and openly discuss cultural ideals, cultural myths, and social realities, and to establish a view of the family as a system that is impinged upon by external forces. The strong inclination to blame alcohol rather than to see a deviant pattern in interaction between family members is largely due to the belief that the individuals are not to blame if alcohol "made them do it." If viewed in social/historical context, families can be perceived as troubled and as being in need of help, while individuals can still be freed from direct blame and guilt.

The patterns of disruption associated with rapid social change which have been discussed above are culturally specific in detail. However, the existence of family disruption and childrearing problems following situations of rapid acculturation and industrialization are found in other third and fourth world cultures.

As Margaret Mead (1978) stated, child abuse and neglect cases reflect the fact that under new social conditions, parents are often confused about how to care for their children, while the traditional back-up system for poor parenting has broken down, leaving many children at risk. In periods of rapid social change, some families experience negative change inside the family as a result of loss of cultural values, norms, and safeguards. The increasing severity of symptoms can be seen across several generations of Navajos, with child abuse and neglect being extreme symptoms of family disruption.

The experience of rapid social change does not in itself mean a family will have problems. Rather, the presence of child abuse and child neglect reflect the rather extreme effects of family disruption in the face of rapid cultural change. In well adapted Navajo families, whether culturally traditional, bicultural, or acculturated, *continuity* in kinship and social values (whether traditional or new) can provide individuals with the skills and support necessary to confront the social pressures and economic stresses they must face in adulthood. Positive self-image, a strong family network, and defined values and beliefs about personal roles and social meaning are all essential for constructive and innovative parenting in traditional, bicultural or acculturated family contexts (Hauswald 1984).

Intervention strategies that have a chance of success must incorporate a knowledge of the roots of disturbance and a realistic assessment of the capacities of the individuals intervening in such cases. Early detection of family problems and assistance in establishing social supports through kinship or religious networks, and an emphasis on the needs of children in both counselling families and in training social workers would change greatly the current emphasis on the needs of the "victim" mother. It is necessary to limit the onus of blame while making parents responsible for making changes that will provide for adequate child rearing.

The passing on of child neglect and abuse from one generation to the next severely threatens the structure of the Navajo family and community. This is often the consequence when DSW cases are put indefinitely on hold and no intervention is made on the behalf of children. The present increase in abuse and neglect statistics may reflect such a pattern, as many of the young parents now mistreating their children were themselves the products of unstable or neglectful families.

## ACKNOWLEDGEMENTS

Preparation for this chapter was supported by a research grant (90–PD–86505) from the Administration for Children, Youth and Families, Department of Health and Human Services through the Diné Center for Human Development, Navajo Community College and by a fellowship from the National Institute on Alcohol Abuse and Alcoholism (5–T32–AA0724–07) through the Alcohol Research Group, School of Public Health, University of California, Berkeley.

## REFERENCES

Aberle, David
  1966 The Peyote Religion Among the Navajo. Chicago: Aldine Press.
Bergman, Robert
  1967 'Boarding School and the Psychological Problems of Indian Children.' unpub. report to the Committee on Indian Health of the American Academy of Pediatrics.
Broudy, D.W. and P.A. May
  1983 'Demographic and Epidemiologic Transition Among the Navajo Indians.' Social Biology 30(1): 1–16.
Callaway, Don
  1977 'The Impact of Industrialization on Navajo Household Organization.' unpublished manuscript.
Chisholm, James
  1981 'Social and Economic Change Among the Navajo: Residence Patterns and the Pickup Truck.' Journal of Anthropological Research 37: 148–57.
Goodman, James
  1982 The Navajo Atlas. Norman: The University of Oklahoma Press.
Harvey, Elinor
  1983 'The Abused, the Abuser, the Helper; a Proposal for Understanding the Needs of All Three.' in Hauswald, L. and Fifield, B. (eds.), Early Intervention and Mediation in

Child Abuse and Neglect Among the Navajos. Tsaile, Arizona: Dine Center for Human Development.

Hauswald, Lizabeth
  1984 The Navajo Way: Continuity and Discontinuity in Contemporary Society. Doctoral Dissertation, Department of Anthropology, University of California, Berkeley.

Kluckhohn, Clyde and Dorothea Leighton
  1946 The Navajo. Cambridge: Harvard University Press.

Korbin, Jill
  1981 Child Abuse and Child Neglect: Cross-Cultural Perspectives. Berkeley: University of California Press.

Kunitz, Stephen
  1973 'Demographic Change Among the Hopi and Navajo Indians.' Lake Powell Research Project Bulletin No. 2.

Lamphere, Louise
  1977 To Run After Them. Tucson: University of Arizona Press.

Leighton, Dorothea and Clyde Kluckhohn
  1947 Children of the People. Cambridge: Harvard University Press.

Levy, Jerrold
  1964 'The Fate of Navajo Twins.' American Anthropologist 66: 883–6.

Levy, Jerrold and Stephen Kunitz
  1971 'Indian Reservations, Anomie, and Social Pathologies.' Southwestern Journal of Anthropology 27: 97–128.

Mead, Margaret
  1978 'Child Abuse.' Presented at the National Conference on Child Abuse and Neglect, Statler Hilton Hotel, New York, New York. April 16–19.

Metcalf, Ann
  1975 'The Effects of Boarding School on Navajo Self-Image and Maternal Behavior.' Doctoral Dissertation, Stanford University.
  1976 'From Schoolgirl to Mother.' Social Problems 23: 535–544.

Shomaker, Dianne
  1984 Fosterage as a Form of Exchange Among the Navajo. Doctoral Dissertation, Department of Anthropology, University of New Mexico.

Topper, Martin
  1985 'Navajo "Alcoholism": Drinking, Alcohol Abuse, and Treatment in a Changing Cultural Environment.' in Bennett, L. and Ames, G. (eds.), The American Experience with Alcohol: Contrasting Cultural Perspectives. New York: Plenum Press.

Topper, Martin and Jackie Curtis
  1984 'Extended Family Therapy: A Clinical Approach to the Treatment of Synergistic Bipolar Anomic Depression among Navajo Agency Town Adolescents.' unpublished manuscript, Navajo Area Indian Health Service, Window Rock, Ariz.

Werner, Elizabeth Emmy
  1979 Cross-Cultural Child Development: A View from the Planet Earth. Monterey, California: Brooks/Cole Publishing.

White, Roger
  1977 'Navajo Child Abuse and Child Neglect Study.' Presented before the Epidemiology Section, American Public Health Association Annual Meeting, Washington, D.C.

Witherspoon, Gary
  1975 Navajo Kinship and Marriage. Chicago: University of Chicago Press.

# CRY BABIES, CULTURE, AND CATASTROPHE: INFANT TEMPERAMENT AMONG THE MASAI

Cross-cultural studies have shown that diversity in the basic characteristics of infant development, cognitive style, and behavior are related to variations in ethnicity and child-rearing practices (Whiting and Child 1953; Geber 1958; Horton 1962; LeVine 1974; Burton and Kirk 1976; de Vries and de Vries 1977; Werner 1979; Super and Harkness 1982). The impact of infant care practices and ecological factors on infant mortality has also been documented, but the infant's own contribution to morbidity and mortality has been more difficult to study (Dickeman 1975; Werner 1979).

In spite of the increasing research interest since the 1970's on the infant's active participation in its own development, most research has been justifiably focused on the impact of the adult world on the infant (Lewis and Rosenblum 1974; Thomas and Chess 1977, 1980). Catastrophic perturbations of the normal flow of life can momentarily lift above the surface of every day social life the contribution made by individual infants to their own morbidity or health. Human reactions to catastrophic events have classically highlighted the broad range of adaptive and maladaptive responses possible from individuals under stress (Lindemann 1944; Bettelheim 1960; Williams and Parkes 1975). The sub-Saharan drought of 1973–74, which added flooding rains at the drought's end to the already damaged grazing lands, provided such an unfortunate "natural experiment". It highlighted the infant's contribution to his or her own development and survival as well as the role that customary child-rearing practices play. Although the devastation was not on the scale of the famine in Ethiopia and Sudan in 1984–85, the drought disrupted pastoral and hunter gatherer life-styles on both sides of the African continent and resulted in mass deaths (Sheets and Morris 1974). Since cycles of drought, famine, and plenty are a recurrent feature in the environments of nomadic and pastoral peoples, observations of the drought's impact on Masai life provided an opportunity to speculate about the interaction of infant characteristics and development, cultural rearing strategies, the physical environment, and infant survival (see Galaty, Aronson, and Salyman, 1981).

The chief orientation of our study was to examine the interaction of the infant's environment with its developmental outcome, in particular the relationship of infant experiences and traits of temperament (de Vries and Sameroff 1984; Thomas and Chess 1977). Thirty years of cross-cultural studies in child development have richly described the various properties of the infant's niche and its relationship to development. For instance, rearing interactions may take place in large polymatric kin networks as well as in isolated monomatric nuclear families (Liederman 1978; Gatere 1980). Available technology and the use of space differ. The caretakers' work requirements, daily routines,

165

Nancy Scheper-Hughes (ed.), Child Survival, 165–185.
© 1987 by D. Reidel Publishing Company.

and social roles as well as their personal qualities, needs, and attitudes differ and affect the quality of caretaker attention (J. Whiting 1977; Sameroff and Chandler 1975; Super and Harkness 1982).

In addition to these more concrete aspects of the environment, the organizational and conceptual framework provided by custom also influences development. It is now axiomatic that cultures bring regularity and stability to the ontogenic process. From birth, the individual's proper passage through the life cycle is a paramount concern of society. The neonate is immediately enmeshed in a net of expectations which strongly shape its rudimentary cognitive and motor capacities. By reinforcing specific infant behaviors and promoting certain relationships over others, each culture, whether its methods are indulgent or severe, controls the learning environment and shapes infant development.

A culture thus enscribes its unique signature on the tasks of infant care. Feeding, ensuring sleep, the socialization of affect, motor and social skills, elimination training, body contact, and monitoring for protection are shaped by a culture's particular folk psychology about children (LeVine 1981). Other cross-cultural studies have suggested that many seemingly biological properties such as temporal patterning of behavior and developmental sequence are, in fact, culturally programmed (J. Whiting and Child 1953; de Vries and de Vries 1977; Super and Harkness 1982). This implies that development follows a peculiarly cultural course based as much on the group's notions of "what a baby is" and how he or she "should" develop as on maturational forces (de Vries and de Vries 1977).

In the first part of this chapter, aspects of the Masai infants' niche are described. Ecological, social organizational and infant rearing factors are related to temperament and health outcomes. The ethnographic material in the second part of the article has been chosen to provide a general picture of Masai life and to underscore aspects of particular relevance to the developmental outcomes of infants. These data were gathered during fieldwork over the period 1973 to 1975 in the Kajiado subsection of Masailand south of Nairobi, where I visited eighteen homesteads: ten in traditional pastoral settings away from Western influence, four adjacent to Amboseli Game Reserve; and four in a relatively modernized, atypical area near Namanga and Bisil. The latter areas represented the new agrarian pattern of domestic life for the Masai. In one modernized and three traditional homesteads I closely observed Masai life over a six-month period. The research in Kajiado was facilitated by the part-time use of a mobile health clinic of the Kajiado Hospital (Van Montfrans 1974). In this clinical setting I worked as a doctor and did not carry out research. The ethnographic, maternal, and pregnancy experiences and specific infant and family data were gathered through spot observation, detailed child rearing interviews adapted from Ainsworth (1967), and other demographic and psychometric instruments that had been tested in Kenyan communities (B. Whiting, J. Whiting and Grawe 1971; J. Whiting

1977). Infants were further assessed with an adapted infant temperament scale (Carey 1973) as well as by a physical examination and anthropometric measurements.

## THE MASAI

The Masai are pastoral, Nilo-Hamitic people who have inhabited the plateau steppe extending from central Kenya south into Tanzania since the fifteenth century (Merkerer 1910; Hollis 1905). They are primarily subsistence herders, whose life is intimately linked with the savanna ecosystem in which they compete for resources with large mammalian herbivores such as elephants, buffalo, and zebras (Western 1973). Most of their activities center on cattle and the search for suitable grazing land. Their settlements of mud and wattle huts are opportunistically placed near available water and grazing land. In 1974, in spite of fifty years of colonial contact and medical service, little modernization had taken place among the Masai of Kajiado District, Kenya, except for a few atypical agrarian social groupings near towns and game reserves.

The population then numbered about 110 000, of whom an estimated 15% are non-Masai. Historically, the Masai have been very warlike, dominating East Africa and excluding slavery from their sphere of influence. In 1974, their warlike propensities had been reduced. Masai values, however, remain deeply entrenched among the warriors. They are the custodians of tribal glory and security and as such are very much an elite group. But today, they are often "rebels without a cause". The Pax Britannica put an end to their raids on the neighboring Bantu, and the Game Department has reduced the opportunity for courageous exploits against lions. Young warriors today, are torn between the choice of school and the modern world, and the free life on the Rift Valley plateau.

Physically, the Masai are a strikingly handsome people. The warrior is "tall, elegant, handsome and walks with a gentle spring of the heel, seemingly proud and indifferent to all but the most necessary external influences" (Sankan 1971). His hair is braided, pigtailed, and dyed with ocher. He carries a spear and is often clothed in a red sheet fastened at each shoulder; he usually is accompanied by a male companion of about his own age. Older Masai retain the sheet and spear but shear their ornamental hair and often add a blanket for warmth, particularly with advancing age. The women, valued by their men for grace and facial beauty, achieve status primarily by the bearing of children. Shrouded in red fabric and often with a leather apron or postnatal belt around their waists, they are richly bedecked with beaded jewelery. Their shaved heads are set off by large necklaces and earrings that accent the eyes and face. Children, who are generally alert and lively, dress alike till age four or six, when with formal naming they assume the dress of their sex. Gait, posture, and subtle jewelery are sexually dimorphic, and although similarly dressed, small Masai boys and girls are easily distinguished at a distance. The piercing of the ears and other scarifications begin at approximately two years and occur again with formal naming.

Masai *social life* revolves around age-sets. For males, age-sets are divided into junior and senior sections and include warrior, elder, and retired elder groupings. The elder group forms the governing council of a kin defined subsection, which guides community organization. A highly democratic group that is seemingly inefficient and non-progressive by design, this gerontocracy governs the patrilineal descent system and age-grade system of the Masai (Spencer 1968). Most social relationships are, however, guided by shared rules, and the elders' council administers justice and levies fines only when disputes arise or rules have been breached.

Traditionally, the Masai diet consisted of milk, with meat at intervals depending upon the state of the herds. In addition, blood drawn from the necks of cattle was taken as a tonic, infant food, or special items of diet. Under conditions of severe drought, when herds were down to an irreducible minimum, blood constituted "survival rations". Vegetable foods were histori- cally considered hardly fit for human consumption, and this cultural prohibi- tion still tends to hold for warriors. Wild animal meat also has had a taboo classification. For all Masai, recently there has been widespread adoption of cornmeal into the diet, bought during periods of drought with the skins of dead animals. Canned vegetable fat, and rice, sugar, and tea are also bought during more prosperous periods.

The Masai live in a variety of social configurations. The most common living unit is a man, his two or three wives, and their children. Variations on this family grouping have evolved over a century of shifts between famine and plenty, often resulting in groups of two to five brothers or friends living together in a homestead. Houses are highly stereotyped, long, oval wicker structures, about 5 feet high and 12 to 18 feet long, thoroughly plastered with cow dung. There are no windows, and entry is by a narrow, light-trapping passage. The furniture consists of two beds composed of a cowhide over a low platform of branches, and stools generally arranged around a three-stone fireplace. The houses line the inner perimeter of a thorn fence, which has one gate for each head of a household.

In addition to the domestic homestead there exist *warrior villages*. Most districts have one warrior village to which all the warriors of that area belong. Outwardly the warriors' village, or *manyatta*, is distinguishable from other homesteads in that it often lacks a containing fence and at ritual or graduation periods a large main warrior house may be constructed at its center. A village is inhabited continuously during ritual periods related to age-grade gradua- tions by fifty to a hundred warriors and sometimes by as many as double that number of young girls and adult women and by a number of warrior younger brothers, who along with the women maintain the houses and tend the cattle.

Due to the shifting nature of grass and water supplies the Masai have been *nomadic*, ready to move according to ecological imperatives. Although a few Masai have taken up farming with the advent of some permanent water supplies, they have no jural or exclusive property rights to land and have shown little tendency to settle down in one area. Nomadism seems a deeply rooted trait which does not easily give way to the scientific range management programs of the last thirty years of Kenyan development. The Masai move their domestic homesteads roughly every six months according to the availability of grass and water. The movements of their cattle follow a definite ecological pattern, of which one feature is the successive occupancy of grazing land with other herbivores such as elephants, buffalo, and zebras. These patterns are, however, disrupted during periods of drought.

Less than a third of Masai homesteads are occupied at any one time, and therefore houses are constantly available for relocation. There is also a direct correlation between the number of Masai settlements and the number of cattle that the land is able to support. Thus, the spacing of settlements follows a pattern of accessibility to both water and grassland (Western 1973). Brown (1977) estimates that 30 to 35 head of cattle, mostly cows with two or three bulls, are required to maintain a pastoral family, or five cattle per person. A reduction in herd number, as occurs in almost any climactic or manmade environmental perturbation, be it drought, rain, gamepreserves, ranches, or overgrazing, presents a direct threat to Masai viability. The delicate ecological balance is further illustrated in this century of shifts between productive periods, 1920–30s and 1960s, and famine and drought periods in the 1940–60s and 1970s. During the period of this study, a 70% reduction of herds had occured in the Kajiado area.

Droughts, social change, and catastrophy are nothing new to pastoral populations. Their livelihood is indeed based on the constant adaptive search for resources and adequate grazing land. Galaty (1981), Jacobs (1980), and Bernstein (1980) all underscore the social arrangements within Masai culture, such as the indigenous social security system that provides breeding stock to kin who have lost their herds, as well as arrangements made with other societies which serve as a safety net for its population. Intermarriage and informal alliances have been created over the years with neighboring societies in order to provide a refuge for Masai women and children during periods of famine, epidemic, or drought. For example, the famines of 1890, 1961, and 1974 were particularly devastating and led to mass migrations into the highland territories of other tribes made safer by these social arrangements.

Since 1970, the rapid social change experienced in Kenya and the environmental stress created by meager rainfull have not been kind to the Masai way of life. The Masai have been beset by drought, famine, agricultural encroachment, and the bear hug of government intervention (Galaty 1981). The advent of ranching techniques and the increasing economic importance of farming have increased self-doubt among the Masai. An entire century of contact with traders and the market system, German and British occupations, and today the press of other rapidly modernizing Kenyan groups, as well as the pull of modern education, is propelling the Masai into the world of modern Africa.

## PREGNANCY, CHILDBIRTH AND MIDWIFERY

The typical Masai woman has approximately six pregnancies in her life-time (Merkerer 1910). As soon as a woman knows that she is pregnant, she and her husband separate until the new baby is weaned at about one and a half to two years after its birth. Officially, neither the husband nor any other man may have intercourse with the wife during this time, but a new pregnancy generally brings the period of suckling to an end. Pregnant women attempt to become as emaciated as possible in order that the birth may proceed more easily. During the last 3 or 4 months of pregnancy the woman abandons her normal diet and exists on a near starvation diet, consisting primarily of a broth of lungs, liver, and kidneys cooked with a bitter bark. The last month, she drinks only milk.

The first birth, if the mother lives near a medical clinic, may take place in a clinic, but this was not often the case in 1974 (Van Montfrans 1974). Generally, the woman is confined in her house, which may only be entered by women or girls, while a midwife provides assistance. Midwifery is in the hands of old women, who practice as professionals and have a surprisingly sophisticated knowledge of anatomy. The midwife makes several prenatal visits to the pregnant woman during the last month of her pregnancy and determines by palpation, the position of the fetus. If the fetus is lying transversely or feet downward, she may try to alter its position by massage. The midwife is sent for as soon as the first contractions begin. The labor position may vary between squatting, sitting, or lying, with resting "on all fours" being the commonly preferred position. If labor does not proceed satisfactorily, walking, massage, or holding the woman upside down is thought to help. During labor other women in attendance may sing supportively in shrill, plaintive cries for divine assistance. A mixture consisting of liquid sheep's fat and a brew of roots is used to reduce labor pains. Very little interference in the birth process is practiced, but episiotomies are often performed. In order to hasten the expelling of the placenta, a laboring women's palate is tickled with a feather to help with contractions. The placenta, which is not an object of particular import, is discared of buried by the midwife.

The infant's umbilical cord is bound round close to the body with a thread of fibrous ox sinew and then severed an inch or so from the body. The newborn infant is then rubbed with liquid sheep fat, a treatment said to be less for cleansing than to strengthen and invigorate the newborn. The infant is then laid on a soft hide, also rubbed with fat, beside its mother. It is given its first bath the following day, in a lukewarm infusion of twigs and stalks, to which is attributed a protective function against illness. The infant is not clothed.

It is said that in the past every newborn boy was submitted to a trial of divine judgment, in order to find out whether by chance his begetter may have been a man belonging to another subsection's kin-group. In the evening, when the cattle came home, the child was laid in one of the entrances to the homestead, so that the whole herd passed over him as they entered. If, in this process, the baby was killed, or so badly injured that he died, he is thought to have been a bastard child (Merkerer 1910). No such ritual was reported in 1974.

The new mother may leave the house as soon as her condition allows, very often on the day following the birth. She is then treated with a series of medications meant to revitalize her organs and maintain good breast milk. She is further required to wear an 8-inch-wide leather belt to help support the organs of her lower abdomen. Until she has fully recovered her health after her confinement, she smears her forehead daily with white clay when she leaves the immediate surroundings of her hut or village. Until the baby can walk, the husband may not partake of any food in the hut in which his wife was delivered, and for the first ten days after her delivery he may not even enter it. He also may not touch the infant the day after he has had sexual intercourse with one of his other wives. If the child's mother dies before it is weaned, another wife suckles it, thereby making it a blood relation of her own children. Foster children are thus held to be related by consanguinity.

In 1910, Merkerer described the great joy and pride at the birth of twins, especially if both were boys. The mother often kept only one of the twins herself, while the other was nursed by one of her husband's other wives or given to a barren relative. The treatment of and perspective on twins is directly related to the social and physical environment. Today, after the encroachments on Masai grazing land mentioned above, I noticed a marked prejudice against twins. Masai mothers selected the stronger male twin for nurturance, giving up the other, male or female, for adoption to a barren relative or occasionally letting it die of neglect, as might be done with twin girls. In other groups such as the Bantu Digo (de Vries and de Vries 1977), the opposite is true. Historically, the Digo considered twins bad luck and neglect as well as infanticide took place. With the advent of Islam, wage labor, and increased prosperity, multiple births and certain congenital malformations are now considered good luck. Among the Digo today, the incidence of multiple births, especially in families of high economic status, is high. This suggests that within a few generations changes in orientation toward offspring can move parallel with economic and resource factors.

In addition to twins in 1974, a Masai newborn was lethally neglected if it was very sick or if it was the illegitimate offspring of an old and sick man. Infanticides such as these at times of environmental stress may be viewed as adaptive, nonpathological maternal strategies (de Vries 1987), a not uncommon practice reported in reviews of the cross-cultural literature (J. Whiting 1977; Dickeman 1975).

## CHILD REARING

Infants, particularly males, are highly valued by the Masai. Mothers are attentive to infant needs and maintain close physical proximity. The baby's first week is spent inside the dark, smoky hut. Gradually the baby is introduced to the outside world, at first carried in the mother's arms and later tied to her back during her daily routine. A nursing mother spends most of her day with her infant, and fewer tasks are expected of her. Young female children relatives and other wives help with child care. The Masai report that the baby learns to get along with everyone in the homestead; since most of the inhabitants are relatives, responsibility for child care is shared. An inconsolable baby is often passed to different women in the area for help. Not much is made of elimination training or motor training, nor do the Masai view their infants as particularly vulnerable or ready to learn when compared to practices in other societies (de Vries and Sameroff 1984).

At one month infant massage, a process of "straightening the mucles of the limbs", begins. A period of body massage together with a fat rub takes place daily for many months. A child will also be placed with his feet in the morning dew to invigorate it and help straighten and strengthen the legs.

The infant sleeps with the mother, and sleep times are not scheduled. The Masai, however, feel that sleep must be controlled; the infant is not to sleep too long. The child must also not sleep on one side in preference to the other for more than a few hours, since this will deform it or cause an uncoordinated growth of the child's musculature. The infant is therefore repeatedly turned during sleep.

Masai neonatal feeding practices are unique. The infant's first food is generally 2 or 3 tablespoons of cream or fat followed by suckling. If the infant does not suckle immediately, butter fat and cow's milk are substituted and may remain as the infant's diet. During the first eight months of life or until the child walks, it is fed approximately a cup of fat a day; after beginning to walk, the child is given a cup every three weeks. Typically, the Masai baby is fed on demand, with the mother offering the breast whenever the infant cries or frets. Since the mother or other lactating female offers the breast only after infant cues, the infant soon becomes responsible for signaling for milk, thus underlining the importance of infant activity and behavioral style in demand feeding.

Weaning usually occurs at the time of a subsequent maternal pregnancy, when the child is approximately two years old. A child is weaned by removing it from its mother to a neighboring hut, or by the mother making her breasts unattractive to it by smearing her nipples with bitter plant juices. A premature drying up the mother's milk is explained by her physicial constitution. A woman tries to restore the secretion of milk by taking a liberal amount of liquid sheep's fat. In the interval the child is fed on cow's milk. As soon as a child is weaned, he is left by himself or with friends inside the homestead the entire day.

In this strong partrilineal society with its admiration for warriors, aggression, and assertiveness in young boys is encouraged. A child is never beaten before it is two years old, and even after that age beatings are rare and never severe. If it is ever necessary to correct a child physically, only its mother may gently spank the child on the bottom.

Naming is extremely complex, especially for boys, who in their lifetime may acquire five or more names that refer to different relationships and life-stages. Perhaps oddly in a strong patriarchal society the boy's mother selects the first name at about the time the first incisors appear. The first name is generally based on a fortunate event that occurred during her pregnancy or the first months of the infant's life or on a physical characteristic, and may be derived interactively as relatives sit around and discuss the infant and the mother. Before that he is usually refered to as *enkerai*, or baby. The day that the name is given is usually celebrated with a feast during which both the child's and the mother's heads are shaved for the first time since her confinement. The hair is placed under the mother's bed, as is the case with all ceremonial hair shavings. At this time, the baby also receives its first ornaments, generally a beaded necklace. Soon after, the father gives the baby a second name, which only he may use. When the child is able "to run", generally about ages 4 to 6, he is given his principal name by the elders of his mother's section. A fourth name may be earned through deeds carried out as a warrior. This name is heralded around Masailand by the ongoing tales of adventure told by wandering warriors as they visit homesteads. A Masai man's last name is acquired after he marries, when he is usually referred to as the father of his eldest child.

Naming has more than just ceremonial importance. For example, in the few deaths I observed, I noticed a difference in maternal reaction between those mothers who lost their infants before naming and those who did so afterwards. The mothers of the unnamed infants tended to show attenuated grief reactions and in conversation acted unexpectedly nonchalant ($N = 3$, including one premature). But the death of a named infant ($N = 2$) seemed to legitimize a grief reaction of massive proportions including screaming, chaotically running about, and self-mutilation that required restraint by other women. One mother, whom I knew relatively well, remained quite detached and calm following the death of a premature infant. The following day she was observed doing normal tasks and in her interaction with others and myself showed little sadness or reactive depression. It is of course difficult to interpret such behavior. Undoubtedly, the Masai stoical attitude to death, marked by avoidance of mentioning the deceased, plays a role. We cannot tell whether these cultural expressions of grief are congruent with the mothers' actual feelings, which perhaps remained undisclosed in these settings. It does suggest the important role of culture in organizing the relationship between mother and neonate and perhaps the psychologically protective function of late naming. Naming gives an infant status as a person. In societies where infant mortality is a regular and common occurrence, late naming may help individual mothers manage their grief reactions. Such a delay in naming may also allow the volitional destruction of offspring at times of scarcity without incurring psychological distress or kin wrath (de Vries 1987; Scheper-Hughes this volume).

## MASAI HEALTH RISKS

Compared with other East African tribes, the Masai are a fairly healthy people. Thanks to their life of isolation, communicable diseases seldom build up to epidemic proportions. The main disease problems are those of respiration, tuberculosis, pneumonia, trauma, venereal and intestinal diseases, and eye ailments. Dental and mental health are good, and birth complications rare. Masai life-style does have endemic conditions created by lack of water and close habitation between animals and man. Manure and fat-anointed bodies attract an enormous fly population, particularly to dranining eyes and nostrils. Eye problems are particularly severe and account for a 40% corneal scoring rate and a 10% monocular blindness rate among the elderly (Vogel *et al.* 1974). Eye diseases due to laceration, wind-blown, volcanic dust, and staphylococcal or trachoma infections are therefore a great threat to Masai well-being.

Infant health risks are many. The Masai habitat is rife with dung and flies, and the incidence of tuberculosis, trachoma, and parasitic disease is high in infants (Vogel *et al.* 1974). Measles, with its complications, is endemic and makes a major contribution to infant mortality during the first year (Morley, Martin and Allen 1967). Protein caloric malnutrition is a major source of infant mortality in Kenya, and the Masai are no exception, as 60% to 70% of their infants are undernourished annually (Blankhart *et al.* 1974). For comparison, Kenya's infant mortality rate is 120 deaths per 1000 live births in the first year, a rather low rate considering that normative infant mortality in developing countries with poor resources ranges from 150 to 200 per 1000 (Vogel *et al.* 1974; Werner 1979). Masai infant mortality was calculated in 1910 under unspecified ecological conditions as exceeding 300 per 1000 (Merkerer 1910). Inclusive of neonatal deaths, 40% of the children died before reaching circumcision age. It is, of course, difficult to report accurately on life history and epidemiological statistics in a nomadic population for which census data are poor, but the baseline Masai infant mortality rate probably falls between the present general Kenyan rate and the 1910 figure.

### 1974

In 1974 the ten year drought that ravaged Masailand was at its height. Throughout Africa the previous year had been a particularly dry one. The Kajiado Masai economy had been virtually devastated, and some families had lost as much as 98% of their herds. Cattle loss is particularly damaging to human infants, since pregnant cows and their suckling calves starve first, impoverishing the milk supply for almost a year until the surviving cows give birth and begin to lactate again. Although there are no precise records, district health workers reported that infant mortality soared under these conditions (Van Montfrans 1974). Massive starvation was avoided through missionary famine relief and by the survival oriented communalism of the Masai, which allowed those in areas receiving sporadic rains to contribute cattle or goats to the vanquished.

Many aspects of social life were, however, disrupted. Family residence patterns shifted as the group searched further for new grazing land. Migration to new areas and contact with unfamiliar kin taxed the traditional polymatric support networks of the homestead and often left mothers isolated in their infant care. The social disruption resulting from severe environmental stress interfered with intergenerational relationships, nurturant activities toward dependents, and social reciprocity among group members, as has been documented among other pastoral groups (Turnbull 1972; Spencer 1968) and uprooted populations (Zwingmann 1978). The Kajiado Masai, then, experienced devastating upheavals in both nutritional and interpersonal aspects of their life style during the drought.

## TEMPERAMENT AND RISK

Infant temperament was first conceptualized as a primarily constitutional characteristic (Thomas et al. 1963). Subsequent models in the West have stressed the complex transactions that shape individual differences in infancy (Brazelton, 1973; Sameroff and Chandler 1975; Thomas and Chess 1980) and credit both genetic (Freedman 1974) and sociocultural (Werner 1979) contributions. These studies have demonstrated the functional significance of infant temperament to development (Thomas and Chess 1977, 1980). Among the subgroups defined in these studies were "difficult" infants – who were less adaptable, more irregular, and more intense and showed greater negative reactions – and "easy" infants – who tended to be more adaptable, more regular, less intense, quieter, and more easily managed. The easy infants had uneventful developmental histories, while the difficult infants had a significantly higher incidence of behavioral problems, possibly because they caused stress in the Western-style family system, leading to "vicious circle" parent-child interactions (Chamberlin 1965; Thomas and Chess 1980). Styles of temperament have also been related to the potential for physical abuse: the incidence of traumatic injury and pediatric illness and longer-term health consequences and, recently, to weight gain in infancy (Kemp et al. 1962; Carey 1972, 1985; Betz 1982). Over the last few years, cross-cultural studies have also demonstrated the significant contributions of individual traits to infant well being and the course of development (Hsu et al. 1981; de Vries and Sameroff 1984; de Vries 1984; Super and Harkness 1982).

In the light of these findings and a suggestion by Geber (1958) that infant traits played a role in the incidence of kwashiorkor in Africa, I postulated that the difficult infant would stress the already compromised Masai mother and family group as the drought worsened and thereby place the infant at particular risk for behavioral and health problems. To test this hypothesis, I selected subgroups of the easiest and the most difficult from a sample of 48 Masai infants and planned to observe them again 3 to 4 months after my initial evaluation of their temperament.

### CLASSIFICATION OF INFANT TEMPERAMENT

Temperament refers to the infant's behavioral disposition. It is the outward manifestation of internal events related to arousal, vigilance, the generation of affect, social bonding, and mobility. Measurement of temperament characteristics traditionally includes an infant's adaptability, activity, mood, temporal patterning, persistence and distractibility of behavior, intensity and threshold of response to stimuli, and mode of managing novel situations.

The proven functional significance of temperament to development (Thomas and Chess 1977) and the availability of the Infant Temperament Questionnaire (Carey 1973), a standardized research instrument initially designed for use in clinical pediatrics, made temperament a natural choice for this study. The use of parental reports such as the temperament questionnaire in assessing infant characteristics, however, introduces some methodological problems (Bates 1982; Sameroff, Seifer and Elias 1982), so it is important that the criteria for establishing reliability and validity in the Masai sample be discussed.

I modified the Infant Temperament Questionnaire after conducting pilot child-rearing interviews and consulting with anthropologists familiar with the Masai (Kirk and Burton 1976). The modified English version was translated into Masai and then back into English by two different translators to compare the accuracy of the translation with the original version. No major differences were found between the original and translated questionnaires. To check the validity of the translation, an item-by-item review was carried out with four families, which demonstrated satisfactory replication of the Western meanings of the questions.

The temperament questionnaire had been standardized in a Western setting and required mothers to describe infant behaviors in common social situations. A number of questions needed to be modified so that they made sense in the context of Masai child care practices while remaining true to the specific behavioral description. The questions about patterns of feeding, sleep, and reactions to illness, play, people, and general sensory stimuli were straightforward and required little alteration. More culturally based questions, such as those about doctor visits, methods of diapering, and methods of dressing and bathing, required modification. For example, questions about doctor visits were changed to requests for descriptions of infant interactions with individuals who had similar roles and access to the infant; the role of the doctor was changed to that of traditional healer, specific ritual leader, or clinic personnel. Infant reactions to soiling, bathing, and dressing were understood, but some items needed to be changed to cultural analogues of these rearing manipulations, such as being carried on the back and being massaged with animal fat. These changes were kept to a minimum to ensure comparability.

Since the mothers were not literates the questionnaire had to be given as an interview. In addition to myself with a translator, the interviewers were a Masai mother who spoke English and a Masai medical student. They were trained in interview techniques, temperament issues, and research methodology in addition to being well versed in the customs of their culture.

## CLASSIFICATION OF DIFFICULT AND EASY INFANTS

Forty-eight 4 to 5-month-old Masai infants (23 males and 25 females) were evaluated with the Infant Temperament Questionnaire. The 70-item multiple-choice questionnaire was scored on a scale of 0 to 2, yielding nine temperament dimensions. High scores indicated the more negative or poor behavior (difficult), and low scores the more positive, or easy behavior. The mean scores listed in Table I are compared with American white and black samples.

TABLE I

Mean temperament scores and standard deviation for Masai infants with comparison scores for black and white Americans

| Temperament | Masai | American[a] White | American[b] Black |
|---|---|---|---|
| N/SD | 48/SD | 200/SD | 70/SD† |
| Activity | 1.01 ± .37 | .52 ± .32* | .55* |
| Rhythmicity | .86 ± .67 | .53 ± .46 | .92 |
| Adaptability | .63 ± .36 | .35 ± .26* | .62 |
| Approach/Withdrawal | .59 ± .47 | .48 ± .35 | .75 |
| Threshold | 1.15 ± .43 | 1.08 ± .39 | 1.35 |
| Intensity | .92 ± .33 | 1.05 ± .32 | 1.04 |
| Mood | .74 ± .32 | .40 ± .25* | .60 |
| Distractibility | .78 ± .40 | .57 ± .32 | .65 |
| Persistence | 1.22 ± .44 | .69 ± .38* | .78* |

[a] From Carey (1972)
[b] From Sameroff et al. (1982)
* significantly different from Masai, p < .05
† Standard deviations not available for American black sample
– Indicates "difficult"/"easy" dimensions

The Masai, black, and white differences are not meant to indicate that temperament is a racial trait, since the diversity of African and American black populations as well as the influence of testing and environmental factors do not warrant such a conclusion. The three-group comparison does depict the variation often found in mean temperament scores across cultures. Although this variation could lead to concern about temperament data, the validity of the scores increases when within-sample comparisons are made and is further strengthened when the extreme difficult and easy ends of the temperament spectrum are used (Sameroff, Seifer and Elias 1982), as was done in this study.

These factors dovetailed with the realities of fieldwork, which rendered the follow-up of all 48 infants unfeasible for medical, financial, and logistical reasons. Instead, two groups, composed of the 10 easiest and the 10 most difficult infants were selected. The criteria for placement in the two subgroups were as follows: of the nine temperament measurements, five items – rhythmicity, adaptability, approach/withdrawal, intensity, and mood – were associated with the definition of difficult or easy. The difficult infants scored highest and the easiest infants scored lowest, in comparison with the total sample of Masai infants, on the five items. By convention (Carey 1973; Thomas and Chess, 1977) infants were assigned to the difficult group if they had scores above the mean on four or five of the items, with one score greater than one standard deviation above the mean, or if they had two or three scores above the mean and two or three of these scores were at least one standard deviation above the mean. The group of 10 easy infants had three or more scores on the five items below the mean, with no scores more than one standard deviation above the mean. The difficult group contained five boys and five girls and the easy group, six boys and four girls.

Chosen in this manner, the difficult and easy groups differed significantly on four of the five items according to the Mann – Whitney $U$ test, one-tailed: adaptability, $U = 2$, $P = 0.001$; approach/withdrawal. $U = 0$, $P = 0.001$; intensity, $U = 7$, $P = 0.01$; and mood, $U = 4$, $P = 0.001$. They did not differ on rhythmicity, $U = 24$, n.s. These results statistically confirmed the descriptive assessment that the two groups were behaviorally distinct.

## FOLLOW-UP STUDY

Near the end of 1974, the infants we had studied were 6 to 8 months old, the drought had worsened, food stores had been depleted, grazing land had diminished, and the migrations in search of better grazing land, with their inherent social upheaval, had begun. Under these circumstances, it was difficult to find the Masai families we had selected for follow-up. By searching former habitats and areas of possible migration, we were able to locate the families of seven of the easy and six of the difficult infants (13 of the 20). At this time, further psychometric tests and an exploration into family adjustment to infant characteristics had been planned, but only mortality outcomes will be reported here.

## RESULTS AND DISCUSSION

On follow-up, a tragic and unexpected picture emerged: of the 13 infants whose families we could find, seven had died. Although high infant mortality rates are common among pastoral and hunter-gatherer peoples (Howell, 1979) and a doubling of these mortality rates during the first year of life may be expected at times of nutritional compromise (Lechtig et al. 1975), the greater than 50% mortality in this subsample was unexpected. Furthermore, although it had been hypothesized that the difficult infants would be at greater risk, five of the seven easy infants had died but only one of the six difficult infants.

The association of difficult and easy temperaments with mortality approaches statistical significance on the Fisher exact test ($P = 0.07$), a highly suggestive finding considering the small sample and the extreme nature of the outcome variable, death. Under the conditions of this study, the adaptive advantage of easy infants that had been found in Western studies had been reversed; the easy, not the difficult, infants seemed ill-suited to the harsh Masai environment.

Although a larger sample size would be required to argue convincingly for the generalizability of these findings as well as to definitively rule out other possible influences, a number of factors known to affect mortality and morbidity were investigated to determine whether the difficult infants differed from the easy infants, or the survivors from the nonsurvivors, on measures other than temperament (United Nations 1971; Sameroff and Chandler 1975).

Did the difficult and easy groups differ? No significant demographic differences or variations in maternal attitude or in level of family modernization were found between the difficult and easy infant groups. During the initial temperament evaluation, problems that the mothers experienced during pregnancy and poor family histories did correlate with the more difficult infants' temperament scores ($r = 0.29$ and $r = 0.36$, respectively, $p < 0.05$). However, these increased risk factors for the difficult infants, while interesting, cannot explain the higher mortality of the easy infants. The difficult infants in the original sample of 48 were also larger (a factor derived from weight, height, and head circumference adjusted for age) than the easy infants ($r = 0.43$, $p < 0.05$). This size disparity lends one to speculate about the interplay of Masai feeding practices, since illness histories did not differentiate the two groups (de Vries and Sameroff 1984; de Vries 1984).

Did the survivors differ from the nonsurvivors? The infant's sex, its age at testing, whether it was a wanted child, whether it was troublesome, its birth order, the age of the mother, her assessment of her milk supply, and the type of family all failed to differentiate the survivors from the nonsurvivors. The mortality histories of older siblings also ruled out the possibility of lethal idiosyncracies in rearing style in the afflicted families. Moreover, the health histories of the infants when they were seen at 4 or 5 months of age did not distinguish the two groups.

Did the located differ from the nonlocated subjects? It is unlikely that the high attrition in the number of families available for follow-up accounts for the results, since no discernible differences (on demographic, environmental, or health variables) were found between the located and nonlocated groups during the first interview session. It must also be noted that the severe ecological stress and social upheaval may have affected the entire sample, as indicated in the mean temperament profile of the Masai infants (Table I). As a group, Masai infants were significantly less active and persistent – traits often associated with malnourishment (Geber 1958; Werner, 1979) – than their better nourished American black and white counterparts.

What, then, contributed to the differential mortality rate? A closer look at the interaction between Masai infant care practices and the nutritionally marginal environment is helpful. Masai and Western child-rearing contexts differ in a number of ways. First of all, in this nomadic group with its admired warrior class, aggression and assertiveness in infants and children are encouraged and expected, not inhibited. Second, the Masai family is not an isolated nuclear unit but a large kin-based living arrangement in which a number of caretakers interact with the infant. In the West, difficult infants, who are more fussy and inflexible, protest more loudly, and require more attention, create family stress and negative parental reactions (Sarett 1975). In the Masai setting, however, it may be argued that difficult infants do not exact the same physical or psychological price from caretakers. Furthermore, the easy, more manageable Masai infant contrasts with the Masai cultural ideal and expectation of assertiveness and boldness, perhaps leading to negative rearing interactions, much as the withdrawn infant in middle-class America, where social adaptability is highly valued, causes familial stress (Thomas and Chess 1980). We may thus postulate that both cultural attitudes and rearing style affect difficult and easy infants differently.

Masai infant feeding practices point to one explanation for these results. The function of infant fussiness in eliciting and competing for maternal attention has been noted (Emde, Gaensbauer and Harmon 1976). In Masai demand breastfeeding, suckling frequently depends on infant activity and cues to the mother, who responds to virtually all cries and fussiness by offering the breast or food. I frequently observed this behavior, and it has been described quantitatively by others in hunter-gatherer populations (Konner and Worthman 1980). Consequently, the difficult, more fussy infant acts as a greater stimulus in the demand feeding situation, thereby spending more time suckling. The "squeaky wheel" hypothesis is supported by the correlation of difficult temperament measures with greater infant size in the entire sample and replicated by the recent finding by Carey (1985) that difficult infants in an American sample also gained weight more rapidly.

The easy infant, on the other hand, is generally quieter and more manageable, and the opposite feeding circumstances may be postulated. Easy Masai infants may provide an attenuated feeding stimulus, thereby getting less milk or food. The problem is exacerbated in a nutritionally deprived mother whose milk supply is already diminished, resulting in inadequate milk production. During the drought, supplementary feedings with dry skim milk mixed with water were added, introducing the enteric health problems that have been associated with bottle feeding in developing countries (Plank and Milanesi 1973). The easy infant may then have been at risk for undernourishment, disease, and perhaps even relative neglect.

This example suggests that the difficult infant may be a problem under normal Masai or Western circumstances, but at times of marginal nutrition the difficult infant may be the one that is fed more because it cries and fusses more. Temperament traits may thus contribute to differential feeding success in the Masai environment and thereby play a role in survival. The unexpected mortality rates underscore the context-dependent nature of developmental outcomes and the mediating influence of infant care practices. These findings may also be interpreted as a possible mechanism for the selection of behavioral traits, thereby contributing to the evolution of biological and even cultural diversity (Plomin, DeFries and Loehlin 1977).

Hypothetically, of course, a factor not examined in the study may have contributed to the result or the mechanism may be slightly different. The endogeneous social security system of the Masai may also serve as a strong intermediary variable in the survival of difficult children. For example, it may be that it is the difficult infant dyad or mother, not the infant per se, that signals the social-kin system for help. It may be that the dyad squeaks and "gets the grease", not the infant. Instead of postulating a mechanism that leads to the infant getting more food directly from the mother, we can postulate a mechanism in which difficulty leads to depletion of maternal resources, which in turn acts as the stimulus to the social system for garnering aid, which then indirectly influences how much the baby is fed.

Since the results and the mechanism that I offer are derived from a mix of quantitative and qualitative field observations of a small number of infants in an exotic setting, I shall reiterate the limitations of the study in closing. The major limitation is that the small sample size does not allow firm etiological conclusions to be drawn. Common problems inherent in cross-cultural research (Brislin, Lonner and Thorndike 1973; Naroll and Cohen 1970), such as the reliability of instrument translation cannot be fully ruled out as influencing the findings. Although much was done to minimize the impact of these factors and produce reliable and valid data, a cautious and modest interpretation of the results remains necessary.

REFERENCES

Ainsworth, M.
    1967 Infancy in Uganda. Baltimore, Md.: Johns Hopkins Press.
Bates, J.E.
    1982 The Concept of Difficult Temperament. Merrill-Palmer Quarterly 4: 299–319.
Bernstein, J.
    1980 The Enemy Is Us. History in Africa, 7: 1–21.
Bettelheim. B.
    1960 The Informed Heart. New York: Free Press.
Betz, B.J.
    1982 Rorschach Characteristics of Individuals of Alpha, Beta, and Gamma Temperament
        Types. American Journal of Social Psychiatry 2(1): 34–40.
Blankhart, P.M. et al.
    1974 Human Nutrition, In: Health and Disease in Kenya. L.C. Vogel et al. (Eds.), Nairobi,
        Kenya: East African Literature Bureau.
Brazelton, T.B.
    1973 Neonatal Behavioral Assessment Scale. Clinics in Developmental Medicine, No. 50.
        Philadelphia: JB Lippincott.
Brislin, R.W., Lonner, W.J., Thorndike, R.M.
    1973 Cross-Cultural Research Methods. New York, John Wiley & Sons.
Brown, L.H.
    1977 The Ecology of Man and Domestic Livestock. Rangeland Management and Ecology in
        East Africa, In: D.J. Pratt and G. Wynne (eds.), Huntington, N.Y., Krieger.
Burton, M., and L. Kirk
    1976 Meaning and Context: A study of Contextual Shifts in Meaning of Masai Personality
        Descriptions. Stirling Award Paper, presented to the American Anthropology Associa-
        tion, Washington, D.C.
Carey, W.B.
    1972 Clinical Application of Infant Temperament Measurements. Journal of Pediatrics 81:
        823–828.
    1973 Measurement of Infant Temperament in Pediatric Practice. In Individual Differences in
        Children. J.C. Westman (ed.), New York: John Wiley.
    1985 Temperament and Increased Weight Gain in Infants. Developmental and Behavioral
        Pediatrics 6(3), 128–131.
Chamberlin, R.
    1965 Approaches to Child Rearing. Clinical Pediatrics (Philadelphia) 4: 150.
de Vries, M.W.
    1984 Temperament and Infant Mortality Among the Masai of East Africa. American Journal
        of Psychiatry 141: 10.
    1987 Alternatives to Mother-Infant Attachment. Studies in Comparative Human Develop-
        ment, Vol. 1. In C. Super and S. Harkness, Eds. New York, Academic Press: in press.
de Vries, M.W. and M.R. de Vries
    1977 Cultural Relativity of Toilet Training Readiness. Pediatrics 60: 170–179.
de Vries, M. and A.J. Sameroff
    1984 Culture and Temperament: Influences on Infant Temperament in Three East African
        Cultures. American Journal of Orthopsychiatry 54: 83–96.
Dickeman, M.
    1975 Infanticide and Demographic Consequences. Annual Review of Ecology and Systema-
        tics 6: 107–137.
Emde, R., T. Gaensbauer and R. Harmon
    1976 Emotional Expression in Infancy: A Biobehavioral Study. Psychological Issues Vol. 10.
        No. 37.

Freedman, D.
1974 Human Infancy: An Evolutionary Perspective. Hillsdale, N.J. Lawrence Earlbaun..
Galaty, J.G.
1981 Masai Pastoral Ideology and Change. *In* Studies in Third World Societies. P. Salyman (ed.), Contemporary Nomadic and Pastoral People. Willamsburg, Va.:.
Galaty, J.G., D. Aronson, and P. Salyman
1981 The Future of Pastoralist Peoples. Ottawa, Canada. International Development Resource Center.
Gatere, S.
1980 Feeding Problems in Children in High Socio-Economic African Families in Nairobi. *In* The Future of Mental Health Services. A. Kieu, W. Muya, and N. Sartorius (eds.), Amsterdam, Excerpta Medica.
Geber, M.
1958 The Psychomotor Development of African Children in the First Year and the Influence of Maternal Behavior. Journal of Social Psychology 47: 185–195.
Hollis, A.C.
1905 The Masai: Their Language and Folklore. London: Oxford University Press.
Horton, R.
1962 The Kalahari World View: An Outline and Interpretation. Africa 32: 197–220.
Howell, N.
1979 Demography of the Dobe !Kung. New York, Academic Press.
Hsu, C–C., W.–T. Soong, J.W. Stigler et al.
1981 The Temperamental Characteristics of Chinese Babies. Child Development 52: 1337–1340.
Kemp, C.H., F.W. Silverman, B.F. Steele et al.
1962 The Battered Child Syndrome. American Journal of Medicine 181: 17–24.
Kirk, L. and M. Burton
1976 Age Estimation of Children in the Field: A Follow-up Study with Attention to Sex Differences. Journal of Cross-Cultural Psychology 7: 315–324.
Konner, M., and C. Worthman
1980 Nursing Frequency, Gonadal Function, and Birth Spacing Among !Kung Hunter-Gatherers. Science 207: 788–789.
Lechtig, A. et al.
1975 Effect of Food Supplementation During Pregnancy on Birth Weight. Pediatrics 56: 508–520.
LeVine, R.
1974 Parental Goals: A Cross-Cultural View. Teachers College Record 76: 226–239.
1981 Anthropology and child development. Paper presented to the Society for Research in Child Development, Boston.
Lewis, I.M., and L.A. Rosenblum
1974 The Effect of the Infant on Its Caregiver. New York: John Wiley.
Liederman, P.H.
1978 The Critical Period Hypothesis Revisited. *In* Early Development Hazards: Predictors and Precautions, F.O. Horowitz, ed. Western University Press.
Lindemann, E.
1944 Symptomatology and Management of Acute Grief. American Journal of Psychiatry 101: 141–148.
Merkerer, N.
1910 Die Masai (translated monograph). Nairobi, Kenya: University of Nairobi (First published Berlin).
Van Montfrans, G.A.
1974 Kajiado District Hospital Annual Report. Kajiado, Kenya: District Hospital.
Morley, D.C., W.J. Marten and I. Allen
1967 Measles in East and Central Africa. East African Medical Journal 44: 497.

Naroll, R., and R. Cohen (eds.)
    1970 A Handbook of Method in Cultural Anthropology. New York, Natural History Press.
Plank, S.J., and M.L. Milanesi
    1973 Infant Feeding and Infant Mortality in Rural Chile. WHO Bulletin 78: 203–210 Geneva:
         World Health Organization.
Plomin, R., J.C. DeFries and J.C. Loehlin
    1977 Genotype-Environment Interaction and Correlation in the Analysis of Human Behav-
         ior. Psychological Bulletin, 84: 309–322.
Sameroff, A.J., and M.J. Chandler
    1974 Reproductive Risks and the Continuum of Caretaking Casualty. In Review of Child
         Development Research, vol 4. S. Scarr-Salapater and G. Siegel (eds.), Chicago:
         University of Chicago Press.
Sameroff, A.J., R. Seifer and P.K. Elias
    1982 Sociocultural Variability in Infant Temperament Ratings. Child Development 53:
         164–173.
Sankan, S.S.
    1971 The Masai: Nairobi. East African Literature Bureau.
Sarett, P.T.
    1975 A Study of the Interactive Effect of Infant Temperament and Maternal Attachment.
         New Brunswick, NJ. Rutgers University, doctoral dissertation.
Sheets, H., and R. Morris
    1974 Disaster in the Desert: Failure of International Relief in the West African Drought.
         Washington, D.C., Carnegie Endowment.
Spencer, P.
    1968 The Samburu: A Study of Gerontocracy in a Nomadic Tribe. Berkeley: University of
         California Press.
Super, C.M., and S. Harkness
    1982 The Infant's Niche in Rural Kenya and Metropolitan America. In Cross-Cultural
         Research at Issue. L.L. Adler (ed.), New York: Academic Press.
Thomas, A., and S. Chess
    1977 Temperament and Development. New York: Brunner/Mazel.
    1980 Dynamics of Psychological Development. New York: Brunner/Mazel.
Thomas, A. et al.
    1963 Behavioral Individuality in Early Childhood. New York: New York University Press.
Turnbull, C.
    1972 The Mountain People. New York: Touchstone. United Nations Department of Eco-
         nomic Affairs
United Nations Department of Economic Affairs.
    1971 Report on Children. New York: UN.
    1975 Demographic Yearbook, Washington, D.C.: UN
Vogel, L.C. et al.
    1974 Health and Disease in Kenya. Nairobi, Kenya: East African Literature Bureau.
Werner, E.E.
    1979 Cross-Cultural Child Development. Monterey, Calif.: Brooks/Cole.
Western, D.
    1973 The Structure, Dynamics, and Changes of the Amboseli Ecosystem. Doctoral disserta-
         tion. University of Nairobi, Kenya.
Whiting, B., J. Whiting and J. Grawe
    1971 Basic Data Forms and Instructions. Child Development Research Unit, University
         of Nairobi, Kenya. Discussed in B. Whiting Changing Life-Styles in Kenya. Daedalus
         106: 2.

Whiting, J.
    1977 Infancticide. Paper presented at the Society for Cross-Cultural Research, Ann Arbor, Mich.
Whiting, J. and I. Child
    1953 Child Training and Personality. New Haven, Conn.: Yale University Press.
Williams, R.M., and C.M. Parkes
    1975 Psychosocial Effects of Disaster: Birth Rate in Aberfan. British Medical Journal 2: 303–304.
Zwingmann, C.H.
    1978 Uprootings: WHO Monograph Series, No. 23. Geneva: World Health Organization.

NANCY SCHEPER-HUGHES

# CULTURE, SCARCITY, AND MATERNAL THINKING: MOTHER LOVE AND CHILD DEATH IN NORTHEAST BRAZIL

> Maternal practices begin in love, a love which for most mothers is as intense, confusing, ambivalent, poignantly sweet as any they will experience.
>
> Sara Ruddick (1980: 344)

This paper is about culture, scarcity, and maternal thinking. It explores maternal beliefs, sentiments, and practices bearing on child treatment and child survival among women of Alto do Cruzeiro, a hillside shantytown of recent rural migrants. It is set in Northeast Brazil, a region dominated by the vestiges of a semifeudal plantation economy which, in its death throes, has spawned a new class: a rural proletariat of unattached and often desperate rural laborers living on the margins of the economy in shantytowns and invasion barrios grafted onto interior market towns. *O Nordeste* is a land of contrasts: cloying fields of sugar cane amidst hunger and disease; a land of authoritarian landlords and libertarian social bandits; of conservative Afro-Brazilian possession cults, and a radical, politicized Catholicism. In short, the Northeast is the heart of the Third World in Brazil – its mothers and babies heirs to the so-called Brazilian Economic Miracle, a policy of capital accumulation that has increased both the Gross National Product and the Gross National Indifference to a childhood mortality rate that has been steadily rising throughout the nation since the late 1960s.[1]

Approximately 1 million children under the age of 5 die each year in Brazil, largely the result of parasitic infections interacting with infectious disease and chronic undernutrition. Of these, few could be saved (for long) by the miracles of modern medicine. Infant and childhood mortality in the Third World is a problem of *political economy*, not of *medical technology*. Here, however, I will discuss another pair of childhood pathogens – maternal detachment and indifference toward infants and babies judged too weak or too vulnerable to survive the pernicious conditions of shantytown life. The following analysis of the reproductive histories of 72 women of Alto do Cruzeiro explores the links between *economic* and *maternal* deprivation, between material and emotional scarcity. It discusses the social and economic context that shapes the expression of maternal sentiments and the cultural meanings of mother love and child death, and determines the experiences of attachment, separation, and loss. It identifies a unifying metaphor of life as a *luta*, a struggle, between strong and weak, or between weak and weaker still, that is invoked by Alto women to explain the necessity of allowing some

187

*Nancy Scheper-Hughes (ed.), Child Survival, 187–208.*

especially their very sick – babies to die *"a mingua,"* that is, without attention, care, or protection. It means to die of want. This same metaphor is projected on to body imagery in mothers' perception of their bodies as "wasted" and their breasts as "sucked dry" by the mouths of their infants, producing the disquieting image of hungry women hungrily consumed by their own children.

Finally, it is argued that maternal thinking and practices are *socially produced* rather than determined by a psychobiological script of innate or universal emotions such as has been suggested in the biomedical literature on "maternal bonding" and, more recently, in the new feminist scholarship on maternal sentiments.

## BACKGROUND/CASE STUDIES

Two events, occurring more or less simultaneously, first captured my attention and started me thinking about maternal behavior under particularly adverse conditions. One event was public and idiosyncratic, the other was private and altogether commonplace. One aroused community sentiments of anger and hostility; the other aroused no public sentiments at all. Both concerned the survival of children in similarly unfortunate circumstances.

### Rosa

During a drought in the summer of 1967 while I was then a Peace Corps health and community development worker living in Alto do Cruziero in the interior market town of Ladeiras (a pseudonym), I was drawn one day by curiosity to the jail cell of a young woman from an outlying rural district who had just been apprehended for the murder of her infant son and 1-year-old daughter. The infant had been smothered, while the little girl had been hacked with a machete and dashed against a tree trunk. Rosa, the mother, became, for a brief period, a central attraction in Ladeiras as both rich and poor passed her barred window in order to rain down slurs on her head: "beast"; "disgraceful wretch"; "women without shame"; "unnatural creature." Face-to-face with the withdrawn and timid girl, I asked her the obvious, "Why did you do it?" And she replied, as she must have for the hundredth time: "To stop them from crying for milk." After a pause she added (perhaps to her own defense): *"Bichinos não sente nada"* – little things have no feelings. Embarrassed, I withdrew quickly, and left the girl (for she was little more than that) alone to ponder her "crime."

### Lourdes and Ze

I lived at that time on the *Alto*, not far from the makeshift lean-to of Lourdes, a young girl of 17, single and pregnant for the second time. Conditions on the Alto do Cruzeiro were then, as now, appalling: contaminated drinking w  r, food shortages, unchecked infectious disease, lack of sanitation, and crowded living conditions decimated especially the oldest and youngest residents of the hill. Lourdes's first born, Ze-Ze, was about a year old and severely marasmic (i.e., malnourished) – toothless, hairless, and unable even to sit up, he spent his days curled up in a hammock or lying on a piece of cardboard on the mud floor where he was harassed by stray dogs and goats. I became involved with Zezino after I was called on to help Lourdes with the birth of her second child, a son about whom a great fuss was made because he was both fair *(loiro)* and robust *(forte)*. With Lourdes's limited energy and attention now given over to the newborn, Zezino's condition worsened and I decided to intervene. I carried him off to the cooperative day care nursery *(creche)* I had organized with the more activist women of the hill. My efforts to rescue Ze were laughed at by the other women, and Zezino himself resisted my efforts to save him with a perversity perhaps only equal to my own. He refused to eat and wailed pitifully whenever I approached him. The *creche* mothers advised me to leave Zezino alone. They said they had seen many babies like this one and that "if a baby *wants* to die, it *will* die" and that this one was completely *desanimado*, despondent, without fight. It was wrong, they cautioned, to fight death. But this was a philosophy alien to me and I continued to do battle with the little boy until finally he gave in: he ate, gained weight, his hair grew in, and his face filled out. Gradually, too, he developed a strong attachment to me. Long before he could walk he would spring to my back where he would wrap his spindly arms and legs around me. His anger at being loosed from that position could be formidable. He even learned to smile. But along with the other women of the *creche* I wondered whether Ze would ever be "right" again, whether he could develop normally after the traumas he had been through. Worse, there were the traumas yet to come since I had to return him to Lourdes in her miserable conditions. And what of Lourdes – was this fair to her? Lourdes did agree to take Zezino back and she seemed more interested in him now that he looked more human than monkey, while my own investment in the child began to wane. By this time I was well socialized into shantytown culture and I never again put so much effort where the odds were so poor.

I returned to the Alto in the summer of 1982, 15 years later. Among the women of the Alto who formed my research sample was Lourdes, still in desperate straits and still fighting to put together the semblance of a life for her five living children, the oldest of whom was Ze, now nearly 20, and filling in as "head" of the household – a slight, quiet, reserved young man with a droll sense of humor. Much was made of the reunion between Zezino and me, and the story was told several times of how I had whisked him off when he was all but given up for dead and had force fed him like a fiesta turkey. Ze laughed the hardest of all, his arm protectively around his mother's shoulders. When I asked Ze later in private the question I asked all my informants – Who has been your greatest friend and ally in life, the one person on whom you could always depend – he took a long drag on his cigarette and replied, "My mother, of course."

I introduce these vignettes as caveats to the following analysis. With respect to the first story, it was to point out that severe child battering leading to death is universally recognized as *criminally deviant* in *Nordestino* society and culture. It is, to this day, so rare as to be almost unthinkable, so abhorrent that the perpetrator is scarcely thought of as human. "Mother love" is a commonsense and richly elaborated motif in Brazilian culture, celebrated in literature, art, and verse, in public ceremonies, in music and folklore, and in the continuing folk Catholic devotion to the Virgin Mother. Nonetheless, selective neglect accompanied by maternal detachment is both widespread among the poorer populations of Ladeiras and "invisible" – generally unrecognized by those outside shantytown culture, even by professionals such as clinic doctors and teachers who come into frequent contact with severely neglected babies and young children. *Within* the shantytown, child death *a mingua* (accompanied by maternal indifference and neglect) is understood as an appropriate maternal response to a deficiency *in* the child. Part of learning how to mother on the Alto includes learning when to "let go."

I also want to point out, with reference to the second vignette, that although the data indicate that Alto mothers do sometimes withdraw care and affection from some of their babies, such behaviors do not invariably lead to death, nor are the distanced maternal emotions irreversible. One of the benefits of returning to the same community where I had previously worked was the chance to observe the positive outcomes of several memorable cases of selective neglect – children, who, like Ze, survived and were later able to win their way inside the domestic circle of protective custody and love. It is also essential to note that selective neglect is not analogous to what we mean in the United States by "child abuse"; it is not motivated by anger, hate, or aggression toward the child. Such sentiments – part of the "classic" child abuse syndrome identified in the United States (Steele and Pollock 1968; Gill 1970; Bourne and Newberger 1979; Gelles 1973; Kempe and Helfer 1980) – appear altogether lacking among women of the Alto who are far more likely to express *pity for*, than anger against, a dependent child, who are disinclined to strike what is seen as an innocent and irrational creature, and who, to the best of my knowledge, never project images of evil or badness onto a small child.

## THE 1982 SAMPLE: THE WOMEN OF O CRUZEIRO

My sample of 72 Alto women was an opportunistic one, comprised of the first women to volunteer for the study following an open meeting I called at the *creche* and social center at the top of the hill. Many more women volunteered over the next several weeks than I could possibly have interviewed during the brief period of my stay (8 weeks). The only criterion for inclusion in the sample was that the woman had been pregnant at least once. All understood that I was studying reproduction and mothering within the context of women's lives on the Alto.

The interviews elicited demographic information, work history, patterns of migration, marital history. This was followed by a discussion of each pregnancy and its outcome. For each live birth the following information was recorded: location of, and assistance with, the delivery; mother's perceptions of the infant's weight, health status, temperament; infant feeding practices; history of early childhood illnesses, how treated, and outcomes, including mortality. Following the reproductive history I asked each mother a series of open-ended, provocative, and evaluative questions, including: Why do so many infants die here? What do infants need most in order to survive the first year of life? What could most improve the situation of mothers and infants here? Who has been your greatest source of comfort and support throughout your adult life? How many children are enough to raise? Do you prefer to raise sons or daughters and why?

As both psychological anthropologist and feminist I was concerned not only with raising questions about *behavior* and *practice* (i.e., *did* some of these women selectively neglect some of their infants and place them at risk) but also with questions of *meaning* and *motivation*, how and why they might do this. I wanted to know what infant death and loss meant to them, and how they explained and interpreted their actions as women and mothers. I wanted to know what were the effects of chronic scarcity and deprivation on women's abilities to nurture, to attend, indeed even to love. And, finally, I wanted to know what were the consequences of continual loss of infants and babies for the world views of Alto mothers, as, at a later stage, I hope to explore the consequences of selective neglect on the personalities, beliefs, and sentiments of those children – like Ze-Ze – who *do* survive in spite of their inauspicious and inhospitable early experiences. What follows here is a discussion of the initial findings from the first and exploratory stage of the research.

I was able to work efficiently during this initial period because I was both known and trusted on the Alto as the *Americana* who had once lived and worked with them. In fact, several of the older women and their adult daughters (now grandmothers and mothers) in my sample were the very same young mothers and toddlers with whom I had worked 15 years earlier (1964–1967) in the construction and operation of a cooperative day care center for working mothers. My previous work and association with the midwives of the Alto and my attendance at numerous home births years ago now gave me access to the homes of young women who gave birth during the research period.

The women interviewed ranged in age from 17 to 71; the median age of 39 meant that most were still potentially fertile. A profile of the average woman in my sample could read as follows. She was born on an *engenho* (sugar plantation) where she grew up working "at the foot of the cane." She attended school briefly and while she can do sums with great facility, she cannot read. After marriage she moved several times always in search of better work conditions for her husband or a better life for the children, preferably a *vida na rua* (a life on urban streets) rather than in the *mata*, the rural backwaters. Her husband or present companion is a "good" man, but described as *meio-fraco*, on the weak side, unskilled, unemployed, or worse, sickly and dependent or, a *cachaceiro*, a drunkard. They have been separated from time to time. She works at least part time in the marketplace, as a domestic, or taking in laundry, or even, seasonally, hiring herself out in the fields. The combined weekly household income in 1982, Cr$5000 ($25.00), put the family on the borders between *pobreza* and *pobretão* – poverty and absolute misery. The nuclear family is counted from above and below – including the little dead angels in heaven, and *os desgraçados*, the living but sinful children on earth.

REPRODUCTIVE HISTORIES

The 72 women reported a staggering *686* pregnancies and 251 childhood deaths (birth to 5 years). The average woman (speaking statistically) experienced 9.5 pregnancies, 1.4 miscarriages, abortions, or stillbirths, and 3.5 deaths of children. She has 4.5 living children. Many infants and toddlers were, however, reported by their mothers to be sick or frail at the time of the interview, and at least some of these could be anticipated to join the mortality statistics in the months and years ahead (see Table I).

Alto babies are at greatest risk during the first year of life: 70% of the deaths had occurred between birth and 6 months, and 82% by the end of the first year. No doubt contributing to high mortality in the first year is the erosion of breastfeeding which, the interviews with my older informants reveal, had begun on the plantations long before commercial powdered milk was available. All Alto infants are reared from birth on *mingaus* and *papas*, cereals of rice or manioc flour mixed with milk and sugar. The breast, when offered at all, is only a supplement to the staple baby food, *mingau*. Central to the precipitous decline in breastfeeding among Alto mothers[2] is not so much a positive valuation of commercial powdered milk as a pervasive devaluation of

TABLE I
Reproductive histories summary

| | |
|---|---|
| Total pregnancies | 686 (9.5/woman) |
| Total living children | 329 (4.5/woman) |
| Miscarriages/abortions | 85 ⎤ 101 (1.4/woman) |
| Stillbirths | 16 ⎦ |
| Childhood deaths (birth–5 yrs.) | 251 (3.5/woman) |
| Childhood deaths (6–12 yrs.) | 5 |

*N* = 72 women; ages 19–71; median age 39.

breastmilk related to the women's often distorted perceptions of their bodies, and breasts in particular, to be discussed below.

### Sex, Birth Order, and Temperament

I probed the circumstances surrounding each pregnancy, birth, and death, and I elicited infant care practices and mothers' theories of infant development and infant needs. In addition, I probed for patterns of preferential treatment or neglect, and I asked the women to share with me their thoughts and feelings about motherhood, family life, about joy and affliction, about loss and grief. Neither the reproductive histories nor the interviews revealed a strong sex or birth order bias.

The 72 mothers reported a total of 251 deaths of offspring from birth to 5 years: 129 males and 122 females (Table II). Despite a fairly pervasive ideology of male dominance in Brazilian culture, the women of the Alto expressed no consistent pattern of sex preference, and virtually all agreed that a mother would want to have a balance between sons and daughters. Both sexes were valued in children, although for different reasons. Boys were said by mothers to be "easy" to care for and were independent from an early age. Sons could be sent out to forage in the market and were unashamed to beg or steal, if necessity came to that. Sons were also enjoyed for their skill in street games and sports, an important aspect of community life on the Alto. But daughters were highly valued as well: they were not only useful at home, but were a mother's lifelong friend and intimate. Alto mothers and daughters strive to stay in proximity to each other throughout the life cycle; distance, dissension, and alienation between mothers and daughters occurs, but is considered both tragic and deviant. "Obviously," Alto mothers would conclude, a woman would want to have at least one *casal* (a boy-girl pair) and preferably two pairs, spaced closely together.

With respect to birth order among the subset of completed families, the most "protected" cohorts were those children occupying a middle rank,

TABLE II
Sex and age at death (birth–5 years)

| | Male | Female | Total | | |
|---|---|---|---|---|---|
| Postpartum | | | | | |
| (1–14 days) | 21 | 12 | 33 | | |
| 15 days–7 weeks | 18 | 8 | 26 | 175 | 205 |
| 2 mos.–6 mos. | 57 | 59 | 116 | (70%) | (82%) |
| 7 mos.–1 year | 13 | 17 | 30 | | |
| 13 mos.–2 years | 12 | 15 | 27 | | |
| $2\frac{1}{2}$ yrs.–5 yrs. | 8 | 11 | 19 | | |
| Totals: | 129 | 122 | 251 | | |

$N = 251$.

neither among the first or last born. Although childhood deaths often occurred in runs, this usually reflected external life circumstances of the mother during that period of her reproductive career, and there were no strong correlations between birth order and survivability. However, the *casula*, the last born child to survive infancy, was particularly loved and indulged.

Far more significant with respect to maternal investment was the mother's perception of the baby's constitution and temperament – the infant's qualities of readiness for the uphill struggle that is life. The mothers readily expressed a preference for babies who evidenced early on the physical and psychological characteristics of "fighters" and "survivors." Active, quick, sharp, playful, and developmentally precocious babies were much preferred to quiet, docile, passsive, inactive, or developmentally delayed babies. Mothers spoke fondly of those babies who were a little *brabo* (wild), who were *sabido* (wise before their years), and who were *jeitoso* (skillful with objects, words, tasks, people). One young mother explained:

I prefer a more active baby, because when they are quick and lively they will never be at a loss in life. The worst temperament in a baby is one that is dull and *morto de espirito* [lifeless], a baby so calm it just sits there without any energy. When they grow up they're good for nothing.

The vividly expressed disaffection of Alto mothers for their quieter and slower babies was particularly unfortunate in an area where malnutrition, parasitic infections, and dehydration artificially produce these symptoms in a great many babies. A particularly lethal form of negative feedback results when some Alto mothers reject and withdraw their affections from their passive and less demanding babies whose disvalued "character traits" are primarily the symptoms of chronic hunger. This pattern is revealed in the mothers' explanations of their children's causes of death.

### PERCEIVED CAUSES OF CHILDHOOD MORTALITY

Although uneducated and, for the most part, illiterate, the shantytown mothers interviewed were all too keenly aware that the primary cause of infant mortality was gastroenteric and other infectious diseases resulting from living in, as they so graphically phrased it, a *porcaria*, a pig sty. When asked why, *in general*, so many babies and young children of O Cruzeiro die, the women were quick to reply: "they die because we are poor, because we are hungry"; "they die because the water we drink is filthy with germs"; "they die because we can't keep them in shoes or away from this human garbage dump we live in"; "they die because we get worthless medical care: 'street medicine,' 'medicine on the run'"; "they die because we have no safe place to leave them when we go off to work."

When asked what it is that infants need most in order to survive the first year of life, the Alto mothers in my sample invariably answered "good food,

TABLE III
Causes of infant/childhood deaths (mothers' explanation)

| | |
|---|---|
| I. *The Natural Realm* (locus of responsibility: natural pathogens) | |
|    A. Gastroenteric (various types of diarrhea) | 71 |
|    B. Other Infectious, Communicable Diseases | 41 |
|    C. Teething (*denticão*) | 13 |
|    D. Skin, Liver, Blood Diseases | 13 |
|    Total: | 138. |
| II. *Supernatural Realm* (locus of responsibility: God, the saints) | |
|    A. *De Repente* (taken suddenly by God, saints) | 9 |
|    B. *Castigo* (punishment for sin of the parent) | 3 |
|    Total: | 12 |
| III. *The Social Realm* (locus of responsibility: human agency is directly or indirectly implied) | |
|    A. Malignant Emotions (envy, shock, fear) | 14 |
|    B. *Resguardo Quebrado* (postpartum or illness precautions broken) | 5 |
|    C. *Mal Trato* (poor care, including poor medical care) | 6 |
|    D. *Doença de Crianca* ("ugly diseases" involving benign neglect) | 39 |
|    E. *Fraqueza* (perceived constitutional weakness that involves maternal under-investment) | 37 |
|    Total: | 101 |

proper nutrition, milk, vitamins." I soon became bored with its concreteness. The irony, however, was that not a single mother had stated that either a lack of food or insufficient milk was a primary or even a contributing cause of death for any of her *own* children. Perhaps they must exercise this denial because the alternative – the recognition that a child is slowly starving to death – is too painful.

Table III offers a condensed rendering of these women's perceptions of the major pathogens affecting the lives of their children. Certainly naturalistic explanations predominated in which biomedical conceptions of contagion and infection blend with aspects of humoral pathology and belief in the etiological significance of teething. While *a vontage de Deus*, God's will, was understood as the ultimate cause of all human events (including the death of one's children), in very few instances did mothers attribute particular deaths to the immediate action or will of God or the saints. Human agency (although not necessarily guilt and responsibility) was imputed to the deaths of 101 of the children. This includes deaths attributed to poor care (*mal trato*), to uncontrolled pathogenic emotions (such as anger or envy resulting in evil eye, or fear resulting in the folk syndrome *susto* [magical fright]), and to breaking of customary precautions (*resguardas*) surrounding childbirth and the 40 days following, and attached to common childhood ailments. Finally, the interviews revealed a pattern of passive selective neglect expressed in the medium of the folk diagnoses of *doença de crianca* (sickness of the child) and of *fraqueza* (weakness) implying in both cases a will toward death in the child.

Underlying and uniting these etiological notions is a world view in which all of life is conceptualized as a *luta*, a power struggle between strong and weak. Death can be stronger than young life, and so mothers can speak of a baby whose drive toward life was not sufficiently strong or well developed, or who had an aversion (*desgosto*) to life. A pregnant woman who is "used up" (*acabado*) from too many previous pregnancies is said to transfer this weakness to the fetus who is then born frail and skinny, unfit for the *luta* ahead. Conversely, when a mother says that her infant suffered many crises during its first year but *vingou* (triumphed) in any case, she is giving proud testimony to the child's inner vitality, his or her will to live, to *lutar* (to fight). If an infant succumbs to *denticão* (teething) it is understood that she died because the "force of the teeth" overwhelmed the delicate little system. The folk pediatric illness *gasto* is almost always fatal because the infant's alimentary canal is reduced to a sieve: whatever goes into the mouth comes out directly in violent bouts of vomiting and diarrhea. The baby becomes *gasto* (spent, wasted), his vital fluids and energy gone. Most disquieting , however, is the image mothers convey of those of their babies who were said to have died of thirst, their tongues blackened and hanging out of their mouths because their mothers were too weak, ruined, or diseased to breastfeed them. One young mother said:

They are born already starving in the womb. They are born bruised and discolored, their tongues swollen in their mouths. If we were to nurse them constantly we would all die of tuberculosis. Weak people can't give much milk.

When I challenged a young and vigorous Alto woman about her inability to breastfeed, she responded angrily, pointing to her breast, "Look. They can suck and suck all they want, but all they will get from me is blood." Once again we have the metaphor of *a luta* – the struggle between weak and weaker over scarce resources. Another reason given by Alto mothers for their failure to breastfeed their babies for more than the first few weeks of life was that their infant had rejected the breast. And why not? For I was told repeatedly by mothers of newborns that their breastmilk was "foul" or "worthless" and for many different reasons. The milk was said to be either "salty" or "bitter" or "watery" or "sour" or "infected" or "dirty" or "diseased." In all, their own milk was rejected as unfit for infants and little more than a vehicle of contamination.

I do not know to what extent mothers' perceptions of breastmilk insufficiency is a function of their nutritional status or of their reliance on supplementary infant feedings of *mingau*, which surely interferes with the mother's own milk production. But I do know that once the breastmilk falters Alto mothers are quick to interpret this as a sympton of their own *fraqueza*, their physical and moral weakness. Similarly, when these young women refer to their breastmilk as scanty, curdled, bitter, or sour, they are also speaking metaphorically to the scarcity and bitterness of their lives as women of the Alto. What has been taken from these women is their faith in their ability to give. As the mothers stated earlier "We have *nothing* to give our children" and "Weak people can't give much milk."

In all, the etiological system and body imagery can be understood as a projection, a microcosm of the hierarchical social order in which strength, force, and power win out. It is a response to, a defense against, and a reflection of the miserable conditions of Alto life. It is these survivor values and perceptions that make Alto mothers reluctant to care for those infants and babies seen as deficient in vital energy, in *animacão*. Multiple births fare poorly on the Alto: few twins and triplets survive infancy. An obstetrical nurse in Ladeiras reported that poor mothers will take the stronger of a set of twins and leave the smaller or frailer for the hospital staff to dispose of as they see fit. All the mothers agreed that it is best if the weak and the disabled die as infants and that they die without a prolonged and wasted struggle. Celia, for example, could speak of her two infants having given her "no trouble" in dying. They just "rolled their eyes to the back of their heads and were still." It is the more gradual, protracted deaths – the deaths of *doença de crianca* – that Alto mothers particularly fear.

## DOENÇA DE CRIANCA: ETHNOMEDICAL SELECTIVE NEGLECT

The Alto mothers spoke frequently and covertly of a cluster of childhood illnesses that are both greatly feared and from which they withdraw treatment and care. They used a euphemism, "sickness of the child," in order to avoid discussing the many anxiety-provoking symptoms and conditions subsumed under the term. The women volunteered that a child with a *doença de crianca* was best left to die *a mingua*, meaning a child allowed to slowly wither away without sufficient care, food, love, or attention. It meant, quite simply, a death by neglect. The women did not like talking about this subject, but neither did they deny or conceal their own behavior or their feelings.

*Doença de crianca* was used to refer to any serious childhood condition which, while not necessarily life-threatening, was believed likely to leave the mother with a permanently disabled, frail, or dependent child. Various paralyses, epilepsy, childhood autism, and developmental disabilities were discussed in this context. The symptoms that mothers particularly feared and which they were likely to label as symptoms of a "sickness of the child" included deliriums from high fevers, fit-like convulsions, extreme passivity and immobility, retarded verbal or motor skills, disinterest in food, play, social interaction, changes in skin color, loss of body liquids and body fat, sunken eyes. The etiology was multicausal; many things caused *doença de crianca* including frights (*pasmo, susto*), germs and other microbes, evil eye, and complications resulting from otherwise normal childhood illnesses.

Measles, diarrhea, even a common cold could, without taking proper precautions, "turn into" (*virar*) a dreaded sickness of the child, thereby marking the child as beyond hope of a normal recovery.

The expansiveness and flexibility of the folk diagnosis allows an Alto mother a great deal of latitude in deciding which of her children are not favored for normal development and from which she may withdraw her attentions. The woman does not hold herself responsible for the death, nor is she blamed by the immediate female community (men seem to have little knowledge of the matter); the cause of death is a perceived deficiency in the child, not a deficiency in the mother. Thirty-nine babies were said to have died of a sickness of the child, but the same behaviors are implied in an additional 37 deaths attributed to *fraqueza* (innate weakness of the child). The following statements of mothers are illustrative:

There are various "qualities" of *doença de crianca*. Some die with rose colored marks all over their body; others die black colored. It's very ugly – with this disease it takes a very long time for them to die. It takes a lot out of the mother. It makes you sad. This sickness we don't treat. If you treat it the child will never be right. Some become crazy. Others are just weak and sickly their whole life.

They die because they have to die. If they were meant to live, it would happen that way as well. I think that if they were always weak, they wouldn't be able to defend themselves in life. So, it is really better to let the weak ones die.

There are two diseases we don't like to talk about because they are the ugliest things in the world. So we just say *doença de crianca* and leave it at that. One of these is what some people call *gotas de serena* [literally "evening mist"] which is a kind of madness, like rabies in a dog. The other is *pasmo*, a terrible paralysis that the child gets from a bad shock. His skin turns black and he just sits there still and dumb in the hammock, really lifeless. We are afraid of these sicknesses of the child. It is best to leave them die.

(*Doença de crianca*)can come from many different things. It can come from a fright the child has, but also from dirty laundry, or from strong germs that enter through the fingernails. Look, we don't like talking about all this. We don't mention its name. We are afraid of calling it up.

It became painfully apparent that Alto mothers were often describing the symptoms of severe malnutrition and gastroenteric illness further complicated by their own selective inattention. Untreated diarrheas and dehydration contributed to the baby's passivity, his or her disinterest in food, and developmental delays. High fevers often produced the fit-like convulsions that mothers feared as harbingers of permanent madness or epilepsy. Because these hungry and dehydrated babies are so passive and uncomplaining, their mothers can easily forget to attend to their needs, and can distance themselves emotionally from what comes to appear as an *unnatural* child, an angel of death that was never meant to live. Many such babies are left alone in their hammocks while their mothers are out working, and not even a sibling or a neighbor woman is within earshot when their feeble cries signal a final crisis, and so they die alone and unattended – *a mingua* as people say. A mother speaks of having "pity" for such a child, but her grief is as attenuated as her attachment to a baby who never demonstrated more than a fragile hold on life. The dead baby is washed and dressed in white satin and covered with sweet-smelling flowers. The coffin is simple: a cardboard or inexpensive wooden box decorated with a lining of purple tissue paper and a silver paper cross. Alto children form the funeral procession. In this way they are socialized to accept as natural and commonplace the burial of siblings and playmates; as later, perhaps they will have to bury their own children and grandchildren.

## BONDING THEORY AND THE BIOLOGICAL BASIS OF MOTHER LOVE

In recent years there has been considerable interest in exploring the biological components of mother-infant attachment. The observations of species specific maternal behavior patterns such as nesting, grooming, and retrieving which have been studied in animal mothers immediately after birth led a number of ethologists, human biologists, anthropologists, pediatricians, and developmental psychologists to posit the parallel existence of a sequence of largely *innate* behaviors in human mothers' responses to their newborn. Such maternal behaviors as smiling, gazing, cooing, nuzzling, sniffing, fondling, and enfolding the newborn immediately postpartum have been observed, recorded, and quantified in order to demonstrate the existence of a universal psychobiological script referred to as "mother-infant bonding" (Klaus and Kennell 1976, 1983).

Maternal bonding (or loving and attentive, if somewhat mindless, attachment to the newborn) is said to be "triggered" in mothers in response to instinctual infant behaviors, especially crying, sucking, clinging and smiling. The automatic "milk let-down" reflex in lactating mothers' responses to hungry infant cries is often cited as evidence of the unlearned and innate components of mothering. Klaus and Kennell and their associates have identified a "critical" or "sensitive" period for maternal bonding that is said to occur immediately postpartum:

There is a sensitive period in the first *minutes* and hours of life during which it is *necessary* that the mother and father have close contact with the neonate for later development to be optimal. [Klaus and Kennell 1976: 14]

If the mother and infant are separated during this time (as is customary in hospital delivery), maternal bonding may be inhibited, suggest Klaus and Kennell, with consequences as serious as maternal indifference toward, or even rejection of, the infant when the two are reunited. Unlike other mammals, however, rarely are these consequences irreversible in *human* mothers:

The process that takes place during the maternal sensitive period differs from imprinting in that there is not a point beyond which the formation of an attachment is precluded. This is the *optimal* but not the sole period for an attachment to develop. Although the process can occur at a later time, it will be more difficult and take longer to achieve. [Kennell, Trause, and Klaus 1975: 88]

Support for the evolutionary genetic basis of human bonding has come from recent studies of hunter-gatherer populations. Research by Draper, Howell, and Konner (see Lee and DeVore 1976) indicates that the relationship between mother and infant in such small, mobile social groups is characterized by: a high degree of physical skin-on-skin contact (for over 70% of the day and night in the early months of life); continuous and prolonged nursing (up to 4 or 5 years); close, attentive, and seemingly "indulgent" maternal behavior. These behaviors "typical of most primate species living in large groups [and of most] hunter-gatherers known today . . . probably represents the usual social environment for development in our species going back millions of years" (SSRC Committee on Biosocial Science n.d.:2). Maternal bonding, therefore, is thought to be part of our human evolutionary inheritance.

Alice Rossi suggests that while "biologically males have only one innate orientation, a sexual one that draws them to women, women have two such orientations, a sexual one toward men, and a reproductive one toward the young" (1977: 5). Human mothering has a strong unlearned component, argues Rossi, because of the precarious timing of human birth. The extremely immature and dependent human neonate requires particularly close attention and care in order to assure its survival. Therefore, it was particularly advantageous for a "maternal instinct" to become genetically encoded in women's evolutionary psychology.

The by now extensive maternal-infant bonding literature[3] has had, among other effects, a profound influence upon changes in the obstetrical management of pregnancy, labor, and delivery in this country and elsewhere. Many hospitals now have "birthing rooms" and rooming-in wards in order to enhance early mother-infant interaction and maternal bonding. Unfortunately, however, some of the "disciples" of Klaus and Kennell enlarged the claims made for the significance of early bonding. This lead to the naive belief among some health professionals that if early contact was *necessary* to ensure *optimal* parenting, perhaps this was *all* that was needed to ensure *competent* parenting. A number of hospital-based intervention programs, based on this shaky assumption, were launched during the 1970s when belief in the critical importance of early bonding was at its height (see Lamb 1982b). Some programs identified high-risk populations for "inadequate" parenting (usually this meant the poor, nonwhite teenage or single mothers, mothers of low birthweight infants, previous child abusers) and manipulated the hospital environment in order to "promote" bonding in the high-risk mothers who were sometimes observed against a matched control group. Rarely was there any attention paid to providing a supportive environment for the mother and child once they left the hospital. Similarly, the child abuse literature is replete with references to abuse and neglect as the consequence of failures in early maternal bonding.[4]

Recently, the scientific basis of bonding theory has been called into question,[5] and several longitudinal studies have not supported claims for any *long-term* effects of early mother-infant interaction (Ali and Lowry 1981; Rutter 1972; Chess and Thomas 1982; Curry 1979; deChateau 1980; deChateau and Wiberg 1977). As the scientific status of maternal bonding has receded, however, a view of womanhood positing the powerful effects of reproduction and mothering on females has arisen among some feminists (Rosaldo and Lamphere 1974; Ortner 1974; Chodorow 1978; Marks and de Courtivron, eds. 1980; Ruddick 1980; Gilligan 1982; Greer 1984). Sara Ruddick, for example, in a widely cited article published in *Feminist Studies* (1980: 346–347) posits certain

features of the mothering experience which are *invariant* and nearly *unchangeable*, and others, which, though changeable, are nearly *universal*. It is therefore possible to identify interests that appear to govern maternal practice throughout the species.

These *interests* concern demands for the *preservation*, *growth*, and *acceptability* of offspring. Ruddick refers to women's experience of a "social-biological pride in the function of their reproductive processes" (1980: 344) and of a "sense of well-being" when their children flourish. Although she acknowledges that some economic and social conditions, such as poverty and isolation "may make [maternal] love frantic" (p. 344), she nonetheless maintains that these "do not kill the love." And she adds, "For whatever reasons, mothers typically find it not only *natural* but compelling to protect and foster the growth of their children" (1980: 344). In stating her strong case for a *generalized* mode of "maternal thinking" Ruddick does specify that her model is based on her "knowledge of the institutions of motherhood in middle-class, white, Protestant, capitalist, patriarchal America" (p. 347) and she does call upon others "to correct her interpretations and to translate across cultures."

This is precisely what I shall do for the remainder of this paper in response to both the "bonding" and the "maternal sentiments" literature.

## CULTURE, SCARCITY, AND HUMAN NEEDS

> I have seen death without weeping
> The destiny of the Northeast is death
> Cattle they kill
> To the people they do something worse
> Traveling *repentista* singer, Brazil

Whenever we social and behavioral scientists involve ourselves in the study of women's lives – most especially thinking and behavior surrounding reproduction and maternity – we frequently come up against psychobiological theories of *human* nature that have been uncritically derived from assumptions and values implicit in the structure of the modern, Western, bourgeois family. Theories of innate maternal scripts such as "bonding," "maternal thinking," or "maternal instincts" are both culture and history bound, the reflection of a very specific and very recent reproductive strategy: to give birth to few babies and to invest heavily in each one. This is a reproductive strategy that was a stranger to most of European history through the early modern period,[6] and it does not reflect the "maternal thinking" of a great many women living in the Third World today where an alternative strategy holds: to give birth to many children, invest selectively based on culturally derived favored characteristics, and hope that a few survive infancy and the early years of life. This reproductive strategy requires a very different conception of maternal thinking, and just as surely elicits different kinds of maternal attachments, feelings, and sentiments – such as, for example, those implicated in the selective neglect of "high-risk" babies on the Alto do Cruzeiro. Since this reproductive strategy is characteristic of much of the world's poorer population today, it would seem that some revision of maternal bonding/maternal thinking as a universal human script is in order.

As might be expected, women whose cumulative experiences lead them to resignation with respect to high fertility *and* to an expectation of frequent failure to rear healthy, living children will respond differently to their new-born than middle-class mothers with both greater control over their fertility *and* a high expectation for the health and viability of their children. Infant life *and* infant death carry different meanings, weight, and significance to Alto women than to the mothers generally studied in "bonding" research. Despite the fact that the birth and neonatal environment on Alto do Cruzeiro should be optimal for intense, early bonding to occur, mother-infant attachment is often muted and *protectively distanced*.

The traditional birth environment among Alto women is a home birth attended by a lay midwife and by several supportive female friends or relatives, especially the woman's mother. Virtually all the mothers in my sample over 40 gave birth at home with a traditional *parteira*; half the younger women still prefer home to hospital delivery, although "charity cases" are accepted in the maternity wing of the town hospital. Even those who do give birth in the town *maternidade* stay for less than 2 days and keep their newborns in a small crib next to the hospital bed.

Alto mothers and infants sleep together until the baby is considered old enough to sleep in its own small hammock or cot next to the mother's bed. Co-sleeping lasts from 1 month to 6 months. Breastfeeding, although greatly attenuated, is the norm for the first few weeks (generally 1 month to 6 weeks in this sample). Although Alto infants are not tied to the mother's person in shawl or sling, the infant spends a good many hours of the day in the arms or, when slightly older, balancing on the hip of the mother or any one of a number of convenient mother surrogates: siblings of both sexes, neighbors, visiting anthropologists. There is a great deal of physical affection expressed toward infants who are frequently stroked, tickled, teased, sniffed (kissing is thought inappropriate), and babbled to by all in the household. In short, all the conditions conducive to "bonding," as described in the medical and psychological literature, can be said to obtain in O Cruzeiro.

Nonetheless, Alto mothers protect themselves from strong, emotional attachment to their infants through a form of nurturance that is, from the start, somewhat "impersonal," for lack of a better word. Many Alto babies remain not only unchristened but *unnamed* until they begin to walk or talk *or* until a medical crisis (and the possibility of death) prompts a hurried, emergency baptism. In such cases (and I have been present at several of these) the name given the child is incidental. In some cases I or another casual onlooker was asked to pick a name spontaneously. Often the infant simply inherits the name of the last infant to have died in the family. Unnamed babies are simply called *ne-ne* (baby) or given a Brazilian generic name, Ze (Joe) or Maria. Adult affection for the *ne-ne* is diffuse and not focused on any particular characteristics of the infant as a little person.

The circulation of babies through informal adoption or abandonment is commonplace on the Alto. Mothers in dire straits will sometimes ask a current or former employer to take their baby as a foster child or even as a future household servant. Young and unmarried women will sometimes leave a 5- or 6-month-old baby on the doorstep of an Alto woman known to be particularly tender-hearted. This happened to a dear friend and key informant during the summer of my stay in 1982, and brought back poignant memories to us both of the occasions during 1964–1967 when we had to cope with several babies abandoned at the cooperative day care center we had organized on the hill.

Given the extraordinary incidence of infant mortality on the Alto, child funerals are an almost daily occurrence and are dispatched with a quality of *la belle indifférence* that outsiders sometimes find quite shocking (see, for example, Scrimshaw 1978). The infant coffin-maker is a village-level specialist found in every community of Northeast Brazil. He sometimes works in the medium of cardboard, papier mâché and scrap material. A brief wake is held in the home when an infant over 6 months dies. Household visitors are expected to admire the sweet angel, but not to grieve. Mothers are scolded by other women if they shed tears for an infant, and few do. There do exist cases of Alto women who refuse to forget the death of a particularly favored baby, but their emotions tend to be dismissed as inappropriate or even as symptomatic of a kind of insanity.

The mundaneness and the high expectancy of infant death is shared by physicians and politicians of the town. In pointing out to the mayor of Ladeiras the rather extraordinary rate of child mortality for the community, he replied that he was aware of the problem and that he had, in fact, fulfilled a campaign promise in that regard: a free baby coffin to all registered voters according to their family's needs.

In all, what is constructed is an environment in which loss is anticipated and bets are hedged. "Mother love" with its attendant emotions of *holding, keeping,* and *preserving* is replaced by an estranged and guarded "watchful waiting." What makes this possible is a cultural conception of the child as human, but significantly less human than the grown child or adult. There is socialized in the Alto mother an emotion of estrangement toward the infant that is protective to her, but potentially lethal to the child. Maria Piers (1978: 37) refers to this state of primitive unconnectedness as "basic strangeness":

Basic strangeness precedes basic trust. It marks the beginning of life and its end. In the intervening years, however, many situations occur that drive us back partially or wholly into that state. Basic strangeness denotes the opposite of empathy. It is a state in which we "turn off" toward others and are unable to experience them as fellow human beings. Instead, we may value them as inanimate objects.

Piers suggests that the single most frequent cause of such total estrangement is "abject poverty" leading to physical weakness and hopelessness. In such a condition, "even one's own child may appear as a competitor" (1978: 39). In human parenting nothing can be taken for granted, least of all that the parent would sacrifice her life and resources for her child. Human mothers who reach the limit of their endurance can and often do become both estranged from and indifferent toward their children. Certainly Piers's concept is worthy of further refinement and investigation.

However, I do not wish to suggest by the foregoing that Alto mothers never suffer the loss of their infants. Indeed, amidst the generally passive and emotionally flat narrations of their lives as women, workers, and mothers, the pain of a particularly unresolved or poignant loss would break through and shatter the equanimity and resignation that is the norm. There would be memories of a *particular* baby in whom a mother's hopes for the future *had* been invested, and she would weep in the telling of *that* death of all the deaths and losses she had endured. In the presence of so "deviant" a response I would be at a loss for how to proceed or, indeed, whether to proceed at all. But invariably my Alto assistant, Irene, or another woman would come to the rescue. "No, Dona Maria," she would scold the grieving woman, "of course you will not go mad with grief. You *will* conform. You will go on. You have *your own life* ahead."

The reproductive and life histories of these shantytown women lead me to question the validity of such ill-defined terms as maternal bonding, attachment, maternal thinking, critical period, and separation anxiety that fill the literature on mother-infant interaction. The terms and concepts seem inadequate to convey the experience of mothering under the less than optimum conditions that prevail throughout much of the world today. The classical maternal bonding model focuses altogether too much attention on too few critical variables and on too brief a period in the mother-child life cycle. The model grossly underestimates the power and significance of social and cultural factors that influence and shape maternal thinking over time: the cultural meanings of sexuality, fertility, death, and survival; mother's assessment of her economic, social support, and psychological resources; family size and composition; characteristics and evaluation of the infant – its strength, beauty, viability, temperament, and "winsomeness."

The bonding model has neither relevance to, nor resonance with, the experiences of the women of O Cruzeiro for whom the life history of attachments follows a tortuous path marked by many interruptions, separations, rejections, and losses reflecting the precariousness of their own existence and survival. But it is also important to note that an early lack of attachment, an indifferent commitment, or even a hostile rejection of an infant does not preclude the possibility of an enfolding drama of mother-child attachments later on, as some of the memorable survivors of early and severe selective neglect, like Ze-Ze, would indicate. That there must be a biological basis to human emotions is not disputed. It is argued, however, that the nature of human love and attachments is a complex phenomenon, socially constructed and made meaningful through culture. A more contextualized model of maternal thinking and sentiments is needed.

Finally, in concluding this paper, I wish to make it abundantly clear that there are many conditions on the Alto do Cruzeiro that are hostile to child survival. Most serious are the ones I scarcely mentioned: contaminated water, unchecked infectious disease, food shortages, the absence of day care facilities, and grossly inadequate medical care. I have focused instead on maternal thinking and behaviors that may also contribute to childhood mortality in order to address the indignities and inhumanities forced on poor women who must make choices and decisions that no woman should have to make. In the final analysis, the selective neglect of children must be understood as a direct consequence of the "selective neglect" of their mothers who have been excluded from participating in what was once called the Economic Miracle of modern Brazil.

## ACKNOWLEDGMENTS

This chapter first appeared under a different sub-title in *ETHOS*, Winter 1985, 13(4): 291–317. The editor acknowledges the kind permission of the American Anthropological Association to republish the article in this volume.

Research for this study was supported by grants from the Southeast Consortium for International Development and the Duke-UNC Women's Studies Research Center, and by an R.J. Reynolds Faculty Development Award. I wish to express my appreciation to D. Michael Hughes, whose own work in and commitment to child welfare have inspired me, and to Irene Lopes da Silva of Alto Do Cruzeiro, who is an invaluable field assistant, a gifted informant, and a dear friend. Carol Stack, Sandra Morgen, and Jaan Valsiner made insightful comments and suggestions on an earlier draft. Discussions with Marten de Vries found their way into this analysis.

NOTES

1. See Paim, Netto-Dias, and De Araujo 1980. Also, see Wood 1977. A recent PAHO investiga- tion of childhood mortality in a dozen urban and rural sites in eight Latin American countries found the City of Recife in Pernambuco, Northeast Brazil, to have the highest infant mortality of all urban centers sampled.
2. See Goldberg, Rodrigues, Thome, and Morris 1982; Grant 1983; Berquo, Cukier, and Spindel 1984. A recent UNICEF report noted that in Brazil the percentage of babies breastfed *for any length of time* has fallen from 96% in 1940 to under 40% in 1974. This same report cites another study which found that among a large sample of children of poor parents in the South of Brazil, bottlefed babies were between three and four times more likely to be seriously malnourished than breastfed babies.
3. See, for example, Klaus and Kennell 1976, 1983; Kennell, Voos, and Klaus 1979; Klaus, Jerauld, and Kreger 1972; Lozoff, Brittenham, and Trause 1977.
4. See, for example, Hurd 1975 and Schwarzbeck 1977.
5. See, for example, Svedja, Campos, and Emede 1980; Lamb 1982a, 1982b, and 1982c; Korsch 1983. Klaus and Kennell (1983) responded to these critiques.
6. Contemporary historians of European and American family life in the early modern period have described child-rearing practices that were at best harshly pragmatic, and at worst sadistic and passively infanticidal. See, for example, Aries 1962; de Mause 1974; Fox and Quitt 1980; Laslett 1965; Shorter 1975; Stone 1977).

REFERENCES

Ali, Z. and M. Lowry
    1981 Early Maternal-Child Contact: Effect on Later Behavior. Developmental Medicine and Child Neurology 23: 337–345.
Aries, Philipe
    1962 Centuries of Childhood: A Social History of Family Life. New York: Vintage.
Berquo, Elza, Rosa Cukier, and Cheywa Spindel
    1984 Caracterizacạo e Determinantes Do Aleitamento Materno na Grande Sạo Paulo e na Grande Recife. CEBRAP – Centro Brasileiro de Analise e Planejamento, Nova Serie, No. 2.
Bourne, Richard, and Eli Newberger (eds.)
    1979 Critical Perspectives on Child Abuse and Neglect. Lexington, MA: Lexington Books.
Chess, Stella, and Alexander Thomas
    1982 Infant Bonding: Mystique and Reality. American Journal of Orthopsychiatry 52(2): 213–222.
Chodorow, Nancy
    1978 The Reproduction of Mothering: Psychoanalysis and Sociology of Gender. Berkeley: University of California Press.
Curry, M.A.H.
    1979 Contact During the First Hour with the Wrapped or Naked Newborn: Effects of Maternal Attachment Behaviors at 36 Hours and Three Months. Birth and Family Journal 6: 227–235.

De Chateau, P.
1980 Post-Neonate Interaction and its Long-Term Effects: Early Experiences and Early Behavior. E.G. Simmel (ed.). New York: Academic Press.

De Chateau, P. and B. Wiberg
1977 Long-Term Effects on Mother-Infant Behavior of Extra Contact During the First Hour Post Partum. Acta Paediatrica Scandinavica 66: 145–151.

De Mause, Lloyd
1974 The History of Childhood. New York: The Psychohistory Press.

Fox, Vivian and Martin H. Quitt
1980 Loving, Parenting and Dying: The Family Cycle in England and America. New York: The Psychohistory Press.

Gelles, Richard
1973 Child Abuse as Psychopathology. American Journal of Orthopsychiatry 43(4): 611–621.

Gilligan, Carol
1982 In a Different Voice: Psychological Theory and Women's Development. Cambridge: Harvard University Press.

Gil, David
1970 Violence Against Children. Cambridge: Harvard University Press.

Goldberg, H., W. Rodrigues, M. Thome, and Morris
1982 Infant Mortality and Breastfeeding in Northeastern Brazil. Paper Presented at the Population Association of America Annual Meeting. San Diego, California.

Grant, J.
1983 The State of the World's Children, 1982–1983. Geneva: UNICEF Information Division

Greer, Germaine
1984 Sex and Destiny: Politics and Human Fertility. New York: Harper & Row.

Hurd, J.L.M.
1975 Assessing Maternal Attachment: First Step Toward the Prevention of Child Abuse. Journal of Obstetric, Gynecologic and Neonatal Nursing 4(4): 25–30.

Kempe, H. and R. Helfer
1980 The Battered Child. Chicago: The University of Chicago Press.

Kennell, J.H., M.A. Trause, and M.H. Klaus
1975 Parent-Infant Interaction. CIBA Foundation Symposium No. 33. Amsterdam: Elsevier.

Kennell, J.H., V.K. Voos, and M.H. Klaus
1979 Parent-Infant Bonding. In J.D. Osfsky (ed.), Handbook of Infant Development. New York: John Wiley.

Klaus, M.H., R. Jerauld, and N.C. Kreger
1972 Maternal Attachment: Importance of the First Post-Partum Days. New England Journal of Medicine 286: 460–463.

Klaus, M.H. and J.H. Kennell, eds.
1976 Maternal-Infant Bonding. St Louis: C.V. Mosby. (Revised Edn.: Parent-Infant Bonding, 1982).

Klaus, M.H. and J.H. Kennell
1983 Parent to Infant Bonding: Setting the Record Straight. Journal of Pediatrics 102(4): 575–576.

Korsch, Barbara
1983 More on Parent-Infant Bonding: Journal of Pediatrics (February): 249–250.

Lamb, Michael
1982a Maternal Attachment and Mother-Neonate Bonding: A Critical Review. Advances in Developmental Psychology, Vol. 2, pp. 1–39. Hillsdale, NJ: Lawrence Erlbaum Associates.
1982b Early Contacts and Maternal-Infant Bonding: One Decade Later. Pediatrics 70(5): 763–768.
1982c The Bonding Phenomenon: Misinterpretations and Their Implications. Journal of Pediatrics 100(4): 555–557.

Laslett, Peter
    1965 The World We Have Lost. London: Methuen.
Lee, R.B. and I. de Vore
    1976 Kalahari Hunter-Gatherers. Cambridge: Harvard University Press.
Lozoff, B., G.M. Brittenham, and M.A. Trause
    1977 The Mother-Newborn Relationship: Limits of Adaptability. Journal of Pediatrics 91:
        1–12.
Marks, Elaine, and Isabelle de Courtivron, eds.
    1980 New French Feminism. New York: Schocken.
Ortner, Sherry
    1974 Is Female to Male as Nature is to Culture? In M. Rosaldo and L. Lamphere (eds.),
        Women, Culture, and Society. Stanford: Stanford University Press. pp 67–88.
Paim, S., C. Netto-Dias, and J. DeAraujo
    1980 Influencia de Fatores Sociais e Ambientais na Mortalidade Infantil. Bon. Of. Sanit.
        Pan-Am. LXXXVIII: 327–340.
Piers, Maria
    1978 Infanticide. New York: W.W. Norton.
Rosaldo, Michelle, and Louise Lamphere
    1974 Introduction. In M. Rosaldo and L. Lamphere (eds.), Women, Culture, and Society.
        Stanford: Stanford University Press. pp. 1–16.
Rossi, Alice
    1977 A Biosocial Perspective on Parenting. Daedalus 106 (2): 1–32.
Ruddick, Sara
    1980 Maternal Thinking. Feminist Studies 6: 342–364.
Rutter, Michael
    1972 Maternal Deprivation Reassessed. New York: Penguin.
Schwarzbeck, C.
    1977 Identification of Infants at Risk for Child Abuse: Observations and Inferences in the
        Examination of the Mother-Infant Dyad. In Child Abuse: Where Do We Go From
        Here? Conference Proceedings, Feb. 18–20, 1977. Washington, DC: Children's Hospi-
        tal National Medical Center, Child Protection Center, pp. 67–69.
Scrimshaw, Susan
    1978 Infant Mortality and Maternal Behavior in the Regulation of Family Size. Population
        and Development Review 4: 383–403.
Shorter, Edward
    1975 The Making of the Modern Family. New York: Basic Books.
SSRC Committee on Biosocial Science
    n.d. Biosocial Foundations of Parenting and Offspring Development. New York: Social
        Science Research Council. Unpublished report.
Steele, Brandt, and Carl Pollock
    1968 A Psychiatric Study of Parents Who Abuse Their Children. In R.E. Helfer and C.H.
        Kempe (eds.), The Battered Child. Chicago: The University of Chicago Press. pp.
        103–147.
Stone, Lawrence
    1977 The Family, Sex, and Marriage in England, 1500–1800. New York: Harper & Row.
Svejda, M.J., J.J. Campos, and R.N. Emede
    1980 Mother-Infant 'Bonding': Failure to Generalize. Child Development 51: 775–779.
Wood, Charles
    1977 Infant Mortality Trends and Capitalist Development in Brazil. Latin American Perspec-
        tives 4(4): 56–65.

# PART IV

## CHILD ABUSE: DEVIANT AND IDIOSYNCRATIC CHILD MALTREATMENT

*Bye-Child*
[He was discovered in the henhouse where she had
    confined him.
He was incapable of saying anything.]

When the lamp glowed,
A yolk of light
In the back window,
The child in the outhouse
Put his eye to a chink –

Little henhouse boy,
Sharp-faced as new moons
Remembered, your photo still
Glimpsed like a rodent
On the floor of my mind,

Little moon man,
Kennelled and faithful
At the foot of the yard,
Your frail shape, luminous,
Weightless, is stirring the dust,

The cobwebs, old droppings
Under the roosts
and dry smells from scraps
she put through your trapdoor
Morning and evening.

After those footsteps, silence;
Vigils, solitudes, fasts,
Unchristened tears,
A puzzled love of the light.
But now you speak at last

With a remote mime
Of something beyond patience,
Your gaping wordless proof
Of lunar distances
Travelled beyond love.

                                        Seamus Heaney, 1980

# SEVERE CHILD ABUSE AMONG THE CANADIAN INUIT.

Irniguluk, aged 14, came into the house from playing outside. As he did so, he knocked over the rifle near the door. His father Ataataluk, called him stupid and knocked him reeling on the floor with a blow to the side of the head. . . . A few day later Irniguluk was complaining to others in the village about his terrible headaches, but he never mentioned the cause, and no one outside of the household knew of the outburst. . . . Someone had shot some caribou and one of the young men, Uvikak brought a frozen carcass to his father, Ataataluk's house, for the usual custom of hospitality and distribution. Relatives and neighbors were invited to come with their knives to carve up and eat the caribou and take some home. As all squatted around the slowly thawing body on the floor, the 14 year old boy and his older sister were playing and eating pieces of frozen meat which were passed to them. In came their mother, Argnakallak with the two year old adopted son, Paatauyuk,[1] whining and with a runny nose, as usual. Irniguluk and his older sister started to tease the toddler Paatauyuk, accusing him of being stupid, of not talking and eating properly, of still being a baby and peeing in his pants.

Paatauyuk cried, gently at first, he did not talk back (he was hardly capable of talking at all) but clung to a table leg and looked at the floor. The older boy then began to trip Paatauyak, bursting with laughter as he fell to the floor, slowly picking himself up, wet with tears, snot and dribble; then they kicked him and knocked him about even as he lay on the floor, and his cries rose to a screaming crescendo. The mother busied herself with household tasks, but kept looking over anxiously, saying nothing, while the men continued with their conversation and the destruction of the caribou carcass. Apirku (the author), who had lived with the family for about two months, said sharply to the two older children "Why do you keep hitting him? He's too small; he only acts stupid because you keep beating him up, and he'll never grow up right if you treat him like that . . .". Hardly had this been said when a tremendous bellow came from Ataataluk across the room. "SILAITUPALUK ANI-LAURUK" (Stupid little thing, get it out of here). He was standing, red in the face, shouting right past Apirku's ear at the bedraggled child. Apirku knew that the imperative was directed as much at him as at the crumpled and whimpering Paatauyuk.

The aging mother caught the youngster by the wrist and dragged him straight outside. Apirku quickly got into his parka and joined them in the whipping icy gale outside. "Why don't you stop them when they attack Paatauyuk?" he asked. "Because when I do, he beats me up too" she replied.

This is a paper I did not want to write because I would be happier if the data did not exist. In fact I wrote a prior version, called the 'The Battered Child Syndrome, Eskimo Style' over fifteen years ago, but sat on it because I had

Nancy Scheper-Hughes (ed.), Child Survival, 211–225.

been quite involved with some cases and because of their rarity, it would have been easy for people in the North to identify the participants.[2] However, time has passed, some of the perpetrators are dead and most of the survivors are adult; futhermore, now that I have lived in nearly twenty Inuit settlements, distributed over a period of more than twenty years, it is much more difficult for readers to identify the personnel involved. Also, with the increased concerns with child-abuse in "the South" and with the present concerns of medical and medical-anthropological authorities[3] in the Canadian North, I accepted the invitation and encouragement of Dr. Nancy Scheper-Hughes to present these data.

The vast majority of ethnographic accounts of the Canadian Inuit (and the Greenlandic and Alaskan Eskimo) bear little evidence of any kind of child-abuse among the Eskimo peoples – at least until the much changed, "urbanized", alcohol-available present. Even today there are relatively few accounts of severe child abuse, even during bouts of alcohol abuse as described by Elaine Schechter (1983). Though there are many accounts of violence between adults, mainly men, in Inuit life, there is very little concerning violence towards children, even in my own earlier writings (Graburn 1960, 1964, 1969a, and b) or in the extremely detailed accounts of Jean Briggs (1970, 1972, 1975, 1978). On the other hand the vast majority of the literature describes and emphasizes the extreme permissiveness of Eskimo child-rearing, their abhorrence of anything like punishment, and their widespread distaste for the common attributes of white people in forcefully expressing their emotions and losing their temper. Typical of such accounts is that of Turner for the Ungava area: "Love for offspring is of the deepest and purest character. Mothers and fathers never inflict corporal punishment on their children . . .". (1894: 191).

Thus the cases which are considered here are extremely rare in my own experience (direct knowledge of four cases in over three years of living in over forty Inuit households in nearly twenty settlements) and even rarer in the extensive literature on the Eskimos. For instance, Thalbitzer (1941: 600) says of Angmagssalingmiut: "The Eskimo does not punish his child. . . . But exceptions were mentioned. Certain women were known not only to have severely scolded their naughty children but also to have beaten them. Here, of course, a good deal depends on the temperament of the woman concerned. . . ." However, there is a definite pattern in the present data and, set in great contrast with the overwhelmingly opposite "normal" behavior, it needs an explanation.

Because of this rarity I was almost afraid that I had collected data which could be refuted by everyone else. I therefore have been in communication with nearly all the other authorities on Canadian Inuit life, asking if they had ever heard of similar cases. In the responses, three patterns have emerged: (1) Those whose experience, sometimes more extensive than my own, had never led them to come across such cases; (2) Those who did not answer the question directly, but seemed to aver that if such cases did exist they were so rare that one should perhaps not report them: and (3) Those who had detailed data on the other cases almost exactly similar to my own, but drawn from other areas and different times. In the latter case, I have included some of their data in my own account below, and I am very grateful for their generosity and directness.

## THE CASES

The cases which provide evidence for this paper were all collected by myself and other ethnographers in the Central and Eastern Canadian Arctic between 1958 and 1976. The communities in which they were collected varied in degree of acculturation though none was purely traditional autonomous Inuit and none were the "new" villages and towns with permanent government housing, many white personnel and institutions, councils, mechanized vehicles, and available alcohol. The hunting camps and settlements were populated by Inuit who were all nominally Christian, though in many cases missionaries were not present, and were dependent on trade with Hudsons Bay Company stores for materials such as ammunition and guns, textiles for clothing and tents, some basic (but not most) foods, and tobacco. Leadership in these communities generally followed the traditional patterns of "wise hunters" (*isumatak*) who exercized quiet suggestive leadership but not authoritarian control. In some cases the leadership was also bound up with the position of catechist in the Church. The vast majority of the adult Inuit were self-employed as hunters and trappers, with very little wage labour (See Graburn 1969a).

The vignette with which I opened the paper is, as far as I know, among the least abusive of the set, and the outcome did less physical harm[4] though I am not in a position to know the long term emotional consequences. Futhermore, it was unique in that more than one person in the family was subject to abuse, whereas in all the other cases there was only one "victim."

Let me quickly summarize the other cases. I should emphasize that these ten cases have been recorded in ten different settlements. This should indicate that we are dealing with a widespread pattern, rather than an odd quirk of regional situation, or acculturative tensions, liquor or economic depression in the more recent period. This summary recounting of the other cases should begin to indicate the common features found in most of the cases.

A young girl, the last in her family of two parents and five siblings, was always teased and thought to be "slow" in growing up. By the time she reached the age of four, she was physically attacked by her parents when they were frustrated by her inability to do the small tasks usually assigned to young girls. Soon, her older brothers and sisters started to beat her up, she "withdrew", rarely ate or spoke, and died. It is not known if her death was a direct result of physical battery or an accumulation of injuries plus sickness.

Another girl, aged about five, was deemed to be stupid by her parents. She was treated badly, given ragged clothes, fed scraps and occasionally hit. Her parents seemed to have given up on her, and they let her grandparents take her over. They too found her difficult to raise, but they did not mistreat her physically. At last report she was alive, but severely retarded socially, though no organic illness was obvious.

A boy, aged five or six, who was similarly maltreated by his parents, appeared to be mentally retarded and undisciplined. Again he was given to his grandparents but could not talk by that age, and couldn't or wouldn't walk. They treated him very kindly, and eventually he began to thrive, learned to talk and walk and grew up to be a "normal" if dull and somewhat non-social teenager.

Another boy was observed in his otherwise normal family by three different anthropologists over a period of years. He appeared to be slightly retarded and would not obey his parent or older siblings in the unquestioning way that Inuit children follow even the subtlest directions of their elders. He was teased and hit and treated very roughly, mainly by his older siblings, but the parents seemed to concur though they only abused him verbally. He was the laughingstock of the household and this behavior was not particularly hidden from visitors to the home. His behavior showed symptoms that might have been labled "hyperactive" in today's psychological parlance. He was a constant source of irritation to those around him.

One little girl (I do not know if she was retarded) was frequently mistreated by the members of her family. Her mother was particularly cruel and used to pull her up by putting hooks in her nostrils (interestingly enough this is the same treatment that was accorded the famous Kaujjajuk in the widespread myth about the boy orphan who was maltreated by his step-family, turned into a polar bear and came back to kill them). White authorities heard about this abuse and took the little girl away to a distant settlement where she was placed in another family. At the age of 13 or 14 she was sent back to her natal family and settlement, but was raped by an older married man and became pregnant, so she was returned to the settlement to which she had originally been sent.

Another girl, aged four, was maltreated and physically beaten, by her mother (a widow). This came to the attention of the Catholic missionary who took her away and looked after her, with the help of an Eskimo woman in his mission. When she seemed to have recovered, physically and mentally, she was adopted into another family where she was well-treated.

A woman was married to the son of the most prestigious family in a village, though she herself was daughter of the least admired family. They had four children and her husband died. She was sent to the hospital along with her baby son a few months old. He was very well treated by the white people at the hospital and became a "favorite" and thrived. However, a year or so later, they were returned to their village where the little boy was very unhappy, could not eat Eskimo-style food and did not know the language. He was teased by his older siblings and regressed; he peed in his clothes and failed to speak. Then all his family started to abuse him, made him sleep in the porch, gave him dog food and even put out cigarettes on his skin. The missionary heard about this and took the boy to the mission where he lived with his family. The mother came in the middle of the night and took the boy back to her home, telling people that the white man had stolen her baby. That same night, coincidentally or not, her younger, unmarried sister (who had taken part in the abuse) rolled on and killed her own baby while it slept. The missionary went and took the young boy again, though only after further tortures, kept him in his house for a few days, and then adopted him out to the boy's grandfather (father's father) and grandmother. It took years for the young boy to recover normal powers of speech and he grew up to be what others called a "delinquent", though he survived to adulthood.

In a similar case a girl had been taken out to hospital when she was a baby and returned to her settlement at about four years old. Her parents and her brothers and sisters often hit her, and only dressed her in ragged clothes. I do not know what happened to her since.

Let me emphasize again the apparent rarity of such phenomena. These are only ten cases out of a population of slightly more than a thousand families (adding up the number of families in all the settlements where these took place). This is a ratio far below any comparable slice of the population in the United States. Child abuse may be more common than this as it might be hidden and therefore unknown to anthropologists, though some missionaries possibly have a fuller knowledge. In some cases anthropologists working in the same villages as some of the above cases, had not learned of them, and we might therefore surmise that other cases have not been reported by anyone. The cases reported do not include the more well-known pattern of infanticide, which usually takes place at, or some time soon after birth. Nor have I included those fairly numerous instances where children have died of unknown causes, i.e. no sickness was known and the child did not bear marks of physical abuse.

## COMMONALITIES

Before attempting any explanations let us consider the apparent commonalities in these few cases, bearing in mind that this is too small a sample for statistical generalizations.

### Age

Though no infants are involved (partly due to the exclusion of infanticide), it appears that severe child abuse does not start in infancy. For boys it tends to start younger, at about two, when the boy is normally expected to become somewhat independent by playing with other boys and going outside. Among girls, no cases were known before the age of four and most are about the age of five when young girls are expected to start to take on female roles by helping around the household, e.g. looking after younger siblings, fetching and carrying and so on. Only in a few cases did the abuse continue much beyond five or six, because the children either died or were taken into other households.

*Abilities*

All the children, as far as it is known, were judged to be socially or mentally disadvantaged before the physical abuse started. Two of these are special cases, when the children returned from hospital "down South" where they had been looked after by white people and partially separated from their mothers; thus the subsequent rejection may have been a protective consequence on the mother's part. These children were unable to quickly readapt to Eskimo-style foods and appropriate role behavior. In the context of the Inuit household, such children were "retarded" in that they were not growing up and meeting the normal expectations of those around. In most cases the children were already withdrawn, passive and uncommunicative, and it is significant that in a number of these, they did not speak at all in marked contrast to the usual loquacious Inuit people. Though a number of the children were physically awkward, only one could be labeled destructively hyperactive.

*Family Background*

In two cases, one boy and one girl, there was only one parent, a widowed mother, but in all but one there were a number of siblings. What is particularly striking is the fact that nearly everyone in the family joined in the abusive behavior. This is very different from the present situation where a high incidence of physical abuse among urban Inuit is usually attributed to drunken fathers (Recent personal communications from the Canadian North).

I have also tried to assess the "social status" of the families. Though it is not often discussed, in nearly all Inuit communities and camps, the families are roughly "ranked" according to status, depending on leadership abilities, econonic success, and moral qualities, and some families are considered marginal or pariah (Briggs 1970; Graburn 1969a). Such ranking is sometimes implicitly hereditary even over three or four generations. In only one case was the abusive family definitely one of the highest ranking people, a recognized leader and moral example. In four cases the family was generally accorded low status, as relatively unsuccessful, people who would be subject of gossip for their moral behavior and the breach of serious norms. In the other cases, the families appeared to be "average" or their status was less well known. Given the fact that in any ordinary Inuit population the proportion of low status, "marginal" families is unlikely to be much more than 10%, these families produce a much higher than expected ratio of child abuse, though I should emphasize that in all cases the assessment of low status was *not* the result of the behavior described here, but was already strongly attributed.

*Outcomes*

Where their later life histories are known, only two of the children remained with their original family, in one case till death, in another with continual abuse. In three cases the family responsible for the abuse gave up the child to another family, though this may have been at the urging of others. In all the others, there was white intervention, especially in the more severe cases where the child might very well have died. Two of these agents were white missionaries who knew the community very well which resulted in adoptions to other family members. And in three of the cases the children were "adopted out" to their grandparents, a not unusual direction for adoption among the Canadian Inuit (Guemple 1979b). Given the nature of the data and the time period required for full reporting, it has not been possible to follow through with assessment of "recovery" of these children, though a number did survive to adolescence but remained poorly functioning individuals.

In all the above cases there was no immediate interference from outside the family except by white people. In two cases the grandparents of the child, i.e. the parents of the abusive parent, stepped in on behalf of the child, and grandparents would generally be the only people to attempt to excercise control in family affairs. This is consonant with the principles of non-interference which governed so much of traditional Eskimo life and which has led to the assertion that Eskimos had no "law" (Graburn 1969b).

### DISCUSSION

Obviously one could start with the simple hypothesis that nearly all of these children failed to develop "normally" and did not progress through the stages of social and linguistic competence expected of those around them, leading to frustration and later to violent outbursts by their families. Although this is part of the picture, we have to consider that *most* Inuit children who exhibit developmental problems are treated with great care and solicitude by their families, with extra love and toleration. For instance, in one of the villages there was a child who was very slow to learn to walk who appeared "slow" or at least unwilling to "grow up" and become independent like other boys. He hung around his mother and whined a lot, but was treated very well by both his parents, who protected him from some the teasing of the other children. He thrived and was a delightful person as a teenager, even though he would probably never be very good at hunting and other adult male tasks.

Thus there must also have been something about the families and the contextual situations which produced this rare and "abnormal" behavior. But at the same time we know that all the families (except one) had children who were treated in the ordinary permissive ways – a relatively common North American pattern that some families are "bad" parents to all their children just does not accord with our data. Even the fact that two of the families were headed by single (widowed) mothers and others were "low" status does not explain the picking on one child among an otherwise well-treated group. In general neither family pattern is known to be associated with child abuse for 99 out of a hundred children.

In traditional and recent Inuit society, it has been fairly common for orphans and certain adopted children to be treated coldly and made to do many of the tasks for the family. Orphans, (*ilijakjuk*) were the subject of neglect and abuse in mythology, and orphans and some adopted children (*tigguak*) may have been treated like "servants" (*kipaluk*). These people, now adults, were adopted (as orphans) in mid-childhood and the normal close family bonds of attachments failed to develop. But in most cases, especially males, the children grew up to be exceptionally competent, and might have become leaders. However, some female orphans are known to have become less than competant, socially integrated adults. In the sample of child abuse cases under consideration, only one child was adopted, none were orphans, and none were treated as servants in the traditional sense; if anything they grew up to be less than competent. In traditional and recent Inuit families, "difficult" children, those who were slow to learn, or were disobedient, were never "taught a lesson" by physical violence; the Inuit do not believe that a child's character can be changed by punishment, but would be taught by constant encouragement and example or, when they are older, by "scolding" *suangajuk* (Briggs 1970: 330–332; Graburn 1969b, Guemple 1979a). Briggs (1970, 1975) aptly demonstrates the lengths which Inuit go to contain their upset emotions and to be subtle in their criticism of an irritating person in their midst. Other, traditional mechanisms which have gone out of use, might have been to change the name (*atik*) and hence the person-soul of a child (or adult) who had bad luck or got into serious trouble.

I think we should look at the wider context of the management of violence in Inuit society to provide a partial explanation of these abuse cases. The normal first response of Inuit to extended or severe social problems is avoidance of withdrawal (*givituk*) whereby the persons offended or upset pretend there is no problem or leave the situation or even move to another social group. (In extreme cases, departure from the social group might have been a form of suicide). We might consider those cases where the child was placed, without white intervention, in another family, to be ways by which the offending family could avoid the problem by a kind of withdrawal. Direct anger (*ningaktuk*) is despised and feared in Inuit society because it might erupt into deadly violence. (According to the Inuit, expressed anger is thought to be characteristic of white people). In spite of this, fear, murder and attempted murder were in fact common in traditional Inuit society, until white authorities became available to solve the problems, i.e. by taking such people out of the community which resulted *de facto* in the more acceptable traditional solution, avoidance (See Graburn 1969b).

However, violence in other forms was quite acceptable. In a way, the hunting of animals, even when ritually surrounded, entailed a kind of violence; I have often seen men laugh at or strike a mortally wounded and terrified animal (see also Briggs 1975: 149). As Turner said of hunting caribou: "Mortally wounded they stand; the limbs gradually diverging to sustain their trembling body; the eyes gazing piteously at the foe, who often mocks their dying struggles or pitches a stone at their quivering legs to make them fall." (1894: 251). Even "closer to home" is the treatment of dogs which, while never treated exactly as pets, were usually given their due and not normally maltreated. However, should a dog disobey, get out of line, or become so injured that it could not pull its weight, it might be treated very cruelly. Men could lash out at a dog with sudden violence, with a whip, stick or boot; dogs which were injured (more than just cut feet) could become the objects of angry ridicule, be beaten mercilessly, and even left behind to starve or be eaten (cf. Briggs 1975: 149). Small animals and birds which had been captured or wounded could be tortured, often by children with the encouragement of adults, until they died (*cf.* Briggs 1975:154). One should also mention another kind of sanctioned violence, this one against humans, though one long past, that is the opportunistic disposal or murder of white people for economic gain. In earlier encounters with explorers and other outsiders, the Inuit were usually seen as smiling, compliant and friendly, willing to trade skins, weapons and toys for the white man's metal, guns and trinkets – except when they weren't! On a number of occasions, the most famous of which was the meeting with the mutineers from Hudson's ship (Asher 1860) when, in the midst of friendly trading, the Inuit suddenly set upon and killed four of the small group of unarmed white people. Such behavior, usually labeled "treachery" by whites, showed that the Inuit were, at a certain point, capable of murder when by surprise or superior strength they thought they could get away with it (Graburn 1969a: 77–93).

Thus I propose three major factors which allow for, but do not totally account for, these outbursts of violence against children.

(1) *The Inuit were capable of great violence under certain circumstances, a feature that stood in marked contrast to their usual peaceful and kind behavior.* In the case of their treatment of animals, we have evidence that they were also capable of deriving pleasure and humour from cruelty, and in all cases the outburst of violence is unpremeditated, rather than a

gradual escalation of anger and hostility. Inuit are extremely patient and tolerant of irritants but, at a certain point this gives way to an extreme expression of violent emotions which are relatively unchecked.

(2) *Although the display of anger and physical violence is rare and is repressed as long as possible, when it does erupt, it does so unchecked by other Inuit who do not interfere.* (Briggs 1970, 1975). Because other Inuit do not immediately interfere (though white agents did in some of the above cases), the feared violence escalates without internal and external control. Even in the much vaunted case of "song contests" (*illuriik*), the normative community settlement of quarrels evaporates immediately violence arises, as was dramatically illustrated in Knud Rasmussen's famous movie *The Wedding of Palo* (1933) (*cf.* Holm 1886). *That the feared and suppressed violence once loosed, may lead directly to murder, confirms the Inuit fear of expressing anger in the first place.*

(3) *The violent and abusive treatment of developmentally delayed or handicapped children was not normative in Inuit culture and society. It seems clear that the perpetrators were somewhat deviant and unusual families whose "abnormal" child's behavior, finallly, brings them to the breaking point – not just a single violent incident but to that point, mentioned above, when violence continues unchecked by internal and external constraints.* In the cases under consideration, we have the extreme instance of violence against one's own children or brothers and sisters, obviously not explicable by gain. Nor could we see these as incidents of *sirnaag*, which Briggs (1975: 143–146) has explained to be the overly aggressive protection of much-loved children; however Briggs has also explained (personal communication) that a wider meaning of the term *sirnaaq* could also include self-protection, in that the mothers may have rejected the children to protect themselves from possible emotional breaks with dying, dull or removed (in hospital) children. The abused children discussed here appear to the family to be "maladapted" to successful life, but we could not explain the cases simply in terms of "selective neglect" or "ethnoeugenics" (Scheper-Hughes 1984: 545) because we know that in most cases such disadvantaged children are treated supportively and lovingly.

In their paper on "The 'Burnt Child Reaction' Among Yukon Delta Eskimos," (1978) Boyer and his co-authors attempt to demonstrate that Eskimos never form really trusting binds with others, even within the family, because of a period of institutionalized severe teasing and "rejection" at about the time of weaning. While I do not believe this to be quite as severe as they claim, it does accord well with the fact that under certain and generally rare circumstances, close and mutually satisfying relationships may be inverted (*mumiktuk* ) into unchecked abuse and violenc from which other parties draw back and allow a downhill course which may end in death.

Jean Briggs is the only other ethnographer I know who has attempted to deal with the complexity, and the ambiguous elements in the relation between Inuit aggression and child-rearing (see especially Briggs 1970, 1975, 1978). While Briggs concurs that the expression of strong emotions, particularly aggression is rare and frowned upon by Eskimos, she also shows at length that aggression to the point of frightening or hurting a child is built into the displays of love which are a normal part of child rearing. This partially supports the statements of Boyer, *et. al* (1978) that parental (and other) relationships are emotionally ambivalent to an unusually high degree. "They are ambivalent about forming close attachments to people, including children." (Briggs 1975: 157). Briggs describes in detail how openly loving relationships are established between parents (and others) and children. Often, but not always, these expressions are accompanied by threats (of violence, death or abandonment) or direct pain (biting, squeezing), but what she does not discuss are instances of violence towards children unaccompanied by expressions of love such as the very rare cases with which we are concerned here. She concludes that there is a "fusion of affection with aggression" in which aggression is masked by affection, and, argues that this kind of behavior "is instrumental in maintaining the non-violent patterns of aggression management in these Eskimo societies." (*idem*) When Inuit are confronted with hostile feelings, their early socialization allows them to transform anger into more benign emotions; however, the same socialization seems to allow for the inverse, as when ordinary tender feelings (for pets, children, vunerable individuals) can, under certain circumstances, be transformed to violent aggression.

## CONCLUSIONS

Briggs (1975) was dealing with two communities in which aggression was well-managed, in which she recounts no severe cases of child-abuse, nor of inter-adult violence, though the latter was known and greatly feared by her informant population. Obviously the present paper is of a wider scope (dealing with a greater number of communities through a slightly longer time period) as it includes several cases of child abuse and considers a context which includes inter-adult violence. In other words, we are concerned with situations in which the usual "non-violent patterns of aggression management" have broken down.

The general structural pattern can be seen: social relationships, including those with animals and the spiritual world, are contracts. When both parties are performing to the expectation of the other, the relationship is smooth, and each party treats the other benignly. When one party feels that their expectations are not being met, they feel resentment, but hide their emotions except perhaps for a slight "withdrawal", hoping that the problem will go away and there will be a return to unstressed "normality" (whether the other party is another adult, a child, an animal, or a white person). In all cases the failure to bring the problem out into the open, except perhaps through tentative teasing or joking, is because the Inuit know that outright breaking of the contract would be irrevocable: there is no forgetting and no one else will intervene . . . an open break leads to a reversal, *mumiktuk*, and consequences that are out of control.

However, the situations which result in violence are not equal for the various categories of *alter* in the implied contracts. In decreasing order we may state: animals are always subjected to violence when hunted, and the behavior of the animal is not the source of the frustration which results in the violence – if anything it is hunger and the needs for skins, sinew, bones and ivory which drive the Inuit to kill, though indeed hunting an animal may be frustrating. Such "violence" (successful hunting) produces satisfaction and occasionally pity for a young, small or weak animal. With pets, often young birds or animals brought in for children to play with, tender feelings are present *along with aggression* which invariably ends in the death of the pet: they may be poked, crushed, kicked, burned or pulled to pieces by children with encouragement and laughter by adults. The pets themselves engender little frustration by their behavior, but obviously pose no threat of retribution either. Briggs has pointed out (1978: 78-80) that there is a further complication: not only are children taught to derive pleasure from being cruel to and even killing animals, but that from the child's point of view the child stands to the pet animal as the mother (parent) does to the child. Thus, at the subconscious level the relationship of the parent to the child may be seen as fraught with ambivalence or even fear of violence, even in the majority situation where the violence does not take place.

Dogs, as Briggs (*op. cit.*) and many others have stated, are much more "human" for the Inuit. They are known by individualizing names, "belong" to families, and are fed, and many stories place dogs as transforming into human beings, or even as the original ancestors of human beings. Dogs are also somewhat human in that they have "sense" (*isuma*) and can learn from threat and punishment to behave and obey. Dogs also generate a lot of frustration for their failure to behave properly and are frequently the targets of aggression to "teach them a lesson", at least in the Inuit mind. Briggs and I and other analysts have also suggested that the violence shown towards dogs may be a "frustration-aggression-displacement" when the Inuit take it out on dogs because of frustrations engendered in the human or ecological spheres, especially since the dogs do not pose a threat of retaliation.

Aggression between adults is most feared, because cultural and personal experience shows that once started, the threat of retaliation and of great violence is ever present. Violence between adults, particularly men, used to be very common between Inuit, though it had become rather rare in those areas subject to Christianity and greater economic stability. Frustration levels between adults have been lowered, due to the lessening of jealousies, mainly between men over women, and because outright starvation had ceased to be a factor in the area under consideration since the late 1950s.

Children are almost considered "sacred" in Inuit society and, next to the supernatural – pre-Christian and Christian – are not the object of expressed anger and aggression. Indeed, children are closely connected with the supernatural, in that at birth they receive a "name-soul" (*atiq*) of a recently deceased relative or camp-mate. Many ethnographic reports state that the Inuit believe that to punish a child would be like hurting your own relative or friend, and some even feared that hitting a child might knock the recently reincarnated sould out of it. Thus, in the cases under consideration, the parents and family members must have been under extreme degrees of frustration to abuse their children for not growing up "properly." Nevertheless, as Briggs has stated, all love is tinged with aggression; and these two related emotions are both part of the Inuit personality, though control of the former over the latter is exercised most completely in relations with children, and least in relation to animals.

The Inuit do not believe that all children should necessarily be treated equally. When a growing child fails in the implicit contract, to a level which is determined by each particular family, the love and caring, and respect can all too quickly turn to hatred, violence, and "giving-up" on the child.

## NOTES

1. Paatauyuk was not an orphan; his mother, a relative, still lived in the village, but his father was in hospital. His mother frequently came to visit. Irniguluk and his older sister were also adopted, as Ataataluk had no children with his second wife Arngnakallak.
2. In the same year I wrote a paper called "Inuariat [The Murders]" in the form of a play, which I have never published in spite of changing all the names. However, short excerpts were included in my published paper "Eskimo Law in the Light of Self- and Group-Interest" *Law and Society Review* 6: 1: 45–60, 1969.
3. In making inquiries about comparable data on this rare phenomenon, I have been told that Inuit and Canadian authorities are presently very concerned with the relatively high incidence of child abuse, perhaps of a different type from my own data, among the contemporary Canadian Inuit.
4. Paatauyuk went to stay in another household for the rest of the visit to the community and still lived elsewhere at the time of a later visit. However, he was the "schlemiel" of the village, always suffering from dire accidents.

## ACKNOWLEDGEMENTS

My gratitude is extended to the following people who have generously discussed their opinions and their data with me in the course of preparing this paper: Lee Guemple, University of Western Ontario; Louis-Jacques Dorais, Université Laval; John O'Neil, University of Manitoba; David Damas, MacMaster University; George and Janet Diveky and Mike Kusugak of

Rankin Inlet, N.W.T. Their contributions have enabled me to present more confirmatory data and have clarified some of the points in the discussion. However, their cases have on purpose been intermingled with my own without regard to settlement and region, in order to ensure strict anonymity and make discovery of personnel as difficult as possible. I am particularly indebted to Dr. Nancy Scheper-Hughes who not only invited me to present my long-hidden data on this topic, but provided thorough guidance and criticism in the analysis of the topic, and to Dr. Jean Briggs of Memorial University, Newfoundland, who spent many hours discussing the data and the analysis at various stages of drafting this paper.

## REFERENCES

Boyer, L.B. et al.
  1978 'The "Burnt Child Reaction" Among the Yukon Delta Eskimos' Journal of Psychological Anthropology 1: 1: 7–56.
Briggs, J.
  1970 Never in Anger: Portrait of an Eskimo Family. Cambridge: Harvard University Press.
  1972 'Issues in Autonomy and Aggression in the Three-year-old: the Utku Eskimo Case.' Seminars in Psychiatry 4 (4): 317–330.
  1975 'The Origins of Non-violence: Aggression in Two Canadian Eskimo Communities.' Psychoanalytic Study of Society 6: 134–203.
  1978 'The Origins of Nonviolence: Inuit Management of Aggression (Canadian Arctic).' pp. 54–93 in Ashley Montagu (ed.), Learning Non-Aggression. New York: Oxford University Press.
Graburn, N.H.H.
  1960 'The Social Organization of an Eskimo Community.' Department of Anthropology, McGill University, Montreal, P.Q. M.A. Thesis.
  1964 Taqagmiut Eskimo Kinship Terminology Ottawa: Northern Coordination and Research Centre, NCRC-64–1.
  1969a Eskimos Without Igloos: Social and Economic Development in Sugluk. Boston: Little, Brown.
  1969b 'Eskimo Law in the Light of Self- and Group-Interest.' Law and Society Review 6: 1: 45–60.
Guemple, L.
  1979a 'Inuit Socialization: A Study of Children as Social Actors in an Eskimo Community.' pp. 39–53. In K. Ishwaran (ed.), Childhood and Adolescence in Canada. Toronto: McGraw-Hill Ryerson.
  1979b Inuit Adoption. Ottawa: National Museum of Man, Mercury Series, Canadian Ethnology Service Paper #47.
Holm, Gustav
  1886 'Konebaads-Expeditionen til Gronlands Ostkyst 1883–85.' Geografisk Tidskrift 8: 79–98.
Schechter, E.
  1983 'Alcohol Rationing and Control Systems in Greenland.' Paper delivered at the annual meetings of the American Anthropological Association, Chicago.
Scheper-Hughes, N.
  1984 'Infant Mortality and Infant Care: Cultural and Economic Constraints on Nurturing in Northeast Brazil.' Social Science and Medicine. 19: 5: 535–546.

Steffanson, Vilhjalmur
1929 My Life with the Eskimos. New York: Macmillan.
Thalbitzer, William
1941 'The Ammassalik Eskimo.' Part II. Meddelelser om Gronland. 40: 530–739.
Turner, Lucien M.
1894 Ethnology of the Ungava District. Washington, D.C.: Bureau of American Ethnology, 11th Annual Report. pp. 167–350.

MARCELO M. SUAREZ-OROZCO

# THE TREATMENT OF CHILDREN IN THE "DIRTY WAR": IDEOLOGY, STATE TERRORISM AND THE ABUSE OF CHILDREN IN ARGENTINA

*DEDICATION*
To the memory of Juan Carlos Anzorena

## INTRODUCTION

This chapter explores the treatment of children in the context of the political developments that occurred in the Argentine Republic during the second half of the 1970s.[1] In the following pages we analyze the use, abuse and meaning of children during the so called 'dirty war.' An aim of the chapter is to identify the socio-atmospheric conditions in which state sponsored abuse of children became an intrinsic part of the political discourse of the *de facto* military regime which ruled Argentina at the time.

The questions we wish to explore include how were the children of suspected "subversives" treated by the Security Forces during the 'dirty war'? Specifically, how were children used, and abused, in the chambers of torture which flourished in Argentina during the second half of the seventies? What was the particular value of children in the context of the engulfing madness? How does the treatment of children in such contexts illuminate a recurring agenda for social consensus through pain? Indeed, Foucault's (1979) curious assertion to the contrary notwithstanding, torture is still very much alive today throughout the world, maintaining prominence in the politics of social consensus [see for example Amnesty International 1984, 1973; Bacry and Ternisien 1980; Ruthven 1978; Vidal-Naquet 1963; Mellor 1961].

An analysis of the instrumental and expressive exploitation of children will take us to the very depths of an eerie universe inhabited by the torturer, the "subversive" and his/her children. In the chambers of the condemned the torturers, armed with electrical prods and other instruments of social consensus, discovered the value of children in the family unit. We shall explore how this social unit of the Argentine society was assaulted and manipulated by the politicians of pain. We shall emphasize that to gain a better understanding of the meaning of the atrocities which occurred, we must consider the "practical" or instrumental as well as the "symbolic" or expressive aspects of the rituals enacted in the Argentine halls of death.

The abuse of children during the nightmare years of the 'dirty war' was tied to the establishment of an elaborate machinery of repression, torture and death. Therefore, in order to *understand and contextualize child abuse as one expression of political violence in Argentina*, we must turn to a consideration,

227

*Nancy Scheper-Hughes (ed.), Child Survival, 227–246.*

albeit brief, of the dynamics of the 'dirty war' and the place of torture within it. A peculiar ritual devised by those running the Argentine death machinery was the torture of children in full view of their parents, or vice versa. We shall explore the meaning of such specific forms of torture. Each time an agent discharges an electrical current through the body of an infant in front of his/her parents, or through the penis or vagina of "subversives," in front of their children, a perverse poly-semantic ritual is enacted. These rituals can be explored as meaningful "texts" telling a horror story about our times.

Our task here is to decode the messages, both hidden and overt, in the historical rediscovery of torture in the Argentine chambers of death. In these ghastly texts, children emerge as valuable commodities to be strategically exploited in a demented 'dirty war' fought between the Security Forces and their phantom, demonic enemies.

THE SOCIO-HISTORICAL SETTING: THE PATH TO THE 'DIRTY WAR'

In the 1970s the Argentine Republic began writing one of the darkest chapters in modern Latin American history. The first half of that decade was characterized by increasing terrorist violence against military and police officers, government officials, diplomats, journalists, industrialists and intellectuals. The Argentine economy was collapsing. Extreme inflation rates made the Argentine *peso* a worthless currency. Unemployment soared. Labor unrest and strikes were daily occurrences. The National University of Buenos Aires became increasingly politicized, losing much of its prestige as a great institution for higher learning.

By the late sixties and early seventies high-ranking members of the military and police hierarchies were kidnapped and/or assassinated in ultra-leftist terrorist operations almost weekly. For example, the chief of the Federal Police, Comisario Villar, a man with as much protection as any head of state, was killed by a bomb that exploded in his boat as he was quietly fishing one week-end. Ex-president [*de facto*] General Aramburo, was kidnapped and executed by a terrorist group, the so-called *Montoneros*, a seemingly unique blend of ultra-leftist internationalist and nationalist Peronists. The heads of major international companies in Buenos Aires were also targets of ultra-leftist terrorist attacks. In one such case the head of FIAT Buenos Aires, an Italian executive was kidnapped by a group of young terrorists in a dramatic operation. He was held for ransom for months and was eventually killed. The *Montoneros* also kidnapped a most influential agro-industrial family, the Born brothers and extracted a reported 60 million dollars for their freedom.

By the early 1970s ultra-rightist paramilitary organizations such as the 'Asociación Anticomunista Argentina' [AAA], began to systematically produce their own brand of terror. Union leaders were executed mid-day in downtown Buenos Aires. Leftists politicians were assassinated in one spectacular operation after another. World renowned academics, such as Professor

Silvio Frondisi, a self-described "theoretical Marxist" and brother of the constitutional ex-president of the Republic, Arturo Frondisi, was kidnapped and executed in public. Journalists also became targets of fire from both the ultra-right and the ultra-left.

In brief, members of all sectors of the society were vulnerable to random flying bullets. The state could no longer monopolize the use of violence. The atmosphere of fear was like a thick fog. No one could feel safe, exempted. The killing became ever more pointless. Bodyguards were in high demand. Paying bribes to terrorist groups for immunity became common practice in the industrial sector. As Timerman reports "monthly sums were paid by companies to right-wing and left-wing organizations simultaneously to assure that their executives wouldn't be assassinated or kidnapped" (1981: 19).

The chaos reached its peak in early 1976 at the hands of Maria Estela ['Isabelita'] Martinez de Perón, then the constitutional President of the Argentine Republic. Terrorist attacks by highly dedicated and efficient groups of both ultra-leftist and ultra-rightist persuasion became daily events. The increasing discontent of the Argentine people with the *status quo*, set the stage for a military take-over of civilian institutions. When the military, promising "order," finally removed 'Isabelita' Perón from the *Casa Rosada* in March of 1976 "the entire country, including the Peronists, breathed a sigh of relief" (Timerman 1981: 26). Instead of order what ensued was one of the most brutal regimes known in a continent already noted for a long history of brutality.

The Argentine Armed Forces had not fought a war during the 20th century.[2] Historically modeled after Germanic ideals, the military has traditionally seen itself as an isolated entity of superior men entrusted with a historical duty to protect the "fatherland" from foreign and, particularly, domestic enemies. According to Timerman (*ibid.*) the degree of the military's segregation from other sectors of the society is remarkable. For example, military men, Timerman notes, would only marry women from military families. A *castelike* segregation of the military from the civilian order must be emphasized.

In the seventies, for the first time in its history, the military came under systematic and vicious attacks from highly efficient terrorist bands. It is important to keep this background in mind in order to explore the subsequent emergence of the ideological matrix in which some very grotesque crimes against humanity were committed – including assaulting children and unborn fetuses with electrical prods. For the purposes of this chapter I would like to slightly modify Elizabeth Colson's plea to anthropologists that we analyze "who can do what with whom and under what circumstances" (Colson 1985: 191) to "who can do what *to* whom and under what circumstances."

It is most likely that active and retired members of the Armed Forces organized, equipped and directed the ultra-right paramilitary groups which began to operate prior to the military take over of March 1976. This was the military's initial response to increasing attacks from the armed ultra-left.

After the March 1976 coup paramilitary gangs, known as *patotas*, began to operate much more visibly under the direct control of the security forces.

On the 24th of March, 1976 the Argentine military installed a *de facto* junta composed of the chiefs of its three branches: the Army, the Navy and the Air Force. The head of the Argentine Army, General Jorge Rafael Videla became the President of the Argentine Republic. Thus "El Proceso de Reorganización Nacional" began [The Process of National Reorganization]. In brief, the self-stated objective of the junta was to "re-organize" the Argentine nation. Their "re-organizational" agenda is of critical importance to understand the fate of families and children in the context of the 'dirty war.' We shall return to this point.

Technically the 'dirty war' against the terrorists began under the constitutional government of 'Isabelita' Perón. As President of the Republic, it was she who signed the orders to unleash military might against leftist terrorism. There is now evidence that this initial military operation against the terrorists was very efficient. In fact, soon after the March military take over leftist terrorist organizations no longer posed any serious threat to the Republic (Cabeza 1985: 170). The armed left had been defeated in the field. Yet the horror continued for years after, haunting largely innocent civilians and children. Once ignited, the technology of death and torture assumes a life of its own, ever broadening its targets beyond any original scope. [For a general consideration of the dynamics of torture growth see, Amnesty International 1973, 1984: 1–102; Bacry and Ternisien 1980; Vidal-Naquet 1963].

As the military grip on civilian institutions became increasingly formalized, a new repressive horror descended upon the Argentine consciousness. After its successful war with the armed left, the security forces turned their 'dirty war' apparatus upon as yet innocent but "potentially dangerous" civilians. What ensued was an unpredictable deployment of terror by the security forces and those working for them. Anyone thought to be sympathizing with the left, or in any way opposing the military regime became a possible target for kidnapping. The term *desaparecido* ["disappeared one"] with its unspoken connotations of death and torture, became part of the new Argentine vocabulary of sorrow. Soon everyone knew a *desaparecido*. All segments of society had become touched by the spreading terror.

Upon the return to democracy in the early 1980s, following the disastrous adventure of the Argentine military in its attempt to take over the Malvinas Islands, the Argentine people began more fully to realize the extent of the crimes committed on the name of "saving" the fatherland from leftist "subversives." Some victims who were allowed to survive told of their ordeals to the world. [For a moving account of his personal nightmare see Timerman 1981]. The Argentine people finally publicly confronted what the rest of the world had long suspected: that thousands of innocent Argentine citizens, including children, had been kidnapped, brutally tortured and ruthlessly executed without any pretense at due process of law.

The military regime had responded to terrorist attacks of the left with one of the most grotesque examples of uncontrollable repression known in recent Western history. The state-controlled terrorist machinery assumed a life of its own. Death squads became autonomous units taking full initiative in seeking out victims. Clandestine detention camps had been set up in military, police and other installations throughout the country to house and torment the kidnapped [see Amnesty International 1984: 143–145; Comisión Nacional Sobre la Desaparición de Personas 1984 and Timerman 1981].

In December of 1983 the democratically elected government of President Raúl Alfonsín responded to the public outcry of horror by creating the Comisión Nacional sobre la Desaparición de Personas [CONADEP]. Prominent Argentines became members of the CONADEP. Ernesto Sabato was appointed the commission's president. Argentine scientists, congressmen, distinguished reporters, business and industry leaders, etc., also were members of the commission.

Their objective was to systematically document the nature and extent of the repression unleashed following the military take over of 1976. For months the commission received and recorded the painful testimony of those who for one reason or another had survived the ordeal of clandestine imprisonment. However, the degree collective fear is still so pervasive that the commission believes that even under present democratic rule the *relatives* of many "disappeared" dare not come forth to relate their cases. In short, not all has yet been revealed.

The 20th of September 1985, the commission presented their report, entitled *Nunca mas* [Never Again], to President Raul Alfonsin. *Nunca Mas* is one of the important documents printed this decade. It presents a detailed, graphic view of a monstrous system for death.

The CONADEP report concluded that *at least* 8960 citizens, including 127 children remain "disappeared" and should be considered dead. (CONADEP 1984: 16). That is not counting the children that were kidnapped, systematically abused by the security forces and then returned to their relatives [see below]. I should point out that many regard the CONADEP estimate of 8960 as much too conservative. Some argue that close to 15 000 persons were disappeared. The assault on children was so systematic that the *Abuelas de la Plaza de Mayo* [Grandmothers of the Plaza de Mayo], formed to find out and make public the savagery inflicted upon children and to help locate those still missing.

Security officers rationalized the necessity of the systematic savage torture "sessions" as the only viable way to combat "leftist terrorism" in an urban setting. [see Timerman 1982; CONADEP 1984: 26–54, Amnesty International 1984: 143–145; El Diario del Juicio vol. I through XV; The Economist 1985: 37–38]. Yet, I emphasize that it is now generally agreed that most of the terrorists died in actual military confrontations with security forces, or committed suicide just prior to capture. In fact, by mid-1976 the terrorists could no longer pose a serious military threat (see Cabeza 1985: 170). In brief, the majority of those brutalized by the repression were sought out and tormented after ultra-leftist violence had been exterminated.

Many of those latter victims were professionals from "suspected occupations" such as psychologists, psychiatrists, sociologists, welfare workers and journalists judged to be "critical" of the regime [see CONADEP 1984: 293–441; Timerman 1981: 93–99]. The irony is that the military specifically sought out these professionals which Foucault (1979) considers to be the "social regulators" which replaced jailers and torturers as consensus agents in post 19th Century Europe. Foucault's model may explain the historical shift in European social control from focusing on the "body" to the "soul," but it obviously fails to account the recurrence of torture in the post-colonial world.

During the 'dirty war' attorneys working of behalf of "disappeared" persons, themselves were made to "disappear" [CONADEP 1984: 416–424]. Members of human rights groups working on behalf of "disappeared" persons, themselves "disappeared" [CONADEP 1984: 424–426]. Students and labor organizers were "disappeared." Other innocent civilians were kidnapped simply "by mistake." Dagmar Ingrid Hagelin, a 17 year old Swedish tourist was mistaken for a "subversive." She was kidnapped by security officers, tortured and then was killed. Others were picked up, tortured and "disappeared" after an anonymous call to the security forces identified them as "subversive." No questions were asked. One such a call could mean a death sentence. The randomness characterizing the 'dirty war' was the key to the establishment of a collective fear.

At the peak of the nightmare entire families were kidnapped [see CONADEP 1984; Timerman 1981]. Pregnant women were kidnapped [see CONADEP 1984: 299–323]. Old men, in some cases over 70 years old were kidnapped [see Timerman 1981: 143]. Children were kidnapped [see CONADEP, *ibid.*; Guthmann 1986: 23–24].

CHILDREN IN THE 'DIRTY WAR'

Let us turn to a more systematic exploration of the various forms of use and abuse to which children were submitted to during the so called 'dirty war.' In order to fully appreciate the meaning of the atrocities committed, as well as the contexts in which these atrocities recur, we also briefly analyze the very nature of torture. Torture today continues to play a central role in the theatrics of political and religious orthodoxy [Amnesty International 1984, 1973; Bacry and Ternisien 1980]. State sponsored torture is an old and widespread phenomena [see for example Mellor 1961; Tomas y Valiente 1973; Ruthven 1978; Foucault 1979]. We will explore the meaning of the torturers assault on children and the family unit in the context of the "re-organizational" fantasies of the *Reorganización Nacional* junta. After delineating the anatomy of terror, and its uses for social control, we turn to explore the ideological blue-print by means of which the atrocities occurred. In certain historical contexts and armed with totalizing ideological agendas human beings have shown themselves to be capable treating other human beings most atrociously. Yet to understand the degree of the madness created in the Argentine torture chambers, we need to explore how a collective delusion could be mobilized in the creation, and subsequent exorcism, of the demonic "subversive." Finally, we turn to a consideration of the instrumental aspects of state sponsored terrorism and abuse as a form of political discourse.

Alicia B. Morales de Galanba related the following case to the CONADEP:

I lived in Mendoza with my children, Paula Natalia and Mauricio. They were a year and a half and two months old. My friend, Maria Luisa Sanchez de Vargas and her two children Josefina, a five year old, and Soledad, a one and a half year old, also lived with us.

On the 12th of June, 1976 at about 11PM, Maria Luisa and I were in the kitchen when we heard knocks and suddenly saw our kitchen invaded by a group of men. Before we could even realize what was going on, they beat us to the floor and blind-folded us. With all the screaming and noise, the children woke up and began crying frantically. The men searched and destroyed each room of the house. As they proceeded, they repeatedly asked me where my husband was. They would also stop and click their weapons as if they were going to kill us. The terror was already within us and would not let me breath. It was a terror that grew with the crying of the little children, increasingly more dementing.

When we could Maria Luisa and I took the children in our arms and tried to calm them down. After about twenty minutes or so, they took us out of the house and shoved us in to a car, probably a Ford. They took us to a place I was later to recognize as Mendoza's Police Headquarters. They put us in an empty room and they took away my two month old baby, Mauricio. I felt that my world was collapsing. I did not wish to live. I soon stopped even crying. I threw my self in the floor and remained in a fetal position. After several hours they returned my two month old baby, Mauricio. Slowly I began to recuperate. For the next two days we kept all four children with us. Josefina and Paula could not tolerate being locked up. They cried constantly, kicking the door, and asking the jailer to let us go.

Then one of the jailers took Josefina [the five year-old] away. Again we felt aware of the terror. We did not know what they wanted to do with the little girl. About two hours later they returned her to us. Josefina told us that they had taken her to the bus terminal to identify people. A while after they came by and took all four children away from us. Eventually the children were taken back to their respective grandparents. After that, they separated Maria Luisa and I, though we were both kept at the same installation. One day the jailer told me that they were going to bring Maria Luisa to my cell. I was happy that I would see her again, although I feared what I would see.

Indeed Maria Luisa was another person. The pain she had suffered made her age. She told me in tears that through a prostitute she was able to see her husband, Jose Vargas, soon after we had been separated. He is now disappeared. When they saw each other Jose told his wife that their daughter, Josefina, was taken to witness a torture session. They had made her witness his torture so that he would talk. This must have been between the 12th and 14th of June, after they took Josefina from our cell. But Maria Luisa's story did not end there. What I heard next was so horrible that even today I feel like I felt then, that of all the tragedies a person may live through, nothing could be worse than this . . . Maria Luisa next told me that a few days before, she was taken to her parents house, in San Juan. She said that she really thought that it was to give her parents the pleasure of seeing that she was alive and to make her renew contact with her girls. Then she said: "But no, instead they took me to a funeral. And you know whose? It was the funeral of my daughter, Josefina," the five year old. When Maria Luisa asked her father, Dr.

Sanchez Sarmiento, a federal attorney, how such a thing happened, he told her that a few days after arriving to their house, the girl took a weapon from her grandfather's drawer and shot herself. [CONADEP 1984: 319-320]

During the years of terror after March of 1976 the children of those who were suspected of "subversive activities" became victims of brutal and systematic abuse. Today 127 children remain "unaccounted for," or in the Argentine vocabulary of terror, *desaparecidos* [see CONADEP 1984: 299–323]. Other children were kidnapped, brutalized and then returned to relatives. As in Josefina's case, the children were often picked up by security officers in the course of capturing the parents [see Slavin 1985: 1–7]. In some cases, if lucky, the children were allowed to remain behind, at times to stay at home all alone through the night. In other cases children were taken to a neighbor who was told to keep them and to keep quiet. Other children died in captivity [see CONADEP 1984: 99–323].

Children became very valuable pawns in the psychotic war that engulfed Argentina into the early 1980s. There is widespread evidence that children were brought into torture sessions to witness how a parent was tortured with electro-shocks, drowning, burning, etc., (CONADEP 1984: 99–323). This is what they did to Josefina, a five year old. She could only erase the atrocities she witnessed by killing herself soon after witnessing the grotesque spectacle involving her father.

Children were tortured in front of the parents commonly to make the adults "talk," sign a confession, or to implicate others in "subversive activities." CONADEP reports a number of such cases [see CONADEP 1984: 20 and 299–323]. The torture of small children, particularly in front of their parents, had been systematic. For example, a doctor who was detained and put to work in a military hospital reported that a renown torturer was very interested in finding out from medical experts how big would a child need to be to survive systematic electric shocks. The torturer asked a military physician, another renown torturer, "how much should a child weigh before we can torture him. Vidal [the Doctor] responded 'after 25 kilos you can run electrical charges through their bodies.'" [El Diario de Juicio 1985: (vol. 12) p. 4]. The Argentine agents of death by no means hold monopoly over the political tormenting of children. For example, Amnesty International's eerie document *Torture in the Eighties* (1984) reports that state sponsored torture of children has been reported in both El Salvador (1984: 155-156) and in Iraq (1984: 99).

In Argentina, family torture sessions were not uncommon [see CONADEP 1984: 20; Timerman 1981: 148–149]. For example, a man reports that after answering a number of questions negatively, security officers began brutally kicking and hitting with a belt his wife and their children, a 13 year old, an 8 year old, and a 3 year old who were witnessing the inferno. Then, he said, the officers turned to their 20 day old daughter and, to their horrified disbelief, they started shaking her violently and holding her head down by her feet, yelling "if you don't talk, we'll kill her." Next they filled the tub with water and submerged the mother several times, drowning her in front of her children (CONADEP 1984: 320).

The children were used for other instrumental purposes. For example, Josefina, a five year old, was taken by the torturers to a bus terminal to identify friends and acquaintances of her parents' (CONADEP 1984: 323). In other words, children were used as "informants" to single out "subversives" to be picked up and tormented. It was apparently easier to make the children "cooperate" after showing them how their parents were tortured.

In other cases children were used as "bait" by the security forces to entrap other "subversives." For example, Fernando, a 13 year old boy, was used to single out friends of his parents. He was then ordered by his captors to set up meeting with two friends of his parents. At that meeting the friends were kidnapped by security forces in front of the boy [see CONADEP 1984: 324].

The abuse of children was thus theatrically organized to force information out of the parents, to have the parents admit to "subversion," and/or to have them sign confessions. In other cases, children became innocent tools in the reproduction of terror. Actively working to capture "subversives" is one such example. The mechanism seemed to work effectively and was based on the fact that the children were induced to expect that by cooperating they would earn their parents' freedom or at least better treatment for them. The scene was so morbid that there are reports that older children, particularly girls, would try to seduce guards in hope that their parents would be treated less brutally (Timerman 1981: 149). Seldom, if ever, did such sexual "favors" result in better treatment.

The instrumental exploitation of children went beyond the immediate "war-related" scenario. Children of *desaparecidos*, particularly babies, were commonly taken as "war booty" [see Chavez 1985a: 19–20; El Diario del Juicio 1985 (vol. 11): 254]. An Uruguayan woman, whose husband and nursing infant disappeared, related:

The 13th of July, 1976 between 11 and 11:30PM, they knocked on the door of our home in Barrio Belgrano in this Capital [Buenos Aires]. At that moment I was breast feeding my baby, Simon. They broke down the door and about 10 to 15 people, in civilian clothing, identified themselves as members of the Argentine Army and the Uruguayan Army. One of the officers introduced himself as Major Gavazzo of the Uruguayan Army. They searched the home and they found written materials which showed them that I worked for the cause of freedom in my country [Uruguay]; then they began torturing me. When they took me away, I asked them what would happen to my baby. They told me that I should not worry about that that they would keep him . . . That was the last time I saw Simon. [CONADEP 1984: 20].

Simon was probably sold in a lucrative black market or placed with a sterile military or upper class couple. The moving film entitled *La historia oficial* treats the plight of a child so "adopted" into an upper middle class family. And the documentary "Las Madres: The Mothers of the Plaza de Mayo," considers the pain of a group of mothers who silently marched around the national plaza for the last 7 years, demanding to know the fate of their sons and daughters who were "disappeared" during the 'dirty war.'

Thus the torturers discovered and manipulated the value of children as the *priceless cathected appendix of the "subversive."* Children became a commodity to be exploited for information in the halls of death and were subsequently placed with families sympathetic to the regime. Yet before a child could be placed with a "proper" family the torturers deemed necessary to radically severe his/her bonds with the "contaminated subversive." Thus assaulting children with electrical prods *in the presence of their parents* should be seen as serving both instrumental and expressive aims.

We have already explored the instrumental aspects of the abuse. Expressively torturing children, or torturing parents in front of the children, can also be seen as a *ritual of separation* in which the torturers proceed to "surgically remove" with electrical prods the subversive's precious "appendix" before turning him/her to a security or upper class family for proper Christian upbringing. We shall return to the implications of this in the following section.

The magnitude of the children's market was such that upon return to democracy the "Grandmothers of the Plaza de Mayo" contacted a number of scientists from the Massachusetts Institute of Technology, the University of California, etc., to identify disappeared children through studies establishing the genetic relatedness between a child and his or her biological relatives [see Slavin 1985: 1–7]. Neighbors who saw a childless couple "adopt" a child under obscure circumstances during the 'dirty war' years are now encouraged to come forth to denounce them.

Pregnant women were treated like all other "subversives." That is they were routinely tortured and often raped [see CONADEP 1984: 299–323]. Some military men eventually were compelled to confess crimes [see also Victor 1981]. A sergeant told the CONADEP that "as a nurse he worked at the Hospital Campo de Mayo [a military installation] between 1976 and 1977. He reported that in the epidemiology wing of the hospital there were a number of pregnant women about to give birth. Their hands and feet were tied and they were given serum to accelerate the delivery. The nurse himself saw four or five women in this condition. He thought they were extremists . . ." (CONADEP 1984: 308–309). He also reported that a guard named Falcon had raped a number of pregnant women (ibid).

Pregnant women, or their husbands, were made to "talk" by placing electric prods inside them, close to the uterus, to discharge electrical currents on the fetus. For example, one pregnant woman who survived her calvary reported that she was brutally tortured during the sixth month of her pregnancy. Subsequent to her release she gave birth to an abnormal child diagnosed as having brain damage (CONADEP 1984: 317–318).

In other cases, the strategy was to keep the mother alive until the birth of her child. The babies were then taken away from the mothers to be sold or placed with sterile couples. The mother could then be executed [see Slavin 1985: 1–7]. The military would fabricate illegal birth certificates, almost always signed by military physicians, in order to place a child with a new couple. Schools are now alerted to report any suspicious birth certificates, particularly if signed by a military physician (*ibid.*)[3]

## THE BODY, CHILDREN AND THE 'RE-ORGANIZATION' OF SOCIETY

The difficult question of why entire families and specifically children entered the stage of terror as key protagonists requires further elaboration. Any satisfactory explanation should relate to both the instrumental and the expressive nature of a terrorist act.

On the instrumental level we have documented how children emerged as priceless commodities to be fully exploited in the politics of pain. Directly torturing a child, or torturing a parent in front of a child, seemed to be a facile way to elicit information from a "subversive." It is much harder to explore the possible symbolic dimensions of the politics of torture. Structural-functional social anthropologists would be quick to point out that the assault on children represents an assault on the generativity and reproduction of the social order itself. Yet this interpretation does not convincingly explain the *specifics* of the spectacle involved. Why not just shoot the children? Why not eliminate them at once following capture? Why were the children tortured? Specifically why were they tortured *in the presence of their parents*? Why were there so many family torture session? Why were so many children *not* killed but rather placed elsewhere, with "proper" families?

A partial answer to *why children* can be explored in the context of the stated wishes of many high ranking officers in charge of the operation. In fact, there are a number of printed reports [see CONADEP 1984: 20] that high ranking officers of the security forces did specifically tell their men that *the war was not on the children* and that children should *not* be taught to grow up to hate the flag and the armed forces [See El Diario del Juicio 1985 vol. v]. Rather, their expressed wishes were that the children be *removed* from the "subversives" and placed in "proper" homes. When a desperate mother asked her tormenters what they would do with her nursing infant as he was being taken away, one said "The war is not on children, we'll keep him" (CONADEP 1984: 20).

Yet we have documented that children of suspected "subversives" were systematically abused regardless of the "official policy." We have also argued that any specific act of torture can be analyzed as a cultural and psychological metamessage conveying a multitude of meanings. I thus argue that the symbolics of political pain underlined the destructive *and re-organizational* agenda on the military operation.

The assault on children and the calculated collective spectacles of torture in which entire families participated are literalization of the military's fantasy of "re-organizing" the Argentine social landscape. The agenda for re-organizing the social landscape was at the heart of why the children had to be removed from "subversive" homes and placed elsewhere. The collective torture session themselves are viewed as a *rite de separation* (Van Gennep 1960). Before a child could be placed with a military or an upper class family for a good Christian education all ties with his/her tainted family had to be severed. Thus collective rituals of pain flourished before placing a child with an acceptable family. A sort of "ideological surgery" was required to sever all bonds.

Indeed, the entire military operation had a very noted re-organizational tone. The very term "Proceso de Reorganización Nacional" under which the military organized its campaign forcefully conveys this imagery. The entire nation needed a "re-organization" according to the military. The assault on children and the family unit represents a most perverse translation of this fantasy of control and the "re-organization" of life through death.

## TERROR AS SOCIAL CONTROL

Thus was forged what Taussig and others have appropriately termed a "culture of terror" (see Taussig 1984: 467–497; Fagen 1985). Thousands of Argentines "were disappeared" by security officers. The term came to capture the power of collective terror as brutal social control. Introducing the word *desaparecido* even in the security of a family discussion, produced a chilling effect. The relatives of *desaparecidos* often knew that a loved one was taken by the security forces. The term itself encouraged a form of pre-rational, magical thinking: just as a son or daughter magically "disappeared" one day, they could so "reappear" another. The networks of horror operated on what soon became a sacred currency, silence. Relatives were often contacted by the captors. Yet these contacts remained in closed secrecy. Money and possessions were extracted from relatives of "disappeared" ones [see CONADEP 1984: 22–23], sometimes even after the *desaparecido* had been killed.

In some cases the *desaparecido* was allowed to talk to his or her relatives, usually over the telephone or through an intermediary. Expectations that the end of the nightmare was possible were thus implanted in the hearts and minds of relatives. The message was monothematic: "be quiet," "don't talk to anyone or for sure she or he will be killed." *Collective silence thus became part of the madness as if it intervened in the causality of events*. Families of *desaparecidos* came to believe that should the rumor begin that a son or daughter was "disappeared," it would mean certain death. In truth, people died regardless of the code of strict silence.

Psychologically it is very hard to mourn without a corpse. Death, in the abstract, can never be as convincing as the body of a loved one. Without concrete evidence of death, there is always hope. Thus the networks of terror and control were firmly established. A collective hysterical denial permeated the atmosphere. In the midst of the horror, many people let themselves believe that there were some minor "abuses," but only of those who were "implicados en algo" [involved in something]. How otherwise could they live with the knowledge that members of the security forces were torturing even children and pregnant women? Such reports were dismissed as part of an exaggerated "international propaganda campaign" against Argentina.

The code of silence was fostered by other fears. To have a *desaparecido* in the family was like having a contagious disease. Life-long friends broke relationships for fear of being caught in the madness. They of course were active participants in the madness. A major fear was that should a person's name be in the private telephone book of a *desaparecido*, that name would become a target. Indeed, many other innocent people were thus recruited to the stage of terror.

## THE IDEOLOGICAL BLUE-PRINT FOR TERROR: PARANOIA AND THE EXORCISM OF INVENTED DEMONS

Terror emerged from the wings and took center stage in a vehement political discourse. The operation was firmly framed on an ideological blue-print. Officers of the Armed Forces saw themselves fighting the final battle for the purest values of the Christian and occidental ethic [see Timerman 1981; El Diario del Juicio 1985 (vols. 4 and 15)].

The paranoid ethos which permeated the operation is unmistakable. According to those responsible for the atrocities, Argentina was the epicenter of a global, final attack on the Western way of life. Children were part of this global plot. If not removed from the polluting "subversive" atmosphere they too could be shaped into godless subversives. The irrational nature of the beliefs is obvious. A Zionist, KGB plot, financed by the American CIA was thought to be behind the terrorist push to finally take over Argentina [see Timerman 1981]. Argentina became a world strategic center for the imminent outbreak of World War III. As Timerman noted: "The Argentine military tapped their vast reservoir of hatred and fantasy so as to synthesize their action into one basic concept: World War III had begun; to enemy was left-wing terrorism; and Argentina was the initial battleground chosen by the enemy" (1981: 101). Terrorist attacks were not seen in a regional frame, but rather a grander script was soon prepared. A historical pattern was sketched out. For example, according to General Viola, the second *de facto* President of the "Proceso de Reorganización Nacional," the country was the victim of an "international Marxist aggression which began to [concentrate on Argentina] at the end of the second World-War." [El Diario del Juicio 1985 (vol. 15): 349].

All atrocities were framed in the context of saving Argentina from the evils of a godless, alien Marxist "infiltration." But the mission was greater than Argentina. The final battle for the Western soul was being fought with electrical prods in the halls of death. The antisemitic nature of the crusade has been treated in some detail by Timerman (1981). In a Kafkaesque dialogue between Timerman and his torturers we get a glance at "political hallucinations" (Timerman 1981: 96) which inflicted the agents of death. The final plot against Argentina was headed by an improbable, comical mixture of Zionist-Marxists working under the guidance of the Soviet KGB and Washington power brokers. The first part of the international plan was to take over Patagonia to create the "Republic of Andina."

Timerman's torturers asked him: "We'd like to know further details on the Andina Plan. How many troops would the State of Israel be prepared to send?" (1981: 73) to invade Argentina! As the torturers explained to Timerman, the final attack on Argentina was orchestrated by three power centers unified by international Jewish solidarity. Israel, in collaboration with "the United States, where Jewish power is evident" And "the Kremlin [which] is still dominated by the same sectors that staged the Bolshevik Revolution, in which Jews played the principal role" (ibid. 73–74) were operating together to invade Southern Argentina, which would eventually function as the food and oil basket in the war to come.

All means were adequate in this momentous crusade. If in order to extract the formidably important name of an "international subversive" it was required to discharge electrical currents through an unborn fetus, so be it. They were saving the western family from a materialistic infection threatening the fatherland. Such perverse reversals characterized much of the operation. If this notable mission required extracting precious information regarding the imminent international invasion from a "subversive" by torturing their children, so be it. The future generations of Argentina were at risk. If the mission required that the small child of a "subversive" witness a torture session to extract key information on the unfolding of history, so be it. Expressively this mad behavior gave to those practicing it a self-righteous view of themselves as sharing with others the sacred mission of saving the fatherland.

### THE ASSAULT ON LIFE: TORTURE AND CHILD ABUSE AS POLITICAL DISCOURSE

Instrumentally torture became an intrinsic part of the military's political mission. Prisoners were routinely tortured before and during interrogation, before execution or before re-gaining freedom. In other cases people were tortured and let go free *without ever been interrogated*. The human body became the canvas in which the "anatomists of pain" (Foucault 1979: 11) dramatized an ancient discourse on power and orthoxy. Indeed a new inquisition was unleashed. The Christian and occidental way of life was to be saved by finally removing all atheist subversives from the landscape. The perverse medical – hygienic and surgical – imagery which accompanied the crusade again point to the paranoid atmosphere that emerged in the midst of the 'dirty war.' An infection had penetrated and was growing, spreading throughout the "fatherland." A 'dirty' war was required to "cleanse" the country of political contamination. Indeed, political killings were commonly referred to as "cleanings." "Los vamos a limpiar" [we will clean you], was a common phrase out of the lips of the torturers. In fact, "limpiar" [to clean] means to kill in Argentine slang, just as "to waste" does in American English slang. It took a 'dirty' war to *limpiar* Argentina.

This imagined growth required radical surgical and hygienic intervention. The enemy must be completely extirpated from the fatherland. The new inquisition was thus framed in medical and sanitary symbolism over political orthodoxy. This metaphorical system also helps explain the prominent role physicians played during the 'dirty war.' In fact, many survivors reported that often during torture sessions, a military or police physician would came in, take their vital signs and proceed to inform the torturers whether to continue torturing, or whether to give the "patient" a break. In fact the torture chambers themselves were known as the *quirofano*, or the "operating room."

The extermination took a very specific, indeed patterned, tone. Again, I argue that we must explain the torture, as well as the *specific* forms the torture took. Torture is never merely an instrumental act. Even when it is routine, as it certainly was in Argentina, each time a torturer discharges an electrical current through his prisoner's body, they become intimate partners in a poly-semantic ritual.

The expressive symbolism of torture is of fundamental importance to explore the unconscious agenda of the torturer. The phallus of men was routinely assaulted with electricity. The castration metaphor is unmistakable. In clandestine *quirofanos* the ideological surgeons thus emasculated godless "subversives", *turning the feared enemy into passive, castrated beings*. The *macho* army men were turning "dangerous subversives," who had given them so much anxiety, indeed for the first time genuine fear, into harmless eunuchs. In the torturer's mind assaulting the penis was always related to the masculinity of their victim. For example, an "ex-torturer" reported a torture session in which an officer ordered him to systematically place the electric prods in the testicles of a victim "to see if he is such a *macho*" (Victor 1981: 67).

Women's generativity was also routinely assaulted. Running electro-shocks through the sources of life, the vagina, uterus and breasts was standard practice. Pregnant women were systematically tortured and raped [see CONADEP 1984: 309]. Systematically electrocuting the symbols of life was necessary to turn the mothers of potential dissidents into helpless beings to be sexually used and discarded. The keepers of the faith were symbolically assaulting the essence of dissident life.

The systematic electrical assault on the genitals is the kind of surgical intervention required for the society the agents of terror wished to carve out: a society of ruling *machos* and obedient, harmless *mansos*, castrated beings, that would not question orders but would just obey. This is the political agenda the repression advocated. In the halls of death, torture became the form through which they created the conforming citizens they wished to govern. In this case the body was the medium in which the "re-organizing" fantasy surfaced.

The "re-organization" of society required "re-organizing" the basic social unit, the family. The family's affective bond was manipulated in skillfull games of horror. Torturing a child may have been done to make a parent talk or sign a confession, but symbolically the torture ritual was the ultimate perversion in the universe of the pain: the surgical severing of the child from the "contaminating" subversive, to violently break the intense affective bond that makes up the Argentine family. In all modern police state – whether rightist or leftist – children are used to get at the parents; as spies, informants or to torture. *Divide et impera* is the rule of thumb. Indeed the torturers in Argentina concentrated on literally and symbolically "dividing" families.

The Argentine journalist Jacobo Timerman who himself was brutally tortured reflected on his encounters with absolute horror in several clandestine prisons. The obscenities enacted in the chambers of death produced the destruction on the units of life:

Of all the dramatic situations I witnessed in clandestine prisons, nothing can compare to those family groups who were tortured often together, sometimes separately but in view of one another, or in different cells, while one was aware of the other being tortured. The entire affective world, constructed over the years with utmost difficulty, collapses with a kick in the father's genitals, a smack on the mother's face, an obscene insult to the sister, or the sexual violation of a daughter. Suddenly an entire culture based on familial love, devotion, the capacity for mutual sacrifice collapses. Nothing is possible in such a universe, and that is precisely what the torturers know.

The fathers' glances: of desperation at first, then of apology, and then of encouragement. Seeking some way to mutually help one another – sending an apple, a glass of water. Those fathers, thrown on the ground, bleeding, endeavoring for their children to find the strength to resist the tortures still in store for them. The impotence, that impotence that arises not from one's failure to do something in defense of one's children but from one's inability to extend a tender gesture. From my cell, I'd hear the whispered voices of children trying to learn what was happening to their parents, and I'd witness the efforts of daughters to win over a guard, to arouse a feeling of tenderness in him, to incite the hope of some lovely future relationship between them in order to learn what was happening to her mother, to have an orange sent to her, to get permission for her to go to the bathroom (Timerman 1981: 148–149).

Torture and death of "subversives" was the magical treatment against the spread of an infectious way of life. To simplify their thinking and to focus energy, the armed left, the democratic left, intellectuals, artists, psychiatrists, psychologists, sociologists, children, pregnant women and other deviants were bunched together as representatives, or potential representatives, or sympathizers with an international assault penetrating the from fatherland the outside and growing, spreading within.

## CONCLUSION

In early 1985, following the return to democratic rule, and responding to a world-wide outcry over the horrors committed by the military, an unprecedented phenomena occurred in Argentina. For the first time in Latin American history, members of a prior *de facto* government were brought to civilian justice. For reasons of space, I can only briefly refer to the trail of the 9 commanders [for a full description of this trial see, El Diario del Juicio 1985]. Technically the six man court was a court-martial, although under civilian control.

At the trial the military leaders continued to hide any remorse behind the ideological shield. General Videla dismissed all accusations asserting that "terrorism is a global phenomena which will one day show that Argentina continues to be a priority target" [see El Diario del Juicio 1985 (vol. 15): 351]. The battle goes on, the invisible enemy is everywhere, because it is within. Others, either hysterically or psychopathically deny that any abuses took place and view the trial as the beginning of the end for the Christian and occidental way of life in Argentina.

These military leaders refuse to accept the legitimacy of the trial. According them "corrupted," myopic politicians and civilians lack the moral authority and strength to pass judgement on their righteous crusade against the very essence of evil. General Videla, for example, "ignores the court and reads, apparently from a book of spiritual meditations" (The Economist 1985: 38). In fact, right-wing military and paramilitary groups have already been found putting bombs to simulate a major leftist guerrilla came back, and thus create the atmosphere in which another military take over would be possible. The more recent revolts by younger officers in Campo de Mayo, Cordoba and Salta over the jurisprudence and legitimacy of civilian courts over crimes committed during the 'Dirty War' again point to the military's castelike attitude of depreciation of civilian institutions. Heuristically, it might prove fruitful to approach these new 'dirty wars' in reference not just to older models relating Latin authoritarianism to oligarcho-militaristic alliances to international interests, but also in terms of an internal structural logic of castelike stratification and depreciation of the civico-democratic order.

On the 9th of December 1985, the civilian court found five of the former top military leaders of crimes committed during the 'dirty war' [see Chavez 1985b: 1–2; Montalbano 1985: 1–2]. General Jorge Videla, President of the first junta and Admiral Emilio Massera, also a junta member were given life sentences. General Roberto Viola, President of the second military junta, received a 17 year sentence. Admiral Armando Lambruschini, the second junta's Navy representative received 8 years; and Brigadier General Orlando Agosti, head of the Air Force and member of the first junta received a four-and-a-half year sentence. Four other military heads were acquitted (Chavez 1985b: 1–2).

Although the trail is a historical event in Latin America and the world, the fact remains that a death machinery of such magnitude was not the exclusive responsibility of the top military leaders. Indeed, over 1,700 legal cases for human rights abuses are pending against other officers. Adolfo Perez-Esquivel, winner of the 1980 Nobel Peace Prize and himself a victim of the repression during the 'dirty war,' has argued that the democratic government must now turn its energies to see that all other officers and security personnel involved in the 'dirty war' be brought to justice. We must await to see the outcome of these proceedings.

The Argentine case is destined to become a textbook example of the madness inherent in collective punishment and the "superorganic" growth of institutionalized terror. The military, with its legendary Nazi orientation, came under serious attack and perceived itself increasingly vulnerable to the terrorists. The armed left, which itself justified terrorism in the name of "humanity," awoke a sleeping monster that acted out its most perverse fantasies. The entire civilian population [even military men which refused to participate in the dirty war] became feared suspects to be eliminated.

We have argued that any machinery of death of this magnitude must receive its energy from obscure unconscious processes as well as from "rational" motives. We identified the specific atmosphere in which these monsters of the unconscious were unleashed. It is unsatisfactory to interpret torture, abuse and extermination in entirely instrumental or class terms. For as Foucault (1979: 3–69) has brilliantly shown, torture is part of the "theatrics" of power. As such it is a deeply symbolic act.

Indeed, we have shown that in the modern "medical" chambers of death the torturers, armed with electrical prods and other artifacts of terror, manufactured their own brand of ideological surgery in their attempts to re-organize the landscape. The torturers thus forged images of the "ideal" compliant, castrated citizen. The specifics of torture underline the unconscious inquisitional agenda of torturers and their supervisors. The busy market locating children with acceptable families also reflect the *reorganizacion* fantasy. Yet before placing children in "proper" homes, the affective bonds with the parents had to be surgically removed. Family torture sessions were interpreted in this context.

In the military's hallucinatory system a final assault on the Western way of life was under way. Argentina became a central focus of this ultimate battle for control. This required an absolute response. The response was a perfect binary opposite of their very fear: a "final" and total assault on the life of the "other." For this reason, the politicians of pain concentrated their obscene skills on the sources of life: the penis, testicles, the vagina, the uterus, the breasts, pregnant women and finally on children themselves.

## NOTES

1. If the language used throughout this article appears unorthodox from the standpoint of traditional social science literature, I wish the reader would keep in mind that the subject matter itself is far from orthodox. This paper has benefited, a great deal I think, by the wise editorial work of Nancy Scheper-Hughes. To her I extend a sincere *gracias*. Carola Suarez-Orozco, Michael Taussig and George A. DeVos also offered their critical comments. To them I extend my gratitude. All errors of fact or interpretation are, of course, my own.
2. The Malvinas conflict was after the 'dirty war.' Argentina was sympathetic to Germany throughout the Second World War and only declared war on Germany on the eve of the German surrender to the Allies.
3. A number of children have been reunited with their biological families through blood typing, see CONADEP 1984; Slavin 1985: 1–7.

## REFERENCES

Amnesty International
    1973 Amnesty international report on torture. London: Gerald Duckworth & Co. Ltd.
    1984 Torture in the eighties: an amnesty international report. London: Amnesty international publications.
Bacry, Daniel and Michel Ternisien
    1980 La torture: la nouvelle inquisition. Paris: Fayard.
Cabeza, Carlos
    1985 Entrevista a Jose Deheza, Ex Ministro de Defensa. El Diario del Juicio. Anō I – No 7. July 9th. pp. 170–171.
Chavez, Lydia
    1985a Argentine Children Who Became 'War Booty.' The San Francisco Chronicle. September, 10th. pp. 18–19.
    1985b Five from Juntas are Found Guilty in Argentine Trial. The New York Times. December, 10th. pp. 1–2.
Colson, Elizabeth
    1985 Using Anthropology in a World on the Move. Human Organization 44, 3: 191–196.
Comisión Nacional Sobre la Desaparición de Personas [CONADEP]
    1984 Nunca Mas: Informe de la Comisión Nacional Sobre la Desaparición de Personas. Buenos Aires: Editorial Universitaria de Buenos Aires.
El Diario del Juicio
    1985 Volumes I through XV. Buenos Aires.
Fagen, Patricia W.
    1985 The Culture of Fear: Responces to State Terrorism in the Southern Cone. Paper Presented at the Center for Latin American Studies, University of California, Berkeley. October 28th.
Foucault, Michel
    1979 Discipline & Punish: The Birth of the Prison. Translated from the French by Alan Sheridan. New York: Vintage Books.
Gennep, Arnold van
    1960 The Rites of Passage. Translated from the French by Vizedom and Caffee. Chicago: The University of Chicago Press.
Guthmann, Edward
    1986 'My Child is Missing.' The San Francisco Examiner. January, 12th. pp. 23–24.
Mellor, Alec
    1961 La torture: son histoire, son abolition, sa reapparition au XXe siècle. Paris: Mame.
Montalbano, William
    1985 Argentina's Ex-Leader Gets Life. Los Angeles Times. December 10th. pp. 1–2.

Ruthven, Malise
1978 Torture: The Grand Conspiracy. London: Weidenfeld and Nicolson.
Slavin, J.P.
1985 Argentine grandmothers seek lost kids. The Daily Californian, vol. XVII, No. 112. Monday, July 15th, pp. 1–7.
Taussig, Michael
1984 Culture of Terror – Space of Death. Roger Casement's Putumayo Report and the Explanation of Torture. Comparative Study of Society and History.
The Economist
1985 Argentina discovers its past, with horror. London, September 28th. pp. 37–38.
Timerman, Jacobo
1981 Prisoner without a name, Cell without a number. New York: Alfred A. Knopf.
Tomas y Valiente, Francisco
1973 La Tortura en España, Estudios Historicos. Barcelona: Editorial Ariel.
Victor, J.
1981 Confesiones de un torturador. Barcelona: Editorial Laia.
Vidal-Naquet, Pierre
1963 Torture: Cancer of Democracy. Baltimore, Maryland: Penguin Books.

JILL E. KORBIN

# CHILD SEXUAL ABUSE:
# IMPLICATIONS FROM THE CROSS-CULTURAL RECORD[1]

This chapter offers an exploratory survey of child sexual abuse based on a review of the cross-cultural record and the literature on child sexual abuse in Euro-American nations. Anthropological complacency about the rarity of incest and sexual conduct within the family has been seriously challenged by recent epidemiological, sociological, and clinical data (e.g. Finkelhor 1979; Herman 1981; Mrazek and Kempe 1981). Conventional wisdom has supported a scientific assumption that the incest taboo was strong enough to preclude such behavior. This complacency fostered reliance on data about norms, values, and beliefs rather than on actual behavior. Rather suddenly, in the mid-to-late 1970s, child sexual abuse, while not a new phenomenon, emerged as a problem of significant professional and public concern in the United States and European nations. Anthropology, as the purveyor of cross-cultural knowledge, has been limited in its ability to contribute meaningfully to current discussions of the universality or cultural specificity of child sexual abuse. Because anthropological efforts have been devoted primarily to explaining the origins and persistence of incest taboos, attention has been distracted from the equally significant issue of the circumstances under which proscribed sexual conduct within the family occurs. This chapter examines definitions of child sexual abuse and incest, surveys the state of current cross-cultural knowledge concerning sexual conduct between adults and children, and suggests directions for cross-cultural research based on knowledge generated in Euro-American nations.

## DEFINITIONS

Literature on child sexual abuse in the United States has fostered conceptual confusion by using the terms "incest" and "child sexual abuse" synonymously (Finkelhor 1985). While definitions of "incest" vary among societies, the term refers to proscribed sexual conduct between culturally-specified relatives. Proscriptions may extend beyond the nuclear family to other consanguineal relatives and to classificatory and fictive kin. "Child sexual abuse," has been defined by the National Center on Child Abuse and Neglect as, "Contact or interactions between a child and an adult when the child is being used for the sexual stimulation of that adult or another person" (1981). "Child sexual abuse," therefore, may be encompassed within a definition of "incest" if the child and the perpetrator are kin. Both biological and classificatory kin tend to be included. However, all child sexual abuse is not incest, and the interchangeable use of the terms is misleading.

The lack of specificity and operational criteria in definitions of "incest" and

247

*Nancy Scheper-Hughes (ed.), Child Survival, 247–265.*
© *1987 by D. Reidel Publishing Company.*

"child sexual abuse" create an array of problems for cultural analysis. Neither incest nor child sexual abuse refer to homogeneous categories of events. In the cross-cultural literature, incest encompasses sexual relations with an array of individuals beyond the nuclear family. Incest is not necessarily restricted to sexual intercourse, but in some societies includes intent and desire to have sexual relations, or behaviors such as sharing food or engaging in suggestive banter (Schneider 1976). Incest also is not restricted to individuals prohibited from marriage. While restrictions on marriage and sexual relations often overlap, in some societies, such as the Tallensi and the Trobriands, individuals who are prohibited from marrying may still engage in sexual relations (Schneider 1976).

Similarly, child sexual abuse is not a unitary phenomenon (Summit and Kryso 1978). Depending on the clinical, the research, or the legal definitions employed, behaviors include exposure, fondling, oral-genital contact, and intercourse. Perpetrators include strangers, neighbors, step-fathers, biological fathers, uncles, brothers, mothers, aunts, and sisters (Finkelhor 1985; Russel 1984). Statistics on child sexual abuse most often lump these diverse behaviors and perpetrators, thereby obtaining the highest possible prevalence figures to underline the magnitude, and thus the seriousness, of the problem. However, the meaning of conclusions about etiology or outcome, for example, must be questioned when a single sexual encounter with a stranger is counted equally with sustained sexual relations with a father. The necessity for precise operational criteria is crucial enough within any society but it is even more imperative when moving into the arena of cross-cultural comparisons.

## TOWARDS CULTURALLY-INFORMED DEFINITIONS

From a cross-cultural perspective, child sexual abuse can be defined as proscribed *sexual conduct* between an adult and a *sexually immature* child for purposes of the adult's *sexual pleasure* or for economic gain through child prostitution or pornography. Because the underlined concepts are culture-bound, further refinement is required.

Even a cursory examination of the cross-cultural literature yields differences in what is defined as *sexual conduct*. A man or woman grasping the testicles of an adult male would be construed as sexually motivated or an affront in the United States, while this same behavior can be a form of non-sexual greeting among Highland New Guinea peoples (Langness 1981b). Sexual conduct, in the context of this definition, must involve seeking sexual stimulation or pleasure. Sexual crimes, such as rape, may involve power and aggression as an alternative to sexual stimulation or pleasure.

*Sexual maturity* is defined differently by societies according to their values and needs. In general, sexual conduct with prepubertal children is not considered appropriate. In preindustrial cultures, menarche, the appearance of secondary sexual characteristics, or the ability to independently perform necessary subsistence tasks most often signal sexual maturity and readiness to take one's place as an adult and a parent. Sexual maturity is not acknowledged in some societies until formal initiation rites have been successfully completed. Such rites may or may not coincide with physiological puberty. In industrialized societies such as the United States and many European nations, sexual maturity is not socially or legally acknowledged until the age of majority at 18 or 21, unless a "teenage pregnancy" occurs.

*Sexual pleasure* also is not a simple concept to define cross-culturally. Pleasure may include feelings of sexual arousal or stimulation, including but not exclusively orgasm.

To emphasize definitional difficulties, not all behaviors that are sensual or involve sexual organs would necessarily be defined as sexual abuse. In some societies, children's genitals are fondled to amuse and please them, calm them or lull them to sleep (Ford and Beach 1951). This would not constitute "abuse" if in that society the behavior was not proscribed and was not for the purposes of adult sexual satisfaction, even if the adult tangentially experienced some degree of pleasure.

From a cross-cultural standpoint, caution would be advisable in the use of the term "abuse." The terminology "child sexual abuse" grew out of its association with physical child abuse and child protection efforts. "Abuse" is clearly an emotionally-laden term that served to draw professional, public and legislative attention to the issue. To label conduct "abuse" necessitates a value judgement prior to analysis. Simply avoiding the term "abuse" will not suspend all judgements of what is optimal or detrimental to child development. While the term "child sexual abuse" can be used as shorthand, efforts should be directed to the long-delayed examination of sexual conduct with children cross-culturally rather than with *a priori* assignments of labels.

While it is difficult to define validly child sexual abuse within a single culture, the problems are multiplied when attempting to standardize definitions for the purposes of cross-cultural comparison. As has been discussed with respect to physical and emotional child abuse, what is considered "good" for children in one society may be regarded as "bad" for proper child rearing and development in another (Korbin 1981). Definitions that rely solely on cultural acceptance of behavior are amorphous, thus reducing the question to a simplistic level of relativity that is as distorting as ethnocentrism. The following criteria may prove helpful in delineating culturally-appropriate definitions. These criteria overlap but are useful as guidelines, with some more readily amenable to operationalization than others.

(1) *Violation of Family Roles/Statuses*: Child sexual abuse is best conceptualized as the disruption of expected roles, relationships, and behaviors, similar to Lévi-Strauss' (1969) conception of incest. The precise sexual act is likely to be less important than the nature of the relationship that was violated. Schneider asserts that incest can be best understood in cultural terms, as "the wrong way to act in a relationship: as father-son, as father-

daughter, as mother-son, as mother-daughter, as brother-sister, as cousins . . ."
(1976: 166) On Ponape, a term referring to sexual relations between parent
and child can be translated as "not understanding being a parent" (Fischer *et
al*. 1976: 200). When sexual conduct with adopted or classificatory kin is
proscribed, the explanation also tends to involve a distortion of the relationship (Marshall 1976; Monberg 1976).

(2) *Coercion*: Children must often be coerced to participate in even the
most appropriate activities. A measure for assessing sexual abuse is the
degree to which force, threat, or deceit must be brought to bear in order to
obtain a child's compliance. In Euro-American nations, a variety of strategies
are employed to obtain children's acquiesence to inappropriate sexual conduct. Sexually abused children may be physically coerced or threatened with
harm to themselves or others. Sexually abused children may be accorded
"favorite" status and provided with material benefits for their compliance and
silence. Some sexually abusive parents use manipulation and deceit, claiming,
for example, that all fathers teach their daughters about sex. It is well to
remember that in most societies children are taught to obey adults, whether
or not they wish to comply.

(3) *Consent*: Sexual abuse may also be determined by the extent to which a
child is capable, by virtue of age, power differentials, and the nature of the
relationship to freely consent. Finkelhor (1985) has argued that children are
simply unable to comprehend, and thereby consent to the change in a
relationship that sexual activity with an adult implies. A lack of physical or
verbal resistance by a child does not necessarily imply consent. As noted with
respect to coercion, children are taught to obey adults.

(4) *Secrecy*: While societies differ in their openness regarding sexuality,
most sexual activity takes place in private. Proscribed sexual conduct with
children is likely to occur in extreme secrecy. If small children's genitals are
fondled openly, with other adults present, this must be considered differently
than fondling of children that takes place secretly, with warnings to the child
not to reveal what has transpired.

(5) *Age discrepancy*: If there is an age discrepancy such that the child and
the adult could not be considered appropriate marriage and/or sexual partners, the sexual conduct can more appropriately be categorized as abusive.
Cultural practices such as child bethrothal and marriage, however, complicate
this issue (Kapadia 1966; Poffenberger 1981).

## METHODOLOGICAL ISSUES

If cross-cultural definitions are resolved, methodological constraints nevertheless remain to be considered. Cross-cultural information on sexual behavior is notoriously difficult to obtain. Researchers generally are limited to
reports of behavior, not direct observations. Ethnographers may be hesitant
to intrude on areas that are private in their own societies. For example,

Caudill and Plath (1966) asked their Japanese informants to draw maps of where they slept instead of asking to observe night-time behavior associated with conjugal relations in the United States. These constraints hold for accepted behaviors, let alone those that are negatively sanctioned.

Even in nations with legally mandated reporting systems, child sexual abuse is considered vastly underreported. Child sexual abuse takes place in such extreme secrecy and privacy that more often than not it goes undetected. There is a psychological resistance among professionals to acknowledging that sexual abuse occurs, even in the face of undeniable evidence. Sgroi (1977) found it necessary to argue that very young "kids with the clap" could only have contracted venereal disease in the same manner as adults, through sexual contact. The Freudian legacy also has contributed to disbelief of children's accounts of sexual molestation by known adults (Masson 1984; Rush 1980). Children who are sexually abused frequently do not disclose their abuse. In Finkelhor's (1979) survey of college students, two-thirds of those who had been sexually victimized as children did not tell anyone of the encounter. Parents also may be hesitant to report the sexual victimization of their children because of the potential stigma, family disruption, and risk of iatrogenic harm as the child negotiates the requisite medical and legal systems. Perhaps only one of every five cases comes to professional attention (Finkelhor 1985). The sample on which clinical and research findings are based is therefore biased.

Anthropological interest in child abuse, as with other forms of deviance, has been slow to develop. Anthropology has tended to devote far greater research attention and theoretical emphasis to the regularities of cultural behavior than to deviance (Edgerton 1976, 1978). The underside of human behavior, then, is not often confronted by anthropologists. Further, it is difficult to conceptualize and therefore to seek out information about behavior that is virtually "unthinkable" in one's own society unless that same behavior is normative in an "exotic" culture. Hence, ritualized homosexuality with prepubescent boys, while at odds with practices in the United States, is more likely to find its way into the ethnographic literature than a few seemingly aberrant and individual cases of homosexual abuse of sons by fathers or mothers' brothers. Low base rate behaviors, such as child abuse, may seem too aberrant from the cultural pattern to warrant ethnographic description (Graburn this volume).

Child sexual abuse simply may be outside the ethnographer's frame of reference as within the repertoire of human behavior. Until recently there has been little reason to suspect that sexual conduct with children occurred with any frequency in our own society. If child sexual abuse also occurs in secrecy in other cultures, it is also unlikely to come to the ethnographer's attention. Rapport in the field is difficult to establish and fragile to maintain. Ethnographers may have been hesitant to risk their fieldwork in order to seek out information about behaviors they assumed unlikely to occur, but highly likely to offend or anger. Gathering genealogies that require naming forbidden relatives has threatened the continuity of fieldwork, as well as life and limb (Chagnon 1968), without going further and asking about sexual conduct with those relatives. Anthropologists have pursued research on such topics as witchcraft, drug use, and cannibalism with intellectual enthusiasm, even when these lines of questioning threatened rapport or continued permission to work in the host country. One can speculate that sexual deviance, particularly with immatures, touches unconscious mechanisms of denial and projection (Devereux 1967). It may be the ultimate forbidden topic to contemplate.

Information about proscribed sexual conduct may not come to light and is likely to be anecdotal when it does. Ethnographers may only become aware that such a liaison has occured when it is flagrant enough to become public, for example when an unintended pregnancy occurs or when a relationship changes from being sexual to involving marriage. Samoan women may reveal proscribed sexual relations prior to giving birth or during a difficult labor because they fear death in childbirth if the true paternity remains concealed (Shore 1976).

A major difficulty with the ethnographic literature is that information is presented in overly generalized terms of: "The X regard incest with great horror and believe that only animals would do such a thing." "The X masturbate their children." "The X set incest offenders adrift in boats to die." There is rarely information on actual cases or intracultural variability. A degree of skepticism is obviously warranted.

Despite these limitations, the ethnographic record indicates that sexual conduct with children occurs in a range of cultures. The next section of this chapter will explore the available evidence.

THE CROSS-CULTURAL EVIDENCE

*Incest*

A complete discussion of incest in the cross-cultural record is the subject of a substantial literature and is clearly beyond the scope of this chapter.[2] Nevertheless it is useful to review the cross-cultural record on incest and its implications for sexual conduct with children. Incest is but one manifestation of child sexual abuse. As noted above, incest and child sexual abuse often are used interchangeably in the European and American child abuse literature. The ethnographic literature frequently does not distinguish incestuous behavior between consenting adults and incestuous behavior between adults and children. If, for example, an ethnography reports that "father-daughter incest is known," information may be lacking on the age of the daughte Incest between adults, in addition to its sexual component, also may involve marriage for the purpose of maintaining control of property, or procreation for the purpose of insuring purity in the blood line. In contrast, between children and adults is less likely to serve other purposes and more likely to be limited to sexual contact.

Virtually all societies have proscriptions, whether formal or informal, on sexual behavior among related individuals. Cultures differ with respect to extensions of incest proscriptions beyond the nuclear family and in the severity with which transgressions are regarded or punished (Murdock 1949; Schneider 1976). Murdock's (1949) classic *Social Structure* included among the empirical findings regarding incest the recognition that:

Despite the strength of cultural barriers and their internalization in the consciences of individuals, sporadic instances of incestuous intercourse are reported in most of our sample societies for which ethnographers have investigated the subject. There is, of course, abundant clinical and criminological evidence of the actual occurrence of incest in our own and related societies. It is clear . . . that even the strongest of cultural restraints are only imperfectly successful (1949: 288–289)

Cultural practices have been documented in which incest occurs openly, in exempted situations and/or by exempted individuals. Exempted situations include religious and ceremonial occasions or special circumstances such as prior to battle. Exempted individuals include specific classes such as royalty or nobility. Hawaiian ali'i and Inca royalty were allowed brother-sister incest for the purposes of maintaining purity of the blood line. Among the Egyptians, both nobility and commoners are reported to be permitted to marry within the nuclear family (Hopkins 1980, Middleton 1962). Twins in Bali (Schneider 1976) and Ponape (Fischer *et al.* 1976) were exempted from restrictions on brother-sister incest because they were presumed to have been intimate previously in the womb. These cultural exceptions and exemptions do not diminish, but rather underline the rules (Schneider 1976).

While the ethnographic literature has described cultural practices and cross-cultural variation with respect to incest, information on transgressions of these rules, beliefs and norms is largely anecdotal and limited to those cases that came to public notice. Much of this literature applies to same-age children engaging in sex play as they mimic adult behavior and learn about acceptable and unacceptable partners (e.g. Shostak 1981), or to cases of sexual behavior between consenting adults that is either punished or eventually accepted by the community (Kiste and Rynkiewich 1976; Pospisil 1958; Turnbull 1961; Weinberg 1955).

The hierarchy of seriousness among incestuous relationships within any culture must be considered. Among Samoans, for example, brother-sister incest was regarded as the most serious potential incest violation, and was surrounded by strict rules and prohibitions. However, father-daughter incest was considered the most serious actual transgression because of the presumed protective nature of the parent-child relationship, ". . . incest between father and daughter is worse than between brother and sister because it is less expected, or less comprehensible" (Shore 1976: 278–279). Both brother-sister and father-daughter violations were known to occur. While instances of mother-son incest could not be recalled, it was rated as equally as serious as father-daughter, again because of the nature of the parent-child relationship (Shore 1976).

Violation of proscriptions concerning incest and sexual conduct with children does not mean that such violations carry no cultural meaning to the perpetrators. Recognition of the "grisly horror" of incest is often well within the rationalizations and defenses of sexually abusing fathers and step-fathers in the United States. Biological fathers may stop short of full sexual intercourse, claiming that while their behavior was not exemplary, it was then not "really" incest. They may even explain their behavior as sex education or as "protecting" their daughters from inexperienced adolescent boys. Step-fathers often plea that even if their behavior was wrong, it wasn't "really" incest because of the absence of a biological relationship (Phelan 1981). Biological and step-fathers alike may adhere to biological definitions of inbreeding and refuse to see sexual molestation of their sons as "incest."

## Sexual Conduct Between Adults and Children

Three conceptual levels have been utilized in the cross-cultural consideration of child abuse: (1) cultural variation in perception of practices as abusive; (2) idiosyncratic departure from cultural norms and values; and (3) societal-level conditions that promote deleterious circumstances for children that are largely beyond individual parental control (Korbin 1981). These three levels also can be applied with respect to sexual conduct with children. At the first level, the ethnographic literature contains evidence, however limited, of normative cultural practices that include sexual conduct between adults and children that may be regarded as abusive in one society but not in another. At the second level, ethnographic information, however sparse, exists on idiosyncratic cases of sexual conduct with children that falls outside of cultural norms. And, at the third level, international child protection movements and media exposés have contributed accounts of sexual misuse of children, most notably in child pornography, prostitution, and in public and private institutions. Examples of these three levels will be discussed in the following sections.

### Cultural practices

Sexual conduct with children can occur in the context of religious or ceremonial events. Ritualized homosexuality as a component of male initiation rites has been well documented in some New Guinea societies (Herdt 1982; Kelly 1977; Shiefflen 1976). These rites reflect a belief that masculinity is acquired, and is dependent upon the intake of semen through the prolonged practice of fellatio with older, sexually mature males. Other practices, such as older males rubbing semen on the boy and sodomy also occur. The intake of semen to insure masculinity is symbolically equated with the necessity of mother's milk for development. Despite the emphasis on growth and gender develop-ment, the sexual component of such rites also is suggested. In the equation between mother's milk and semen, one would predict that the father would be the most appropriate donor/nurturer of the growth-inducing substance for his offspring. However, the same constraints on incestuous relations apply between fathers and sons as would apply in heterosexual relations (Herdt 1982; Kelly 1977; Schiefflen 1976), thereby suggesting a recognized sexual component in this ritualized behavior.

Ceremonial defloration and insemination of young brides at menarche also has been reported in New Guinea. The cultural meaning of this behavior was that the girl should produce a "goblin child," a child of the collective, before beginning conjugal relations with her young husband. Again, an implicit sexual component occurs alongside the more explicit ritual purpose. Ideally, the inseminator should be the young groom's father. However, he is "too ashamed" to engage in sexual relations with the girl who is to become his daughter-in-law and so most often asks a sib mate to perform the function for him (Langness 1981; Thurnwald 1916).

Sexualized behaviors with children also occur in the context of daily normative child rearing practices. In some societies, adults may fondle the genitals of their very young children (Ford and Beach 1951). In Turkey, Olson (1981) reported that adults kiss and praise the genitals of young children, celebrating their eventual fertility. The ethnographer was encour-aged to be a good mother and do likewise with her young daughter. Pona-peans acknowledge the attractiveness and pleasure of children's sexual organs with the saying, "Is there no one who lifts up his child and sniffs?" referring to the "widespread custom of playing with a baby affectionately by lifting it up and sniffing or blowing on the genitals" (Fischer *et al.* 1976: 203).

Sexual relations between adults and prepubescent children may occur in the context of marriage. In India, for example, child marriage that paired very young girls with adult men was an accepted and valued marriage pattern. It guaranteed the girl's virginity and assured a marriage that would benefit her family. It was recognized, however, that the prepubescent girl was subject to the sexual attentions of her husband, despite her immaturity and lack of physical readiness for sexual intercourse. Consumation prior to the menarche was prohibited by law, but was frequently violated (Kapadia 1966, Poffen-berger 1981).

In societies that are repressive of childhood sexual behavior, such as masturbation, punishments or threats thereof may be harsh. Among the Kwoma of New Guinea, an adult woman may beat a boy's penis with a stick if she observes an erection (Ford and Beach 1951). In rural India, parents may threaten to burn a young boy's penis with a stick if he is found mastur-bating (Poffenberger 1981). In Euro-American nations, it is well to remember that into the present Century, extreme measures were taken to prevent children from masturbating. Between 1850 and 1900, surgical procedures were imposed on children whose parents were concerned about masturbation. These included clitoridectomy, sometimes without anesthesia, cutting or infibulation of the penis, or cauterization of the penis and clitoris. After 1900, physical restraints to prevent masturbation, which were sometimes quite elaborate, became more popular. Until the 1920s, some parents sought and some physicians performed clitoridectomies on young girls to prevent masturbation (Schultz 1982).

In the United States, organizations such as the Rene Guyon Society, the Childhood Sensuality Circle and the North American Man/Boy Love Association (NAMBLA) openly defy cultural proscriptions against sex with children. They claim that restricting childrens' sexual expression is itself harmful and abusive. The Rene Guyon Society, for example, advocates its view of healthy child development with the motto, "Sex by year eight or else it's too late." These groups seek to legitimize their pedophillic orientation. They claim an overarching "pro-child" ideology, asserting that children should exercise self-determination in all facets of their lives, including sex with adults. These groups further attempt to legitimize their sexual conduct with children by requiring the child's consent and opposing coercion, and by imposing their own rules, such as establishing the minimum age for full intercourse and the necessity of using condoms (deYoung 1984). As noted above, Finkelhor (1985) and child protection advocates argue that children, by virtue of their immaturity and the power differential between children and adults, are incapable of informed consent to sexual behavior with adults.

In areas of Sub-Saharan Africa and the Middle East, children are subjected to genital surgery ranging from clitoridectomy to infibulation for females, and from circumcision to subincision for males. It is a matter of extremely controversial debate whether these practices, which are normative and positively valued in the societies in which they occur, should be identified as either physically or sexually abusive. These operations are frequently, but not necessarily, part of initiation rites (Hayes, 1975; Kennedy 1970; Langness 1981; LeVine and LeVine 1966; Lyons 1981). The Gusii of East Africa are willing to relinquish traditional genital surgery, or to have it performed in clinics with anesthesia and under sterile conditions, but only if legitimate adult status in the group is otherwise assured (LeVine and LeVine 1981). Understanding the context and meaning of these practices does not diminish the attendant physical or psychological suffering which they entail (Keesing 1982). However, eradication imposed from outside the culture is unlikely to be successful since a single practice cannot be separated from larger cultural meanings and context (World Health Organization 1979).

*Idiosyncratic violations*

The cultural and normative behaviors discussed in the preceding section would not necessarily conform to the criteria discussed earlier for child sexual abuse. They nevertheless indicate that, cross-culturally, children are not precluded from all sexualized behavior. The ethnographic record also contains limited evidence that sexual conduct with children occurs outside of culturally accepted contexts.

Among the Gusii of East Africa, sexual relations between prepubescent girls and their classificatory or biological fathers were reported to occur and were most often treated as religious offenses. Sexual molestation of young girls by unrelated schoolteachers in Nigeria and Kenya, however, was a cause of public outrage and scandal that often resulted in the extrusion of the teacher from the community (LeVine and LeVine 1981). The Ponapean saying noted earlier with respect to the allure of young children's genitals, may also refer to intercourse between children and biological or classificatory parents, and be employed as an explanation for such proscribed incidents. In a community of rural Hawaiian-Polynesians, the pregnancy of an adolescent girl aroused suspicion on the part of her biological father that she had been sexually molested by her step-father. While this proved not to be the case, it was considered a legitimate parental concern within the community. Another man had a sexual relationship with a teenage foster daughter. When discovered, his behavior was condemned and the girl emotionally supported as the victimized party. Nevertheless, the community regarded the behavior as a matter of private shame and not something to be reported to the authorities (Korbin 1976).

Sexual relations with children also have been reported to be perpetrated by individuals outside of usual social control mechanisms. Goldstein (1964) reported on a category of Tibetan monks, the *Ldab Ilobs*, who engaged in a range of rule-breaking behaviors, including the kidnapping of both adults and young boys for homosexual purposes. Schoolboys tried to protect themselves by moving in groups and carrying small knives. Families did not complain because of fear of retaliation by the *Ldab Ilobs*. Also, as is the case in Euro-American societies, there is a stigma attached to having been sexually victimized. The monks were generous with material goods for their homosexual partners, which was some compensation as well as an enticement to "voluntary" partners.

In the United States, estimates of the incidence and prevalence of child sexual abuse vary due to methodological and definitional differences in existing research. Some definitions include exhibitionism (Finkelhor 1979) while others require physical contact (Russell 1984). Nevertheless, indications are that between one-fifth and one-third of all females and approximately 9% of all males will have a sexual encounter with an adult before the age of 18. The nature of the sexual conduct, the age of the child, and the identity of the perpetrator are usually combined in available statistics, making comparison between studies problematic. Within the parent-child dyad, approximately one in twenty females will have sexual contact ranging from fondling to full intercourse with a father or step-father before reaching the age of 18 (Finkelhor 1985). Recent cases of sexual victimization of preschoolers in day care centers in California, Colorado, New Jersey, and numerous other states have added fuel to the fire of public concern about the vulnerability of children to sexual assault. There has been a rash of autobiographical accounts of childhood sexual abuse (e.g. Armstrong 1978; Bass and Thornton 1983; Brady 1979, Morris 1982) and television, newspaper, and radio documentaries and reports. Self-help groups such as Parents United and sexual assault teams have multiplied.

Thus, in a decade, child sexual abuse in the United States has been transformed from a virtually unrecognized issue to a problem of major public and professional concern. Since its identification in the United States, child sexual abuse has been recognized as a significant problem in a number of nations, including, but not exclusively, Britain (Mrazek, Lynch and Bentovim 1981), Japan (Ikeda 1982), Sweden (Ronstrom 1985), Malaysia (Nathan and Hwang 1981), The Netherlands (Doek 1981), and Canada (Badgley 1984).

*Societal conditions*

Child prostitution and sexual exploitation have been reported throughout history and across cultures (Mrazek 1981; Schultz 1982). International child protection literature supplements the ethnographic record in documenting the sexual abuse of children, particularly in pornography and prostitution (Anti-Slavery Society 1985; Herrmann and Jupp 1985). In pre-revolutionary China, young girls could be sold into prostitution during famines or when there was an excess of "unfortunate" female births in a family (Chow 1978; Korbin 1981b; Smedley 1976). In conditions of poverty, children in Third World countries may be enticed by the material rewards provided by prostitution and pornography, fueled by national and international pedophile organizations (Perpinan 1985; Salayakianond 1985). Child prostitution also has been documented in the United States and Europe (Sereny 1985; Weisberg 1985).

## ANTECEDENTS OF CHILD SEXUAL ABUSE

Information on adherence to, and deviation from cultural proscriptions regarding sexual conduct with children is woefully inadequate for comparative purposes. As a generally disapproved, and therefore covert behavior it is not realistic to expect valid and reliable incidence or prevalence rates for cross-cultural comparison. Statistics are elusive even within nations that have mandatory reporting systems. At present, cross-cultural research may be most fruitfully devoted to the circumstances under which sexual conduct with children occurs and whether those circumstances conform to what has been identified in Euro-American nations. The factors that cross-cultural research can address can be grouped as follows:

## Cultural Values

What cultural values promote or preclude proscribed sexual behavior with children? Sanday (1981) has identified a cultural constellation of male dominance, gender segregation, and interpersonal violence that is associated with rape. Can such a constellation of cultural values and characteristics be identified for sexual conduct with children? As was discovered in the United States and Europe, cultural values against sexual conduct with children do not necessarily preclude its ocurrence. Child sexual abuse in Europe and the United States tends to be a pervasive family pattern rather than a one-time event, and more than one child in the family may be involved (Herman 1981; MacFarlane and Korbin 1983). Once the cultural prohibition is violated, it may more easily be violated the next time. Samoans have expressed a similar belief about incest violations, ". . . once you have done it, you find that there is nothing wrong with it, and you do it again and again" (Shore 1976: 281).

## Social Networks and Supports

In the United States, child abuse and neglect are more likely to occur in families who are socially isolated, whose behaviors are outside the scrutiny of others and who do not have a network to call upon for assistance in child care (Garbarino 1977). This is supported by the available cross-cultural literature for child maltreatment (Korbin 1981). Incestuous families that are reported in the cross-cultural literature may be marginal to the community (Wilson 1961). However, it must be cautioned that sexually abusive fathers in the United States are frequently the "pillars of the community" and, cross-culturally, individuals of high social status may be provided latitude in violating rules, including incest regulations (Fischer *et al.* 1976; Edgerton 1985; Pospisil 1958).

## Family and Household Composition

Blended and step-families in the United States are at increased risk of child sexual abuse. Girls with step-fathers are five times more likely to be sexually abused (Finkelhor 1980). While step-fathers are more likely to sexually abuse than biological fathers (Russell 1984b), the increased risk is not accounted for by step-fathers alone, but by a series of boyfriends and suitors, and their friends, as the mother seeks a new mate (Finkelhor 1979).

Housing patterns are also important. In traditional Pueblo apartment-style living, congested conditions with co-sleeping provided scant opportunity for clandestine sexual conduct with children. Pueblo informants believed that the movement into government-subsidized dwellings, with separate bedrooms and increased privacy, afforded more opportunity for child sexual abuse, and indeed resulted in more actual cases (Scheper-Hughes 1985). This is in contrast to the stereotype (that is not empirically supported) that poor families in Appalachia who sleep together are prone to sexual abuse of children.

## Vulnerable Children

Even in cultures that greatly value children, some children are more vulnerable to a range of abuses than are others (Korbin 1981), including child sexual abuse. For example, Turkish orphans who do not have extended kinship networks to ensure their welfare are more likely to be sexually abused, after which they have little recourse but prostitution (Olson 1981). An important area for cross-cultural research concerns categories of children vulnerable to sexual abuse.

Beliefs about children's inherent sexuality and the impact of sexual behavior on their development can be expected to have an impact. If female virginity and chastity are closely tied to family honor (e.g. Hayes 1975; Kennedy 1970), does this protect female children from intrafamilial sexual abuse? If female children are protected, do their brothers also benefit from this protection or are they at risk of sexual abuse?

## Adult Perpetrators

In the United States, a consistent profile of sexually abusive adults has not emerged. Individuals marginal to their communities as well as individuals in positions of relative power have been identified as sexual abusers. A distinction has sometimes been drawn between "regressed pedophiles" who turn to their children in times of stress and "fixated pedophiles" who have an enduring and persistent sexual attraction to children (Groth 1979). The presence or absence of pedophilia cross-culturally also should be subject to ethnographic examination. Sexually deviant individuals such as hermaphrodites have been accessible to ethnographic study (Edgerton 1964), and pedophilia similarly may be accessible.

Combining the above factors, the cross-cultural record can be used to test theoretical models for child sexual abuse. One promising framework for cross-cultural research is the ecological model with levels of analysis, from the individual to the cultural, nesting within one another (Bronfenbrenner 1979; Garbarino 1977). Another framework is Finkelhor's (1985) "four preconditions model" that begins with predisposing factors in the perpetrator, moves through internal inhibitors and external constraints, and finally considers resistance in the child. Examining child sexual abuse across cultural contexts may also afford new theoretical perspectives.

## CONCLUDING REMARKS

In the absence of data, conclusions about the cross-cultural prevalence or etiology of sexual conduct between adults and children are premature. While anthropologists have not as yet contributed substantial writings on the issue of sexual conduct between children and adults, ethnographers have nevertheless laid the groundwork for cross-cultural considerations of this behavior. Important implications can be drawn and questions raised utilizing the cross-cultural record. It is hoped that this chapter will further discussion and stimulate needed cross-cultural research. The unanticipated prevalence of child sexual abuse in the United States stimulated professionals and the public to action. It should alert anthropologists to the existence of sexual conduct with children as within the repertoire of human behavior and disarm too facile assumptions that the incest taboo is strong enough to preclude the behavior.

## NOTES

1. Earlier versions of this paper were presented at the Third National Conference on Child Sexual Abuse in 1984 and at the Annual Meetings of the American Anthropological Association in 1985. I would like to thank Nancy Scheper-Hughes for her thoughtful and helpful suggestions on this manuscript.
2. An extensive anthropological literature exists on incest. For an overview, the reader is referred to Devereux (1939), Evans-Pritchard (1951), Lévi-Strauss (1969), Malinowski (1929), Murdock (1949), Parsons (1954), Schneider (1976), Shepler (1983), and Wolf (1970).

## REFERENCES

Anti-Slavery Society
    1985 The Sexual Exploitation of Children: Prostitution and Pornography. Report for UNICEF.
Armstrong, L.
    1978 Kiss Daddy Goodnight. New York: Hawthorne.
Badgley, R.
    1984 Sexual Offences Against Children. Ottawa: Canadian Government Printing Centre.
Bass, E. and L. Thornton, Eds.
    1983 I Never Told Anyone: Writings by Women Survivors of Child Sexual Abuse. New York: Harper and Row.
Brady, K.
    1979 Father's Days. A True Story of Incest. New York: Dell.
Bronfenbrenner, U.
    1979 The Ecology of Human Development. Cambridge, MA: Harvard University Press.
Caudill, W. and D. Plath
    1966 Who Sleeps By Whom? Parent-child Involvement in Urban Japanese Families. Psychiatry 29: 344–366.
Chagnon, N.
    1968 Yanomamo. The Fierce People. New York: Holt, Rinehart, and Winston.
Chow, C.
    1978 Journey in Tears: Memory of a Girlhood in China. New York: McGraw-Hill.

Devereux, G.
    1939 The Social and Cultural Implications of Incest Among the Mohave Indians. Psycho-
       analytic Quarterly 8: 510–533.
    1967 From Anxiety to Method in the Behavioral Sciences. The Hague: Mouton.
deYoung, M.
    1984 Ethics and the "Lunatic Fringe": The Case of Pedophile Organizations. Human Organi-
       zation 43(1): 72–74.
Doek, J.
    1981 Sexual Abuse of Children: An Examination of European Criminal Law. In P. Mrazek
       and C.H. Kempe (Eds.), Sexually Abused Children and Their Families. New York:
       Pergamon Press. pp. 75–84.
Edgerton, R.B.
    1964 Pokot Intersexuality: An East African Example of Sexual Incongruity. American
       Anthropologist 66: 1288–1299.
    1976 Deviance: A Cross-Cultural Perspective. Menlo Park, CA: Cummings.
    1978 The Study of Deviance – Marginal Man or Everyman? In G. Spindler (Ed.), The
       Making of Psychological Anthropolgy. Berkeley: University of California Press. pp.
       442–478.
    1985 Rules, Exceptions, and Social Order. Berkeley: University of California Press.
Evans-Pritchard, E.E.
    1951 Kinship and Marriage Among the Nuer. Oxford: Oxford University Press.
Finkelhor, D.
    1979 Sexually Victimized Children. New York: Free Press.
    1980 Risk Factors in the Sexual Victimization of Children. Child Abuse and Neglect: The
       International Journal 4(4): 265–273.
    1985 Child Sexual Abuse. New Theory and Research. New York: Free Press.
Finkelhor, D. and J. Korbin
    1985 Child Abuse in a Global Perspective. UNICEF Working Paper.
Fischer, J., Ward, R. and M. Ward
    1976 Ponapean Conceptions of Incest. Journal of the Polynesian Society 85(2): 199–207.
Ford, C. and F. Beach
    1951 Patterns of Sexual Behavior. New York: Harper and Brothers.
Garbarino, J.
    1977 The Human Ecology of Child Maltreatment. Journal of Marriage and the Family 39(4):
       721–735.
Giovanni, J. and R. Becerra
    1979 Defining Child Abuse. New York: Free Press.
Goldstein, M.
    1964 A Study of the Ldab Ldob. Central Asiatic Journal 9(2): 123–141.
Groth, N.
    1979 Men Who Rape. New York: Plenum.
Hayes, R.O.
    1975 Female Genital Mutilation, Fertility Control, Women's Roles, and the Patrilineage in
       Modern Sudan: A Functional Analysis. American Ethnologist 2(4): 617–633.
Herdt, G.
    1982 Fetish and Fantasy in Sambia Initiation. In G. Herdt (Ed.) Rituals of Manhood, Male
       Initiation in Papua New Guinea. Berkeley: University of California Press. pp. 44–98.
Herman, J.
    1981 Father-Daughter Incest. Cambridge: Harvard University Press.
Herrmann, M. and M. Jupp
    1985 Commercial Child Pornography and Pedophile Organizations: An International Re-
       port. Response 8(2): 7–10.

Hopkins, K.
    1980 Brother-Sister Marriage in Roman Egypt. Comparative Studies in Society and History 22: 303–354.
Ikeda, Y.
    1982 A Short Introduction to Child Abuse in Japan. Child Abuse and Neglect: The International Journal 6(4): 487–492.
Kapadia K.
    1966 Marriage and Family in northern India. Calcutta: Oxford University Press.
Keesing, R.
    1982 Introduction. In G. Herdt (Ed.), Rituals of Manhood. Male Initiation in Papua New Guinea. Berkeley: University of California Press. pp. 1–43.
Kelly, R.
    1977 Etoro Social Structure. Ann Arbor: University of Michigan Press.
Kennedy, J.
    1970 Circumcision and Excision in Egyptian Nubia. Man 5(2): 175–191.
Kiste, R. and M. Rynkiewich
    1976 Incest and Exogamy: A Comparative Study of Two Marshallese Populations. Journal of the Polynesian Society 85(2): 209–226.
Korbin, J.
    1976 Fieldnotes.
    1981 (Ed.) Child Abuse and Neglect: Cross-Cultural Perspectives. Berkeley: University of California Press.
    1981b "Very Few Cases": Child Abuse and Neglect in the People's Republic of China. In J. Korbin (Ed.), Child Abuse and Neglect: Cross-Cultural Perspectives. Berkeley: University of California Press. pp. 166–185.
Labby, D.
    1976 Incest as Cannibalism: The Yapese Analysis. Journal of the Polynesian Society 85(2): 171–179.
Langness, L.L.
    1981 Child Abuse and Cultural Values: The Case of New Guinea. In J. Korbin (Ed.) Child Abuse and Neglect: Cross-Cultural Perspectives. Berkeley: University of California Press. pp. 13–34.
    1981b Personal communication.
LeVine, R. and B. LeVine
    1966 Nyansongo: A Gusii Community in Africa. New York: Wiley and Sons.
LeVine, S. and R. LeVine
    1981 Child Abuse and Neglect in SubSaharan Africa. In J. Korbin (Ed.) Child Abuse and Neglect: Cross-Cultural Perspectives. Berkeley: University of California Press. pp. 35–55.
Lévi-Strauss, C.
    1969 Elementary Structures of Kinship. Boston: Beacon Press.
Lyons, H.
    1981 Anthropologists, Moralities, and Relativities: The Problem of Genital Mutilations. Canadian Review of Sociology and Anthropology 18(4): 499–518.
MacFarlane, K. and J. Korbin
    1983 Confronting the Incest Secret Long After the Fact: A Family Study of Multiple Victimization with Strategies for Intervention. Child Abuse and Neglect: The International Journal 7(2): 225–237.
Malinowski, B.
    1929 The Sexual Life of Savages. Boston: Routledge and Sons.
Marshall, M.
    1976 Incest and Exogamy on Namoluk Atoll. Journal of the Polynesian Society 85(2): 181–197.

Masson, J.
  1984 Assault on the Truth: Freud's Suppression of the Seduction Theory. New York: Farrar,
      Status & Giroux.
Middleton, R.
  1962 Brother-Sister and Father-Daughter Marriage in Ancient Egypt. American Sociological
      Review 27: 603–611.
Minturn, L.
  1985 A New Look at the Universal Incest Taboo. Paper presented at the Meetings of the
      American Anthropological Association, Washington, D.C., December.
Monberg, T.
  1976 Ungrammatical "Love" on Bellona. Journal of the Polynesian Society 85(2): 243–255.
Morris, M.
  1982 If I should Die Before I Wake. Boston: T.B. Tarcher.
Mrazek, P.
  1981 Definition and Recognition of Sexual Child Abuse: Historical and Cultural Perspec-
      tives. In P. Mrazek and C.H. Kempe (Eds.), Sexually Abused Children and Their
      Families. New York: Pergamon Press. pp. 5–15.
Mrazek, P. and C.H. Kempe, Eds.
  1981 Sexually Abused Children and Their Families. New York: Pergamon Press.
Mrazek, P., Lynch, M. and A. Bentovim
  1981 Recognition of Child Sexual Abuse in the United Kingdom. In P. Mrazek and C.H.
      Kempe (Eds.), Sexually Abused Children and Their Families. New York: Pergamon
      Press. pp. 35–50.
Murdock, G.P.
  1949 Social Structure. New York: Macmillan.
Nathan, L. and Hwang, W.T.
  1981 Child Abuse in an Urban Centre in Malaysia. Child Abuse and Neglect: The Interna-
      tional Journal 5(3): 241–248.
National Center on Child Abuse and Neglect
  1981 Study Findings: National Study of Incidence and Severity of Child Abuse and Neglect.
      Washington, D.C.: DHEW.
Olson, E.
  1981 Socioeconomic and Psychocultural Contexts of Child Abuse and Neglect in Turkey. In
      J. Korbin (Ed.), Child Abuse and Neglect: Cross-Cultural Perspectives. Berkeley:
      University of California. pp. 96–119.
Parsons, T.
  1954 The Incest Taboo in Relation to Social Structure and the Socialization of the Child.
      British Journal of Sociology 5: 102–115.
Perpinan, M.S.
  1985 Strategies Against Sexual Trafficking. Response 8(2): 22.
Phelan, P.
  1981 The Process of Incest: A Cultural Analysis. Ph.D. Dissertation, Stanford University.
Poffenberger, T.
  1981 Child Rearing and Social Structure in Rural India: Toward a Cross-Cultural Definition
      of Child Abuse and Neglect. In J. Korbin (Ed.), Child Abuse and Neglect: Cross-
      Cultural Perspectives. Berkeley: University of California Press. pp. 71–95.
Ronstrom, A.
  1984 Child Sexual Abuse in Sweden. Paper presented at Sweden-U.S. Seminar on Child
      Abuse and Neglect. Satra Bruk, Sweden.
Rush, F.
  1980 The Best Kept Secret. Sexual Abuse of Children. New York: McGraw-Hill.

Russell, D.
    1984a Sexual Exploitation: Rape, Child Sexual Abuse, and Sexual Harassment. Beverly
        Hills, California: Sage.
    1984b The Prevalence and Seriousness of Incestuous Abuse: Step-fathers Versus Biological
        Fathers. Child Abuse and Neglect: The International Journal 7: 133–146.
Salayakianond, W.
    1985 Prostitution in Thailand. Response: 8(2): 23.
Sanday, P.
    1981 The Socio-Cultural Context of Rape. A Cross Cultural Study. Journal of Social Issues
        37: 5–27.
Scheper-Hughes, N.
    1985 Personal Communication.
Schieffelin, E.
    1976 The Sorrow of the Lonely and the Burning of the Dancers. New York: St. Martin's
        Press.
Schneider, D.
    1976 The Meaning of Incest. Journal of the Polynesian Society 85(2): 149–169.
Schultz, L.
    1982 Child Sexual Abuse in Historical Perspective. Journal of Social Work and Human
        Sexuality 1(1/2): 21–35.
Sereny, G.
    1985 The Invisible Children. Child Prostitution in America, West Germany and Great
        Britain. New York: Knopf.
Sgroi, S.
    1977 "Kids With the Clap:" Gonorrhea as an Indicator of Child Sexual Abuse. Victimology
        2(2): 251–267.
Sheper, J.
    1983 Incest. A Biosocial View. New York: Academic Press.
Shore, B.
    1976 Incest Prohibitions and the Logic of Power in Samoa. Journal of the Polynesian Society
        85(2): 275–296.
Summit, R. and J. Kryso
    1978 Sexual Abuse of Children. A Clinical Spectrum. American Journal of Orthopsychiatry
        48(2): 237–251.
Thurnwald, R.
    1916 Banaro Society. Memoirs of the American Anthropological Society Volume III, no. 4.
Weinberg, S.K.
    1955 Incest Behavior. Secaucus, New Jersey: Citadel Press.
Weisberg, D.K.
    1985 Children of the Night. A Study of Adolescent Prostitution. Lexington, MA: Lexington
        Books.
Wilson, P.
    1961 Incest: A Case Study. Social and Economic Studies 12: 200–209.
Wolf, A.
    1970 Childhood Association and Sexual Attraction: A Further Test of the Westermarck
        Hypothesis. American Anthropologist 72: 503–513.
World Health Organization
    1979 Traditional Practices Affecting the Health of Women. Khartoum Conference.

# PRELIMINARY REMARKS ON A STUDY OF INCEST IN ENGLAND[1]

Anthropology has largely concerned itself with explaining the incest taboo and has had little to say on its violation, incest itself. This state of affairs has not passed without comment from those concerned with the sexual abuse of children (Forward and Buck 1978, Willner 1983). As early as 1963, Masters remarked, "One should always keep in mind, as anthropologists often do not, that the existence of a formal incest prohibition does not mean that it is enforced, or that people pay much attention to it." (1963: 45) Anthropologists would undoubtedly agree that the existence of prohibitions does not mean that the forbidden behaviour does not occur. Yet there are few discussions of incest to be found in the anthropological literature.

One reason for this may be the paucity of cases and the secrecy which surrounds them. Traditionally, anthropologists have studied small communities, whether these have been societies where the total population was not large, or where the groups studied have been segments of a larger socio-cultural whole. It is possible that during a stay in such a community, no such case might come to light. The famous case reported by Malinowski came to his attention as an instance of suicide and he records that it was only considerably later that he discovered the circumstances surrounding the death (1926: 77). Schwerin sets out the only case on which he obtained information during his field-work. It came to public knowledge because of the girl's pregnancy, otherwise he might never have heard of it (1980).

However, data on incest in Western societies have been available for several decades and anthropologists have largely ignored them. Willner argues, plausibly enough, that the reason for this is the place that the incest taboo holds in anthropological theory. (1983: 135). Its fascination derives from the combination of apparent universality and socially specific diversity. As Willner puts it: "The allure of theorizing about species-wide institutions has survived repeated evidence that incest taboos are neither unitary nor universal". (Willner 1983: 135).

The difficult of reconciling the diversity of sexual prohibitions with the universal fact of their existence in all human societies has divided anthropological opinion. Some anthropologists accept the evolutionary explanations put forward by socio-biologists, which is based on the assumption that breaches of the incest taboo are rare (Fox 1975, 1980; Brain 1979). Incest is something which does not often occur. Human behaviour can thus be compared with that of animal species in which breeding between closely related animals appears to be inhibited. Thus Fox states: "According to these theories, then, human beings are 'naturally non-incestuous', and this is the reason why we don't easily approve of the practice. I think they are right . . ."

*Nancy Scheper-Hughes (ed.), Child Survival*, 267–290.

(1980: 14). The rest of his book is an account of how evolution must have proceeded in order to develop this inbuilt aversion to incest in human beings.

This type of theory rests on certain other assumptions which, unlike the assumption that incest is uncommon, are not made explicit. They are not without significance for a study of incest, although modern evidence drawn from the study of cases of the sexual abuse of children, tends to throw doubt on their validity. In Western society, the sexual abuse of children can no longer with accuracy be described as rare when estimates of its incidence reach as high a figure as $12\frac{1}{2}$% of women surveyed (Landis 1956). The second assumption, that incest may be equated with inbreeding, implies a particular definition of incest: sexual intercourse. Other sexual behaviour, which cannot result in conception, is therefore not incestuous and can be ignored. But, as Schneider has pointed out, in many societies, including those of the West, sexual approaches, revealing an apparent intent to have intercourse, too great familiarity, taking too close a personal interest are all types of behaviour associated with incest and equally forbidden. Case material, drawn from Western societies, makes it clear that incestuous intercourse is the culmination of a period of sexual involvement and contact. Offenders who are caught during this preliminary period would, under this definition, not be guilty of incest.[2] In fact, such behaviour clearly indicates a sexual relation and general opinion would consider all sexual activity equally forbidden and incestuous. In order to justify the comparison with animal breeding behaviour, incest must also be assumed to be sexual intercourse between mature individuals. Homosexual intercourse or sexual activity between immature siblings is thus not considered incestuous.[3] Further, the sexual experience of children is assumed to consist of 'play' and experimentation which occurs 'naturally' where children are brought up in close association and not restricted by parental authority. Fox, for example, argues that such bodily contacts and 'play' develop in the maturing individual an avoidance of such partners when mature, an averson to sibling incest. However, the literature on child sexual abuse makes it clear, as do the data I discuss later in this article, that incest often begins when children are well below puberty. Further, the difference of ages among siblings make one question the characteristic of 'playfulness' with its implications of consensual activity. Some research indicates that sibling incest, in the sense of full intercourse is relatively common (Finkelhor 1979). Finkelhor remarks that "Our findings of a large number of incestuous involvement would suggest, that such a mechanism (the imprinting of aversion) was weak, easily by-passed or non-existent." (1979: 92). In short, the thesis that the incest taboo is an evolutionary development to prevent imbreeding is open to a number of objections, methodological and factual, which cannot be fully dealt with in a short paper (but see Willner 1983). This brief review has merely aimed to show that assumptions about, and definitions of, incest are intimately connected with particular theories. Where they are not made explicit they can seriously confuse the issues.

Not all those who stress the universality of the incest taboo are convinced of its biological function. Many anthropologists such as Radcliffe-Brown, Seligman or Lévi-Strauss or sociologists like Parsons, share the assumption made by the evolutionists that the incest taboo refers to the relations within the family. Radcliffe-Brown defined incest as "sexual relations within the family" (1950: 69), as do the others mentioned. Others, like Malinowski and Murdock, while recognising that the range of such prohibitions may vary cross-culturally, nevertheless associate the taboo primarily with the family and see other prohibitions as extensions outwards of the primary rule. They all interpret the taboo as a means of promoting the stability of the family as a child rearing group. In Malinowski's words: "A group leading a joint life with the intimacy of daily concerns, with the need of an organised authority and unselfish devotion, cannot tolerate within its framework the possibilities of sexual approaches, for these act as a competitive and disruptive force incompatible with the even tenor and stability of the family." (1940: 105).[4] Others have agreed with him that sexual relations between parents and children would subvert parental (paternal) authority and it was generally assumed by these earlier anthropologists that sexual jealousy and rivalry would disrupt family relationships. However, since the incest taboo was defined in terms of the family, the argument that its social function is to maintain family structure is teleological.

The accumulation of detailed field data has since made it clear that taboos on sexual relations rarely refer only to nuclear kin. Even in Western society, they include grandparents and grandchildren, uncles or aunts or persons connected by marriage. A comparison of the range of relationships where sexual relationships are prohibited revealed the wide variation in different societies. This variation extends to the range of persons between whom sex is prohibited, the sanctions said to be invoked in different cases of breach of the taboo and general attitudes to possible offences against it. These elements vary independently (Goody 1956). Even the meanings of terms used to describe such offences may not be strictly comparable. Goody uses the Concise Oxford Dictionary definition of incest as "sexual commerce of near kindred" to point out that to use this as referring to the family is inaccurate and ignores the existence of different definitions of kinship.

Even within one society, the meaning of incest is not standardised. The Shorter Oxford Dictionary defines incest as "The crime of sexual intercourse or cohabitation between persons related within the degrees within which marriage is prohibited by law."[5] This view is that associated with the Christian religion and seems to be the definition underlying the other main social theory of the incest taboo, propounded originally in the nineteenth century by Tyler and not much later in a slightly different form by Durkheim. Its most recent version is that of Lévi-Strauss (1949). This explanation interprets the incest taboo in terms of relations between families, not within them. The ban on sexual relations within the family entails marrying outside it and ensures that the exchange of women in marriage creates social relationships between

families. The incest taboo is thus the basis of human culture as it distinguishes, conceptually, between kin and non-kin, and of society, since it
establishes a system of social linkages. While still stressing the universality of
the incest taboo, this view of it emphasises its socio-cultural quality, asserting
that it is the taboo which differentiates human from animal society. Incest is
thus a fundamentally anti-social act, since it denies this vital distinction. This
theory makes the exactly opposite assumptions to the ethological theory,
based as it is on the idea that it is in the nature of human beings and animals to
avoid sex with their near kin.

The two types of social explanation differ in the priority each gives to one
or other of the relationships covered by the incest taboo (Seligman 1950).
Both ignore any wide range of relations but in one, an emphasis on the
intergenerational ban, between parent and child, leads to an explanation in
terms of authority and the parent's role in socialising offspring, while focus-
sing primarily on the intergenerational taboo governing siblings relations
results in a theory stressing relations with other families. The failure of this
latter theory to distinguish between a ban on sexual relations and a prohibition on marriage was also the basis of criticism from others (Fox 1967, Mair
1980). There are several well-documented cases of societies where it is
possible to have affairs with individuals who are not marriageable.

Dissatisfaction with the early explanations of the incest taboo centred on
their inability to deal with cross-cultural variation and the translation of
indigenous terms in a manner which ignored their differences from the
Western concept of incest and the incest taboo. Goody's review of the
literature pointed out in detail how sexual offences in other societies may be
defined quite differently in relation to different concepts of kinship and
relations by marriage. Among the Ashanti, for example, sexual relations
between mother and child, or between siblings with the same mother,
constitute the offence of *mogyadie* (literally: eating up of one's own blood).
All sexual relations between members of the same matrilineal clan are
*mogyadie*. Another offence, *atwebenefie*, covered sexual relations among a
wide range of persons, related mostly through marriage, among which were
included father and child. *Atwebenefie* did not cover all relationships which
we might term adulterous, for some of those fell under still another classification, so that one could not translate *atwebenefie* by the term adultery. Thus
the Ashanti have no concept of the incest taboo, in the sense of a single
prohibition covering all relationships in the nuclear family. Such relationships
*are* all covered by bans on sexual relations, but only as the result of a
combination of more than one, more inclusive bans, which emphasise wider
categories of relationships, not the family. Goody concludes that "The study
of incest in any society must be related, not merely to the analysis of marriage
prohibitions or preferences, but also to 'adultery' so that it can be seen within
the total constellation of sexual offences within that society." (1956: 36).

Most British social anthropologists today would accept the difficulty of providing a unitary explanation of such a variable phenomenon as the incest taboo, and oppose explanations which assert its unitary nature. The most extreme relativist position today is probably that of an American, Schneider, who lists his 'revisions' of the nature of the incest taboo as follows: "First, the concept is not confined to kinsmen. Second, it is not confined to sexual intercourse. Third it is centred on modes of behaviour, or, more accurately, on kinds of relationships." (1976: 165) Incest, he concludes "is symbolic of the special way in which the pattern of social relationships may be broken" (1976: 168). The problem of explaining the incest taboo becomes a matter of specifying the meaning of sexuality as a symbol of certain social relationships and not others.

While debates of this nature leave little room for considering whether the incest taboo is broken, this study is directly concerned with incest in a Western society, in order to assess the accuracy of our understanding of it in our own society. Taking a relativist, rather than a unitarist or ethological approach, I begin from the social context from which incest takes its significance.

## THE BRITISH CONTEXT

In Britain, sexual activity is generally thought proper only between adults. Strict Christian doctrine, of course, condemns all sexual relations outside marriage, which has the effect of reserving sexual activity to adults, since marriage requires the partners to be mature. Thereafter, spouses are expected to be faithful to one another, though adultery is no longer an offence in law and since the reform of the Divorce Law, is no longer, of itself, grounds for divorce, although it may be taken to prove breakdown of the marriage. Public opinion still regards adultery as serious and damaging to the marital relationship, while recognising that it is likely to happen and that marriages may survive it. The association between a sexual relationship and marriage is still strong, despite the publicity afforded to 'alternative unions'. In fact, the association between a regular sexual relationship and domesticity is not really disturbed by couples who live together without being legally married. It is promiscuity or the commercialisation of sex, both of which are viewed negatively, which form the antithesis of marriage.

The definition of adult status is blurred in modern Britain. The marriage of persons under 18 requires parental consent, but a girl may legally consent to a sexual relationship once she is 16. For a youth to consent, legally, to homosexual intercourse he must be over 21. The law formalises but does not reflect public opinion, being sometimes ahead of it, sometimes behind it. A consideration of the law of sexual offences is, nevertheless, a useful place to begin understanding the context in which incest is placed, for incest is an unlawful act as well as the subject of a social taboo.

## THE LAW AND SEXUAL OFFENCES

In Britain, sexual relations with a girl under 16 are unlawful, for she is deemed unable to give her consent. If she is under 13, this is a separate and more serious offence, carrying the possibility of a life sentence. A boy under 14 may not be prosecuted for either offence because of "the irrebuttable presumption that a boy under 14 is incapable of sexual intercourse." (Howard League Working Party Report 1985: 174).[6] A youth over that age may be guilty of such offences but sentences are often light. As already indicated, a boy under 21 may not give his consent to a homosexual relationship but homosexuality as such is no longer illegal, although it is still not accepted as legitimate by public opinion. Buggery,[7] however, is still illegal, although children under 14 cannot be held to have consented to it, and cannot be prosecuted. Rape also concerns the matter of consent, it being necessary to prove that the woman did not consent, a matter on which there has been much public discussion. In general, then, a legal definition of sexual offences implies lack of consent, with the age of the parties, the question of whether force was used against a victim, whether as violence, threat or by the mere fact of the perpetrator's being older, stronger, or better informed being factors which relate to that main issue. By contrast, the offence of incest is defined in terms of knowledge of certain pre-existing relationships; consent is not possible where this knowledge exists.

There are two laws which enforce the incest taboo. The Incest Act of 1567 made incest illegal in Scotland; it defines incest as sexual intercourse between grandfather/grandchild, uncle/niece, father/daughter, mother/son, and brother/ sister (including half-siblings). Sexual relations between certain categories of affines are also incestuous.[8] These are: parent-in-law/child's spouse, step-parent/step-child, grandparent-in-law/grandchild's spouse, stepgrandparent/step-grandchild. Homosexual relations within these degrees of relatedness are included but not relationships which are not based on marriage. Thus sexual relations between a man and his illegitimate daughter are not incestuous under Scottish Law, although they are illegal if the daughter is under 16.

The Law relative to England and Wales, with which the law in Northern Ireland has been brought into line, was passed some three and a half centuries later, in 1908. Prior to 1857, the offence had been a religious one, under the jurisdiction of the ecclesiastical court. Incest was brought together with other sexual offences under the Sexual Offences Act 1956. The law embodied here differs from that of Scotland in that it does not include uncle/niece but it does include adoptive and illegitimate relationships of the listed degrees of kinship; no affines are specified. Step relations are excluded, where the Scottish law includes them. (Nowhere in Britain are sexual relations between step-siblings banned; they are not forbidden to marry either.) As a result of the differences in these laws, some sexual relationships would be criminal offences in Scotland, although not in the rest of the country, and *vice versa*.

The earlier, Scottish, law is clearly concerned with the incompatibility of sexual relationships and relations of kinship and marriage; the range of persons listed in the Incest Act is identical with the list of prohibited degrees of marriage. This is not the case in the rest of Britain, despite the Shorter Oxford Dictionary's definition. For example, uncle and niece may not marry but sexual relations between them is not incest. The enactment of the 1908 law took place in a social atmosphere in which, increasingly, kinship was being defined as a matter of 'blood' rather than marriage. This may account for the narrow range of relatives listed and the inclusion of illegitimate relationships, but not step-relations.[9] However, when adoption became legal in 1928, adoptive parents and chhildren were made subject to the law on incest, which indicates that the underlying notion of disturbance to important relationships was still strong, although now defined in relation to 'the family'.

## SOCIAL VALUES

General attitudes as to what constitutes incest lack the clarity of the legal rules. They range between strong disapproval of sexual relationships which are not incestuous in law (uncle/niece or step-father/step-child) and the view that there is nothing wrong in sexual intercourse between step-parent and child because they are not 'biologically' related. There is a strong lobby pressing for reform of the law of marriage to allow step-parents and children to marry. But the relation between the law and public opinion is ambiguous. As Sybil Wolfram has pointed out (1983) cousins have been marriageable since 1540 but there is still unease about it (Strathern 1981: 171–2). The perfectly legal marriage of step-brother and step-sister may be opposed by kin who say they are 'too close' to marry. In particular the law requires there to have been full intercourse for the offence to be classified as incest, whereas other sexual activities would generally be regarded as incestuous if they occurred between close kin.

The idea of 'closeness' fuses two distinct concepts: degrees of kinship, with its implications of ties of 'blood' or genetic connection and membership of a domestic unit. The latter is given kinship status by identifying it with 'the family', and this too accounts for the assimilation of relations based on adoption, fostering and second marriages to those based on 'natural ties'. It would come as a surprise to some people to realise that step-fathers who have a sexual intercourse with their step-daughters are not, in law, guilty of incest.

A general feature of incest taboos, now well established by anthropological research, is that public attitudes to them are not uniform, even within one society. Some breaches of the taboo may be regarded as relatively trivial, as ridiculous or demeaning to the individual who commits them, but as deserving of no particular public action. Others evoke expressions of horror at the very idea of a breach. In Western society generally, and also in Britain, sibling incest is viewed far less negatively than parent-child incest, particularly where both participants are children (Renvoize 1982: 120). Indeed, the sexual behaviour of children may be seen as experiments, to be discouraged but not actually incestuous. This attitude is also seen in the anthropological view which defines incest as full intercourse between mature individuals. Where siblings are adult there is more concern but no great revulsion. This general British view lies behind the majority recommendation of the Criminal Law Revision Committee, reported by Michael Zander in The Guardian (6 November 1980) that sexual intercourse between consenting adult brother and sister should become lawful.[10]

The same attitude is found in other writings. An article by Andrew Wilson in The Observer some days earlier than Zander's came out strongly in favour of a change in the law. It drew attention to "the poignant case of two young people who were dragged before a St. Albans Court" and described their respectable characters and devotion to their children. It is noticeable that those who support reform of the law define incest as sexual relations between adult siblings, while those who oppose it describe the sexual exploitation of a young girl by her father. This neatly illustrates the attitudes both to different forms of incest and to sexual relations between consenting adults as opposed to between adult and child.

The action of the courts also mirrors this differentiation of the offence into two, of which sibling incest is the lesser crime. Bailey and McCabe point out that ". . . incest is not shown to be an offence of the first magnitude but punishments are relatively severe" (1979: 751). The severe punishments, however, fall on a particular offender, the older man. Such a person has a 70% chance of being imprisoned, while "women and young men are not usually subject to heavy custodial penalties. Conditional discharge, probation, and, in the case of juveniles, care orders, are frequently used" (1979: 752). The majority of convicted offenders in Hall-Williams' study were "between 30 and 50 with the majority clustering round about 40", mostly convicted of incest with daughters. (Hall-Williams 1974). Similarly, in some States of the United States, father/daughter incest is singled out as 'aggravated incest' or made subject to much harsher penalties than sibling incest or mother/son incest.

The use of the term 'child sexual abuse' includes incest, particularly between the generations' in a wider category of sexual offence about which there are widely held feelings in society generally. The labelling of incest in this way expresses general horror at cruelty to children, but it tends to mask the fact that many of the 'abusers' are parents. Parental love and care is thought of as both 'natural' and the deepest moral imperative. The ideal of the family rests on these ideas so that to recognise that children may not be safe in their own homes is difficult for most people. Men convicted of sexual offences against children must usually be segregated from other prisoners for their own safety. A senior Probation Officer at Wandsworth Prison assured me that many convicts view 'child molesters' as less than human, no matter what the nature of their own offences. (See also Howard League Working

Party Report 1985: 44–46). Yet review of public opinion would be incomplete without a record of the existence in Western societies of pornography involving children (Herman 1979, Renvoize 1981). In Britain there is a tiny minority of people, some of them involved in organisations such as the Paedophile Information Exchange, who argue that sexual experience for children is educational and liberating. Thus even the taboo on sexual relations with children cannot be considered as being completely accepted, despite the wide revulsion with which such acts are regarded.

The effect of such different attitudes to different forms of sexual activity and to incest in particular, is to constitute probable bias in much of the the data available for study. If sibling incest, either between children or consenting adults, is regarded as not meriting concern, it is likely to be under-reported. The assumption among bio-social or ethological anthropologists that sexual contacts (not intercourse) are common among siblings is not uncommon. One or two people have assured me that this is so, but without producing cases to back their assertions. It may be expected to happen but the reported cases are rare; in my total of 96 cases there are only 11 of sibling incest. In general, the evidence is inconclusive.

There is some evidence that sibling incest is relatively rare. Kinsey's rather dismissive remark that "the most frequent incestuous contacts are between pre-adolescent children but the number of such cases among adolescents and older males is very small" (Kinsey 1948) refers to undefined 'contacts' but receives some support from other data drawn, like Kinsey's, from retrospective reporting (Herman 1981, Meiselman 1979). But, while sibling incest may be viewed with less horror than intergenerational sexual relations, it is not approved. Parents discourage such behaviour and, as one would expect, children involved in sibling incest are frequently those who are neglected by parents. In a number of cases, sexual contacts and even intercourse between young siblings was a consequence of the general sexualisation of domestic relations and cannot be considered separately. In seven of the 11 cases in my study a father was also involved.

On the other hand, a recent study by Finkelhor comes to an opposite conclusion. He argues, on the basis of a study of university students, that "although incest itself is touted as the ultimate taboo, what is really most taboo is cross-generational sexual contact, particularly within the family" (1979: 87). He claims that sibling incest is much more prevalent but his figures are not easy to interpret. He states that only 10% of his reported cases of incest involved cross-generational liaisons, but he includes as 'incest' sexual relations with a range of relatives (cousins and step-siblings, for example) who, in Britain would not be considered subject to the incest taboo. He lists 60 males and 151 females as reporting incest under this definition and, presumably, these figures form the basis for his later calculations of proportions of sibling incest. Some of these had multiple experiences but we are not told how many of these involve both inter- and intra-generational sexual experiences. Moreover, as he points out, there are discrepancies in the rate of reporting for men and women; women report many more experiences with brothers and cousins while men report far fewer. He concludes "these figures pose a riddle for which we have no adequate explanation at the present moment. It strikes right at the heart of the very important but inadequately researched subject of the validity of sex surveys. We can assume with some confidence that many people fail to report or under report their sexual experience, but we know very little about what kind of people underreport which kinds of experiences" (1979: 95–96). And, he might have added, we do not know if, and how, people disguise their experiences by reporting sexual contact with a more distant relative, to lessen the opprobrium, or with a closer one to heighten the sense of outrage.

The question of whether inter- or intra-generational incest is the commoner form must remain unsettled for the time being. Estimates are also affected by how the offence is defined: if the legal definition (full penetration) is used, then sibling incest is probably not very common. If however, all forms of sexual contact including touching or examining the genitals, and verbal exchanges, then sibling incest is probably the commonest form. However, as Finkelhor points out, and my data fully confirm, sibling incest is not always consensual, nor a matter of mutual exploration in a relationship of equality. Much sibling incest involves force used on small girls by older boys or on younger boys by older ones. It can be as traumatic as inter-generational sex. All the cases reported by Finkelhor were of this nature.[11] During a phone-in radio programme in Britain recently, a woman telephoned long-distance to emphasise the brutal and aggressive nature of the treatment she had suffered from her two brothers. There are many similar cases reported which make it clear that the unconcern of those who describe sibling incest as childish play or doomed love do so despite the evidence.

## THE AVAILABLE DATA IN ENGLAND

In large-scale, bureaucratically organised societies such as Britain there are a number of different sources of data on incest. Each has its own in-built limitations and bias, so that they are difficult to compare. Usually incest is defined slightly differently in each case. The narrowest definition is the legal: figures on convictions for incest give the lowest incidence. Some cases of incestuous interference which are reported are not prosecuted for lack of evidence that will convince a court; some offenders are charged with lesser offences. In 1938, the recorded offences notified to the police in England and Wales were as shown in Table I.

The figures for convictions are much lower: in the category of incest, the number of cases convicted (100) represents only 41% of reported cases, although the proportion of cases of incest relative to other convictions for sexual offences remains the same (1.5% of the convictions as opposed to

TABLE I
Notifiable sexual offences recorded by the Police

| | % | No. |
|---|---|---|
| Indecent assault on a female | 53.1 | 10 833 |
| Unlawful sexual intercourse with a girl under 16 | 13.6 | 2 773 |
| Indecent assault on a male | 10.7 | 2 178 |
| Indecency between males | 6.7 | 1 362 |
| Rape | 6.5 | 1 334 |
| Buggery | 2.9 | 588 |
| Gross indecency with a child | 2.5 | 511 |
| Unlawful sexual intercourse with a girl under 15 | 1.2 | 254 |
| Incest | 1.2 | 243 |
| Procuration | 0.8 | 161 |
| Bigamy | 0.5 | 92 |
| Abduction | 0.4 | 81 |
| | 100% | 20 410 |

*Source*: Home Office Statistical Bulletin 5/84 cited in *Unlawful Sex*, Howard League Working Party Report 1985, pp. 13–14.

1.2% of reports). But it must be borne in mind that the criminal statistics list offences, not offenders, and some offenders are charged with more than one offence. Other incestuous offenders are undoubtedly recorded in other categories of sexual offence.

Other published information concerns victims rather than offences. Voluntary child-care agencies, such as the National Society for the Prevention of Cruelty to Children and the British Association for the Study and Prevention of Child Abuse and Neglect publish figures from time to time. BASPCAN's 1981 report suggested "an absolute minimum of 1500 cases of sexual abuse (including incest) a year in Britain with a strong indication that this was merely the tip of the iceberg." (Henshaw 1982). The NSPCC also published figures of sexual abuse in a volume entitled *Trends in Child Abuse* (Creighton 1984). In 1982, of 783 children on their registers, 40 (5.1%) were victims of child sexual abuse.

Research specifically designed to discover the prevalence of incest in Britain has hardly started. Most estimates are "guesstimates". Surveys in the USA are usually based on specific populations (often college students) who are asked to report their childhood experiences (e.g. Finkelhor 1979). The cases reported are drawn from segments of the total population and have features which make them difficult to use as a basis for estimating national prevalence. In Britain, a recent survey commissioned by Channel Four Television attempted to take a national survey. The interviews were carried out by a firm of professional opinion pollsters, using sophisticated techniques to provide a sample which would be representative of different classes and regions in Britain, in a manner similar to that designed to estimate voting behaviour. 2019 Men and women were interviewed and asked to report on a "wide range of experiences from being talked to about sex in an erotic way or exhibitionism (no physical contact) to being fondled/masturbated (physical contact) to sexual intercourse which had taken place before they were 16." (Baker and Duncan 1985: 458). The response rate was high (87%). The results showed that girls were significantly more at risk than boys as far as incestuous abuse was concerned (0.85% of all woman and 0.3% of men). The report also makes clear that sexual intercourse is only a small proportion of incestuous activity experienced as abuse (0.25% of the sample). Unfortunately, since the survey was specifically concerned with the sexual abuse of children by adults, it seems to have excluded sexual experience between children and therefore may have nothing to contribute to the debate about the prevalence of sibling incest.

Such a study, based on retrospective reporting by adults of childhood experiences, is vulnerable to the objection that the reports could not be verified in any way and might include false allegations or fantasies. However, great care was taken with the design of the survey, informants were assured of anonymity and in the absence of any obvious motive for misleading interviewers, it remains for the critics to prove their case. In addition many of the conclusions seem to be consistent with other data. A more serious limitation which this survey shares with all retrospective reporting by adults of different ages is that it covers a long time-span and we cannot tell what factors may have affected reporting rates for the different age-groups. The results cannot tell us whether the prevalence of abuse is increasing or decreasing.

However, the retrospective survey is the only method so far devised of obtaining information on the prevalence of incest or child sexual abuse. All other data must be recognised as being haphazardly drawn from the total number of cases. They represent only the cases which come to the attention of the agencies concerned, in a number of different ways. This can be shown most clearly where voluntary agencies offering support to the victims are concerned. The people who contact Incest Survivors groups, Rape Crisis centres, in person or on the telephone, are self-selected, characterised by a willingness and an ability to take this action.[12] In this they differ from the apparently large number of victims who remain silent, or from those whose abuse is disclosed in other ways. Any case material provided by these specialist groups or agencies is difficult to relate to the total field of such cases, not because it is unreliable but because we have, as yet, no clear understanding of the process which result in cases coming to light.

In short, each type of data has its own limitations, which make comparisons fraught with difficulties (Meiselman 1979). For example, while it seems clear that only a proportion of cases of incest come to the attention of the police, we cannot say how few or how many. The police figures are not obtained in the same way as those of the general survey; cases which are referred for treatment are not always reported to the police, nor are all cases of which an agency has knowledge referred or reported. It is essential to keep in mind the characteristics which are built into the data by the purpose for which they have been collected and by the methods used. If this is done, however, the data do yield results, however rough and ready; indeed, to obtain any sort of overall picture, different sorts of data must be used in combination. Too great a dependence on one source of information is likely to bias the enquiry.

## THE LONDON STUDY

For the social anthropologist the major defect in all the available data is the lack of information on the social circumstances surrounding the case. A therapeutic setting with a focus on family therapy seemed to offer the most detailed information. If the basis of therapy is 'the family', then it would be likely that there would be a broader knowledge of the social context than in agencies concerned with either victims or offenders. Police reports and Social Services files are not normally open to research by outsiders.

The Department of Psychological Medicine in which my study is located is part of a children's hospital in London. It contains within it a team specialising in child sexual abuse, established as a special unit in 1980. The patients are all under 18 and, in practice, even some 17 years olds may be referred elsewhere. This limitation is less serious than it seems, for all the accounts indicate that incest which begins when both partners are adults is very rare indeed.

The CSA Unit, as I shall call it,[13] receives referrals, not merely from the London Metropolitan area but from the Home Counties which surround it and, on occasion, from even further afield. While it is not the only source of treatment for these cases, it is pre-eminent in the field and many of those who work in other hospitals were once part of this team. The cases are referred mainly by social work departments of local government authorities, but sometimes the police, general practitioners or psychiatrists may refer cases. They thus represent a proportion of cases occurring in London but what proportion it is impossible to say. This study is not primarily concerned with the prevalence or incidence of incest but with an analysis of cases of incest in reference to anthropological work on the subject. However, the data show similarities with other data so that the cases are not particularly unusual but resemble others reported on elsewhere.

So far I have identified 196 cases, distributed by date of referral[14] as follows:

| | |
|---|---|
| pre-1984, undated | 5 |
| 1980 (from September only) | 2 |
| 1981 | 8 |
| 1982 | 25 |
| 1983 | 52 |
| 1984 | 104 |
| Total | 196 |

The increase in the volume of referrals is mirrored in other data: for example, the NSPCC reported that, during 1977–81, 68 cases of sexual abuse were reported to them, while in 1982 there were 38 cases in one year alone. The dramatic rise in reports to all agencies represents, in the view of those concerned, not a rising rate of abuse but greater public awareness and willingness to report. Staff in the CSA Unit noticed that television programmes on the subject shown in 1983 and 1984 and in which members of the Unit took part, had noticeable and immediate effects on referrals, some of them by individuals involved in a case, rather than agencies.[15] The 196 cases concern child sexual abuse, defined implicitly as physical contact. The Unit's definition thus covers a variety of sexual offence, as far as the law is concerned, but legal intervention is not always involved.[16] Some cases are referred for diagnosis, others for consultation and court reports, all of which involve only one or two sessions; others come for treatment over a period of time. Cases may be referred at various points after disclosure of the abuse: during police investigations or court proceedings, or at the point where a convicted offender is about to be released from prison and there is doubt about whether he should be allowed to return home. The cases are, therefore, far from homogeneous in nature and the amount of information in the files varies a good deal.

Most of the cases involve one offender and one victim; in just under a third (29%) there are several victims and in a few (9%) there is more than one offender. A total of 259 children is involved, 208 girls and 51 boys. Over half the boys (28) were involved in cases with multiple victims, but only a quarter of all the girls (52). (In 6 cases it was not clear whether there were other abusers or victims.) It is generally recognised that the sexual abuse of boys is underreported, and the figures indicate that it is more likely to be reported where several children are involved: only 11 cases where the only victim was a boy as against 28 where boys were involved with other children, either boys (7) or both boys and girls (21). There is no indication, though, whether the under-reporting occurs in the referral process or whether boys tell someone less frequently than girls.

Only 98 of these cases of sexual abuse involve incest, using that term to cover all forms of sexual contact between tabooed kin, but in the vast majority victim and offender were known to each other. Only 3 offenders were strangers and 23 were either neighbours, friends of the children's parents or known in other capacities; the rest were either relatives or members of the children's own households. By far the commonest perpetrators of incest were fathers (86 men); sibling incest accounts for only 11 cases and in six of these there was more than one offender, always a senior kinsman, usually a father.

The pattern of non-incestuous abuse is very similar: step-fathers are the offenders in 56 cases, 6 of them cases of multiple offenders, father substitutes in a further 8. Only 37 of the offenders in the category of step-father were legally married to the victim's mother so that it would be possible to report these categories as 37 step-fathers and 27 father-substitutes. Thus offenders are most commonly fathers, step-fathers, and father substitutes, in that order.

This is not an unexpected result. Authorities on incest and child sexual abuse in America (Herman 1981, Meiselman 1979), in Germany (Maisch 1973) and in Western society generally (Renvoize) single out these relationships as being most commonly the source of child sexual abuse. However, most of them focus on the kinship relationship as the model for the other types, referring to 'fathers' in general, whether they are step-fathers or 'natural' fathers. This lack of distinction is also found in the social workers' reports for the CSA Unit cases. It may only be a casual reference which indicates that the offender is a step-father; in one or two cases the victim herself did not know she was not the natural daughter of the man who abused her.

The general stress on the kinship relationship seems to me to be misplaced. Despite the much-publicised frequency of divorce, there are still many more households in which children are living with both their 'natural' parents than with only one or with adoptive or foster-parents. One would therefore expect that the relative proportions of 'fathers' and father-substitutes of all sorts would reflect their incidence in the population. If it were the kinship relationship that were the predominant factor, then more fathers would be among the offenders. Unfortunately, the CSA Unit data does not allow us to draw firm conclusions, for the pattern may merely reflect the greater willingness of child victims to disclose abuse by men who are not their 'real' fathers. I have good evidence that some offenders who abuse step-daughters think their action less heinous than 'true' incest; several are on record as declaring that the victim was 'only' a step-daughter or they would 'never' have had sexual relations with their own daughter. It is possible that the taboo *is* weaker in the case of step-fathers or father-substitutes because so much social emphasis is placed on the 'biological' tie as the source of 'real' parenthood. Nevertheless, it must also be noted that there are some cases in this study of men who abused both their own daughters and their step-daughters. Moreover there seems little difference in the nature of the abuse of daughters and step-daughters. From a preliminary analysis of the case-material it does not seem that offenders are more likely to have full intercourse with a step-daughter than a daughter; the impression given by these cases is that those which involve a father do not differ at all, in their details, from cases where the offender is a step-father or father-substitute.

What is more significant than the type of relationship between offender and victim is their membership of a common household. Only 5 out of 98 cases of incest concerned kin who are not living together; in one case (father/daughter) it was unclear whether the sexual abuse had not started before the parents separated and in the others the victims were spending long periods regularly in the offenders' households. 63 of the non-incestuous abusers were also living in the same house as their victims. 21 were not members of the child's household but this includes some neighbours and kin. (In 13 cases either the identity of the abused or the residential arrangements were unclear.) Only about 15% of these cases involve outsiders. The sexual abuse of children is predominantly a domestic crime. The ideals of privacy and autonomy which inhibit neighbours, friends or kin from 'interfering' in what goes on behind the closed door, which marks the household territory, are strong; so is the fear of gossip and public shame which prevent members of the household seeking help.

## EXPLANATIONS

A common stereotype of the incest offender, or of the child sexual abuser, is that he is socially defective or marginal in some way. It is common to find incest associated with isolated rural areas (in Britain the Fen country, Ireland, and more remote backwaters are often cited) or with poor slum areas of cities. It is said to be a 'way of life' among the poor or minority groups who have little social prestige. The individuals themselves may be thought to be lacking in the qualities which make an individual a responsible social being: they are to be of poor intelligence, of criminal background or to be alcoholics. These qualities indicate the uncontrolled, brutish image of the offender. The explanations implicit in these stereotypes is that incest is a failure of social institutions to socialise certain individuals: their deviant behaviour is caused by ungoverned 'animal-like' behaviour or with practices which diminish the hold that social precepts have over this. The association of incest with other deviant behaviour, with alcoholism, crime, mental illness or low intelligence, is entirely consistent with this general view. An association with poverty, overcrowding and the circumstances characteristic of people who are marginal in social terms and of low social prestige follows the attribution, common in all societies, of higher moral worth to the upper strata of society.

The data do not give strong support to these current explanations. As others have noted (Maisch 1973, Hall-Williams 1974) alcoholism and crime are only weakly associated with incest or the sexual abuse of children. There *are* cases which fit the stereotypes but they form by no means the majority of cases, which they would have to do to supply a convincing explanation. Maisch also argued that there is no clear association with the lower social classes (1973: 113–4) but the CSA Unit cases do not seem to support this but, rather, to fit a popular stereotype of child sexual abuse as a result of social conditions. A closer examination will make clear that the bias in the data is only superficially what one would expect if the popular myth were accurate, but the problem is complex.

Table II shows the occupational categories into which the male members of the household of abused children in my study have been divided. Only 119 cases provided sufficient information to use and there was too little about the employment of women to include. Women living alone with their children are classified as cases where the classification is not applicable (N/A). The categories used are those of market research, in order to facilitate comparison with the prevalence survey carried out by MORI for Channel Four Television.

TABLE II
Occupational classes of male household members in CSA Unit cases

| | Not Incest | | Incest | | Total CSA | |
|---|---|---|---|---|---|---|
| | No. | % | No. | % | No | % |
| A. Higher managerial/professional | 0 | 0 | 2 | 3.1 | 2 | 1.7 |
| B. Lower managerial/professional | 5 | 9.1 | 2 | 3.1 | 7 | 5.9 |
| C1. Skilled supervisory/lower non-manual | 6 | 10.9 | 8 | 12.5 | 14 | 11.8 |
| C2. Skilled manual | 14 | 25.5 | 21 | 32.8 | 35 | 29.4 |
| D. Unskilled manual | 10 | 18.2 | 11 | 17.2 | 21 | 17.7 |
| E. Residual, including retired and casuals | 2 | 3.6 | 4 | 6.3 | 6 | 5.0 |
| U. Unemployed | 9 | 16.4 | 12 | 18.8 | 21 | 17.7 |
| NA. Not applicable | 9 | 16.4 | 4 | 6.3 | 13 | 10.9 |
| Total | 55 | 100.1 | 64 | 100.1 | 119 | 100.1 |

Class C2 is the most heavily represented in the figures, with a third of all cases of incest and a quarter of those where the sexual abuse is not incestuous. The previous occupations of those now unemployed would change that picture very little; they too consist largely of manual labour, jobs either quite unskilled or with skills at the lower range of class C2. By contrast classes A and B are very much under-represented in the CSA cases. There is very little difference too, in the pattern for incestuous and non-incestuous sexual abuse. Both the cases in Class A are cases of incest but with such small numbers, this could happen by chance. Similarly, where classes E and U are concerned, a fairly large percentage difference is due to a rather small difference in numbers of incestuous and non-incestuous cases. Overall, nearly half the cases (47%) are accounted for by classes C2 and D, with only 10% of cases coming from the two professional classes. While this does not confirm the thesis that cases would be more frequent among labourers and the very poorest (class E), it would seem to indicate that child sexual abuse is infrequent in professional households.

By contrast, the MORI survey shows a much more even distribution across all classes of the population. Table III, taken from Table I in Baker and Duncan (1985: 460) shows the difference in pattern.

TABLE III

Class of Victims of Child Sexual Abuse (percentages) (the order of the groups has been changed to facilitate comparison)

|                         | AB | C1 | C2 | DE | No. of cases |
|-------------------------|----|----|----|----|--------------|
| General population      | 16 | 22 | 33 | 19 | 2019         |
| Refused to answer       | 16 | 24 | 32 | 29 | 259          |
| Non-abused group        | 16 | 21 | 33 | 30 | 1553         |
| Abused group            | 13 | 27 | 34 | 26 | 206          |
| CSA Unit cases[17]      | 11 | 16 | 41 | 32 | 85           |

In the survey figures there is very little difference between the percentage of respondents alleging sexual abuse in each class and the proportions of that class in the general population. Classes AB have a slightly smaller abused group and class C1 a slight larger one than their share of the general population would lead one to expect but the difference is small in the first case (3%) though somewhat more significant in the second (5%). The CSA Unit cases are distributed much more unevenly, although it is important to remember that they can be compared with the survey figures only with caution, since the two studies operate with rather different definitions of abuse. That of the survey is much wider, including all forms of sexual contact. The MORI survey found a rate of incestuous abuse of 0.6 (about 12 cases) although if all parental figures were included the rate doubled to 1.3% (26 cases). We do not know these are distributed by class, and the number is too small to be of significance; however, it is clear that referrals to the CSA Unit conform much more to the general idea of where such cases would occur.

Other data, however, show a quite different distribution of incidence. The Incest Crisis Line consists of telephone numbers, freely advertised, which may be called by anyone wanting advice. It is largely a resource for victims whose abuse has not been disclosed but those manning the telephones offer advice to the rare perpetrators who call, as well as others. Richard Johnson gave me the background information[18] on new cases which came to him over a period of three months from 1st May 1985. There were 22, shown in Table IV categorised in the same occupational classes as the other data.

Here the contrast is very striking: 12 of the Incest Crisis Line's 22 cases (54.5%) involve the top two occupational classes, whereas only 4 of the CSA Unit cases do (6.2%). Members of the lower strata hardly figure at all among Incest Crisis Line clients; there are proportionately more among CSA Unit patients, but the bulk of the latter from the skilled manual and lower non-manual classes with a concentration in class C2, whereas 77% of the Incest Crisis Line clients came from household supported by non-manual occupations.

It would appear that the class compositions of a set of cases depends largely

TABLE IV

Occupational classes of households of self-referring clients of the Incest Crisis Line compared with the CSA data on incest

| Class | Incest Crisis Line | | CSA Unit | |
|---|---|---|---|---|
| | No. | % | No. | % |
| A | 7 | 31.8 | 2 | 3.1 |
| B | 5 | 22.7 | 2 | 3.1 |
| C1 | 5 | 22.7 | 8 | 12.5 |
| C2 | 1 | 4.6 | 21 | 32.8 |
| D | 2 | 9.1 | 11 | 17.2 |
| E | 1 | 4.6 | 4 | 6.3 |
| NA | 1 | 4.6 | 4 | 6.3 |
| U | 0 | 0 | 12 | 18.8 |
| Total | 22 | 100.1 | 64 | 100.1 |

on the means by which the data are collected. The hospital referrals come largely from the Social Services, whose work tends to focus on a certain sector of the population. Even so, the cases do not confirm the popular stereotype of incest as being more common the further down the social scale one goes. There is also evidence that incidents of child sexual abuse, and incest among the professional and upper classes are escaping detection. Data from the Incest Crisis Line receive confirmation from anecdotal evidence given me by psychiatrists and other therapists. There are a number of possible reasons for this. First, victims in upper-class households are less likely to disclose their abuse because they are aware that their fathers or step-fathers are influential and they feel they will not be believed. In addition, a sense of 'family honour' may be stronger among members of these households and their fear of public shame consequently may be greater. The effect of public censure is no myth; offenders may lose their jobs and public ostracism and name-calling has been sufficient, in several cases, for households to have to move to escape it.

Alternatively, children in these households do make disclosures, but other mechanisms come into play to prevent the case reaching public record. Referral to a doctor or psychiatrist may be the outcome; or the marriage may break up and divorce ensue without the offence being made public or the offender prosecuted. I have been told of a case where a woman used her knowledge of her husband's incest to force a divorce and a generous maintenance settlement. There is no statutory obligation to report cases of child sexual abuse or incest, at least where medical or legal practitioners are concerned. The advice of these specialists is expensive, so that these means of coping with sexual offences are available mostly to the wealthy. It seems highly likely, then, that there are 'hidden' cases whose disclosure would make it much clearer that popular explanations for incest are inadequate.

## ANTHROPOLOGICAL EXPLANATIONS

The CSA Unit data make it abundantly clear that it is not accurate to distinguish sexual intercourse and other sexual activity between kin, calling the former incest and ignoring the latter. Often sexual activity begins with touching or oral sex but full intercourse takes place after a time. The CSA Unit's own analysis of its cases indicate that about a quarter of cases started when the child was under five years old and two-thirds of the cases when the child was under 10. The duration of the sexual relationship was almost always longer than six months: in 40% of the cases it lasted between two and four years, and in nearly 20% over five years. Clearly, the time at which the relationship was discovered determined whether sexual intercourse had taken place. Breaches of the taboo which involve older girls as they reach maturity do occur but they are not common. A victim may not have the courage to tell someone until she is 16 or 17 but it is almost always shown that the activity started years before. These factors together with the growing realisation that many more boys are also sexually abused by their fathers makes it impossible to maintain the comparison between human sexual activities and the breeding behaviour of animals, to regard the incest taboo as a mechanism which prevents genetic defects in offspring or ensures their evolutionary fitness.

The more 'social' rather than biological theories of the incest taboo fare little better. It is clear that certain domestic groups can tolerate sexual relationships within them for a considerable time. Incest does not appear to unleash an orgy of sexual rivalry among the males of the household nor does it prevent the senior man or men of the household exercising authority over other members. Indeed, the maintenance of secrecy about what is happening is often an index of the degree of power which the offender can exert over other members. As Malinowski observed among the Trobrianders (1926) and Schapera confirmed for the Tswana (1940), there is no action until someone complains of the offence. It is the exposure of what has happened which, in most cases, destroys kinship and domestic relationships. Schneider's thesis that incest is the means by which such relationships are broken receives some confirmation, but only if knowledge of the acts becomes public.

The sexual abuse of children has been associated with isolated households, whether these are conceived as geographically isolated in rural areas (Finkelhor 1979) or socially isolated in the mobile anonymity of modern society. Neither the CSA Unit cases nor the Channel Four survey would confirm these findings for Britain. In many cases, there is evidence of relationships with friends, neighbours and kin. Victims often confide in people outside the domestic group: cousins or friends of their own age, teachers and sometimes social workers. In some cases, it is true, the father or step-father is jealously possessive of his daughter or step-daughter, attempting to restrict her movements and prevent her making friends, particularly boy-friends, of her own age. But such restrictions seem equally directed at preventing the abuse being disclosed and keeping the secret intact. Isolation is in these cases as much a result of incest or child sexual abuse as a cause of it. Moreover, we know from retrospective surveys that victims of sexual abuse do eventually leave the household, and form households of their own. The theory which explains the incest taboo as a mechanism which creates relationships between households receives no clear confirmation from my data.

Anthropological theories which seek to explain the incest taboo in terms of their deleterious social consequences are, in effect, tautologous. They conclude that the taboo exists to prevent the consequences of breaking it, whether these results are conceptualised as the disruption of relations within the domestic group, or the lack of relations outside it. The authors draw their perceptions of the harm caused by the sexual abuse of children within their natal household from within their understanding of their own society; the data show that many of these perceptions are inaccurate. Biological theories are also based on lack of sound empirical studies. The study of the phenomenon is still in its infancy but the research on which these preliminary remarks are based, when complete, will be an initial step towards a better anthropological understanding of incest.

## NOTES

1. The research is being funded by the Economic and Social Research Council whose support I am glad to acknowledge here. I am also indebted to the Institute of Child Health of the University of London, who made me a Senior Research Fellow. A particular debt of gratitude is owed to the members of the Child Sexual Abuse Team of the hospital in which I am working, for their hospitality and help. I do not identify them or the hospital in order to preserve the confidentiality of their records. A draft of this paper was read at a seminar in the University of Rochester, in December 1985. I thank members of the seminar for helpful comments but they are not responsible for what I have written.
2. The law in Great Britain also defines incest as sexual intercourse; penetration must be proved if an offender is to be convicted of incest.
3. The possibility of homosexual incest is not usually considered by writers of this school. The fact that it occurs is another indication that the comparison with breeding behaviour may be misleading.
4. This formulation by Malinowski appears, rather oddly, to include conjugal relationships, unless we are to understand that it is sexual approaches, courtship, rather than sexual relationships, which disrupt the family.
5. This dictionary also notes the loose use of 'incestuous' to mean 'adulterous'.
6. But in 1985, two youths of 14, who had formed part of a group which raped two girls, were found guilty of rape.
7. Anal intercourse (buggery) between husband and wife is also, technically, illegal.
8. Affines are those people connected by a marriage. As anthropologists use the term, it includes more relatives than those covered by the term 'in-law'. Step relations are also affines, although in common speech they are distinguished from in-laws.
9. Wolfram (1983) argues that the eugenic motive behind the Incest Act of 1908 has been exaggerated. Certainly, one of the sponsors of the Bill was the National Society for the Prevention of Cruelty to Children, who actively sought to obtain convictions for incest once the act was passed. (Parr 1910).

10. West Germany revised its laws to exclude sexual relations between brother and sister, when under 18, from legal penalties.

11. His study was concerned with sexually victimised children. He defines victimisation as occurring when the victim was five or more years younger than the perpetrator. He thus excluded sexual activity between children of approximately the same age. (1979: 56).

12. Since the organisations guarantee complete anonymity to those who consult them, they are understandably unwilling to divulge or discuss details of cases.

13. I read all case-files from the establishment of the special unit in 1981 until the end of 1984. This terminal point was chosen, partly not to interfere with the work of the department and partly because information on cases referred after that date was still coming in. While a few files could not be traced I am confident that these cases represent almost all referred in that period. Since writing this article 8 more files have been traced.

14. After a series of three television programmes on incest in 1984, there were 637 calls to the number displayed on the screen as a help-line. 476 were concerned with cases of child sexual abuse. By far the greatest number of these calls was from women abused as children (328–60%), but others were involved in a current relationship. 50 men who confessed to perpetrating the offence also telephoned. Callers were referred to specialist agencies for further help. (Source: BBC Back Up services)

15. Members of the Unit have found that it is difficult to keep clients in therapy if there is no legal constraint, such as a court order, to ensure that they attend. There is a tendency now for them to be reluctant to accept cases for therapy where there are no such sanctions for treatment, although consultations may be given.

16. The General Household Survey of 1982 showed that 82% of children under 16 and 81% of those under 18 were living with both natural parents. Only 6% of children under 16 and the same percentage of children under 18 were living with a natural mother and a stepfather. The remaining small percentage is divided among other living arrangements.

17. The percentages are not the same as in Table II because two categories which do not figure in the survey (unemployed and lone parent) have been removed.

18. I am most grateful to him for recording the information for me. No details which might identify individuals were included.

## REFERENCES

Bailey, V. and McCabe, S.
   1979 'Reforming the Law of Incest', Criminal Law Review, 1979: 749–764.
Baker, A. and Duncan, S.
   1985 'Child Sexual Abuse – a Study of Prevalence in Great Britain'. Journal of Child Abuse and Neglect 9: 457–467.
Brain, J.L.
   1979 The Last Taboo: Sex and the Fear of Death, Anchor Press/Doubleday. New York.
Creighton, S.
   1984 The Abuse of Children. The Nationality Society for the Prevention of Cruelty to Children. London.
Dingwall, R., Eekelaar, J. and Murray, T.
   1983 The Protection of Children: State Intervention and Family Life. Blackwell. Oxford.
Finkelhor, D.
   1979 Sexually Victimised Children. Free Press, New York.
Forward, S. and Buck, C.
   1978 Betrayal of Innocence: Incest and its Devastation. J.P. Tarcher Inc. USA. Penguin edition 1981, London.

Fox, R.
  1967 'Totem and Taboo Reconsidered' *in* The Structural Study of Myth and Totemism, (ed.) E. Leach (A.S.A. Monograph 5) Tavistock, London.
  1975 'Primate Kin and human kinship', *in* Biosocial Anthropology, (ed.) R. Fox. Malaby, London.
  1980 The Red Lamp of Incest. Dutton, New York.
Goody, J.
  1956 'A Comparative Approach to Incest and Adultery' British Journal of Sociology 7: 286–305.
Hall-Williams, J.E.
  1974 'The Neglect of Incest: a Criminologist's View' Medicine, Science and the Law. Jan. 64–67.
Henshaw, D.
  1983 'The child abuse that no one dares mention', The Listener, 13. May.
Herman, J.
  1981 Father/Daughter Incest. Harvard University Press, USA.
Howard League Working Party Report
  1985 Unlawful Sex: Offences, Victims and Offenders in the Criminal Justice System of England and Wales. Waterlow, London.
Kinsey and others
  1948 Sexual Behaviour in the Human Male. W.B. Saunders, Philadelphia and London.
Landis, J.
  1956 'Experiences of 500 children with adult sexual deviants'. Psychiatric Quarterly Supplement 3, 91–109.
Lévi-Strauss, C.
  1949 Les Structures Elementaires de la Parente. Plon, Paris.
Mair, L.
  1971 Marriage. Penguin Books. Harmondsworth, England.
Maisch, H.
  1973 Incest, Andre Deutsch, London.
Malinowski, B.
  1926 Crime and Custom in Savage Society. Routledge and Kegan Paul, London.
  1940 A Sociological Analysis of the Rationale of the Prohibated Degrees in Marriage, *in* Kindred and Affinity as Impediments to Marriage: a Report to the Archbishop of Canterbury.
Masters, R.E.
  1963 Patterns of incest. Julian Press, New York.
Meiselman, K.
  1978 Incest: a psychological study of causes and effects with treatment recommendations. Jossey Bass, San Francisco, Washington, London.
Parr, R.J.
  1910 Flame and Flannelette: Being the Facts concerning the Modern Slaughter of the Innocents. N.S.P.C.C. London.
Parsons, C. Talcott
  1954 'The incest taboo in relation to social structure and the socialisation of the child'. British Journal of Sociology 5: 101–117.
Radcliffe-Brown, A.
  1950 Introduction to African Systems of Kinship and Marriage. (eds.) Radcliffe-Brown and Daryll Forde. International African Institute, London.
Renvoize, J.
  1982 Incest: a Family Pattern. Routledge, Kegan Paul, London.

Schapera, I.
  1940 'The Tswana Conception of Incest', *in* Social Structure: Essays presented to A.R. Radcliffe-Brown. Russell and Russell, New York.
Schneider, D.
  1976 'The Meaning of Incest'. Journal of the Polynesian Society 85, 149–70.
Schwerin, K.H.
  1980 'Incest and Kinship Structure' *in* The Versatility of Kinship, R.M. Keesing (ed.), Academic Press.
Seligman, B.
  1950 'Incest and Exogamy: a Reconsideration', American Anthropologist 52, 305–316.
Strathern, M.
  1981 Kinship at the Core: an anthropology of Elmdon in north-west Essex in the nineteen sixties. Cambridge University Press, Cambridge.
Willner, D.
  1983 'Definition and violation: incest and the incest taboos', Man. n.s. Vol. 18 No. 1: 134–159.
Wolfram, S.
  1983 'Eugenics and the Punishment of Incest Act 1908', Criminal Law Review 508–518.

# PART V

# CHILD SAVING: PROBLEMS AND DILEMMAS IN SOCIAL INTERVENTION

Are there no workhouses? Are there no poorhouses?

Dickens, *A Christmas Carol*, 1843

'Mr. Limbkins, I beg your pardon, sir! Oliver Twist has asked for more!'

There was a general start. Horror was depicted in every countenance.

'For *more*! said Mr. Limbkins. 'Compose yourself, Bumble, and answer me distinctly. Do I understand that he asked for more, after he had eaten the supper allotted by the dietary?'

'He did, sir,' replied Bumble.

'That boy will be hung,' said the gentleman in the white waistcoat. 'I know that boy will be hung.'

Dickens, *Oliver Twist*, 1837

CLAIRE MONOD CASSIDY

# WORLD-VIEW CONFLICT AND TODDLER MALNUTRITION: CHANGE AGENT DILEMMAS

The child lay against her mother's breast. Sometimes she whined, mostly she was quiet. Her eyes were slightly sunken, her skin was hot and dry. The day before, the mother had withdrawn food to help control her diarrhea. Several hours before, the mother had withdrawn fluids to prevent the feverish child from suffering chills. The fieldworker said, "She must have aspirin and water." The mother worried, "No, it will make her cold." But the fieldworker prevailed; the child gulped two cups of water and some aspirin. Soon she began to shake, to drip. Her fever broke and she slept.

- Was the mother neglecting her child?
- Was the mother ignorant of appropriate health-care techniques?
- Did the fieldworker behave ethically?

On another day, a fieldworker lay in her hammock, eyes swollen shut. For three days she hadn't eaten; sometimes she sipped a little water through a straw passed between her massively swollen lips. On both the first and second day of the swelling, other workers had taken her by truck to the biomedical doctor; both times he'd given her injections of cortisone. On this third day she told everyone to go away. Then a village mother came bringing a bowl of green gel. Over the protests of other fieldworkers, the villager slathered the gel over the sick woman's face. Soon drops of liquid poured off her face. In a few hours she could slit open her eyes. With continued applications of gel she was back to normal by the next day.[1]

- Were the fieldworkers neglecting their colleague?
- Were they ignorant of appropriate health-care techniques?
- Did the villager behave ethically?

## INTRODUCTION

Among the many conditions of the Third World poor that have been shown to contribute to the development of protein-energy malnutrition (PEM) in infants and toddlers are a constellation of child-care behaviors variously labeled as "harmful" and as "cultural blocks" (first anecdote above, and Table I). Parents who practice these behaviors, especially after they have been introduced to alternative child-care methods, are often labeled "neglectful." The labelers are mainly professional change agents and other cultural outsiders who perceive themselves as having a stake in the welfare of Third World children.

In contrast, culturally sensitive research aimed at understanding parental motivations often demonstrates that the parents themselves consider their child-care strategies not only as culturally normal but as positively beneficial. Even when their children become malnourished, these parents do not usually label themselves as neglectful.

*Nancy Scheper-Hughes (ed.), Child Survival, 293–324.*
© *1987 by D. Reidel Publishing Company.*

TABLE I

Types of child-care behaviors known to promote toddler malnutrition*

---

Exacerbation of psychological stress during weaning
    Arrival of new infant when toddler is less than 24 months of age
    Abrupt weaning, with or without enforced separation from mother
    Expectation of mature behavior and punishment for dependent behavior
    Deviation of attention to preferred sibling
Food restriction
    Concept of diet "appropriate" to toddlers
    Food taboos
    Dietary adjustments during illness
Food competition
    With elders, siblings and caretakers
    With persons of culturally preferred sex
    With persons of culturally preferred relationship

---

* Adapted from Cassidy 1980, Table 1. There are also children whose own behavior promotes malnutrition, particularly children who are unresponsive or weak (Pollitt 1973, Korbin 1984).

The anecdotes which began this paper and the situations just described are classic examples of world-view (values) conflict: the interveners[2] and their Third World clients begin from different assumptions, and perceive and interpret the same "objective reality" differently.

Development specialists have identified the alleviation of Third World childhood malnutrition as a priority, and yet, according to their own evaluations, their intervention is only partially and occasionally effective. Why might that be? And can anything practical be done about it?

Most efforts to understand why carefully planned interventions have unpredicted or undesired outcomes focus on the target populations ("beneficiaries") or on variables in their environments.[3] Meanwhile, the assumptions of the interveners, and the organizational structures within which they work, have not received the attention they deserve,[4] for both intervener world-view and donor agency structure impose important limitations on the intervention process. Unrecognized world-view conflict can cause interveners to misinterpret client goals, to blame clients for behaving in culturally normal ways, to feel frustrated, and even to experience occupational "burnout." As many professional change agents have told me, these are familiar hazards of their occupations.

In this chapter I focus on child malnutrition because it is a topic with which I am familiar. However, if accurate, my remarks should be generalizable beyond child survival issues. The burden of my argument is that concerned culture change agents can learn to reduce the severity or frequency of problems associated with world-view conflict by becoming more aware of their own roles in causing or perpetuating such conflict. They can examine not so much the "culture blocks" of client populations as their own. The practical ends of such professional self-examination are to help interveners design and implement more effective projects, and to avoid "burnout."

I could perhaps not have written this paper were I not at once an "insider" and "outsider" to the several world-views described. As such I feel close enough to sympathize, but detached enough to analyze. I have been trained both as anthropologist and biologist, but for the last several years have used these academic skills only peripherally as I worked within the development field as manager and change agent. The philosophical nexus of my childhood and early adulthood was altruism and positivism; more recently, like so many others, I have begun to explore ecological approaches to interpreting reality.

## THE MODEL

In Paraguay, mothers do not lose children who die; they gain an angel in heaven who can help the rest of the family prosper by interceding with God (Vega 1985). In Brazil, mothers may find it wrong to fight against the deaths of children who seem weak (Scheper-Hughes, this volume). In Africa, Bariba parents may resist forming strong attachments to small children until the children have sprouted teeth and received a formal name (Sargent, this volume). In India, girl children often receive less food and care than boys (Miller, this volume; Rosenberg 1973; Lindenbaum 1977; Johansson 1984). In Belize productive adults get more and better food than small children who because "they are doing nothing" are surely not as hungry (Cassidy, nd). Other development workers come richly supplied with their own stories of child-care habits that seem, from a Western perspective, at the least startling or puzzling, but perhaps also misguided, harmful, or even outrageously inequitable.

The model that follows is intended to make sense both of the world-view that informs the child-care techniques Westerners have associated with childhood malnutrition and of the stress reactions that typify many Western thinkers. Like all models, this one does not reflect "reality"; it is constructed by abstraction and generalization from my own experience.

World-view[5] descriptions summarize sets of (often unconscious) assumptions and values that permit users to perceive, categorize, and understand events in the world and socialize their children; they are not necessarily "scientific," nor do they describe the beliefs of specific persons, projects, or agencies. For those who hope to communicate cross-culturally, it is inappropriate to ask whether another's world-view is "rational"; all world-views have an internal logic, while "rationality" is a value bias characteristic of particular world-views. It is also counterproductive to judge one world-view as "better" or "worse" than another; each has its strengths and limitations, and each can be approached with a tolerant dispassion. It is useful to analyze world-views because such study shows both how a world-view helps users identify and solve real problems; and also how differences in world-view result in different interpretations of and solutions to the same set of problems. With even partial knowledge of these issues, it is sometimes possible to recognize characteristics of a world-view that inhibit "success." Sometimes these can be changed.

In an earlier paper (Cassidy 1982) I argued that most peoples, whether or not they accept the concept of PEM, do recognize many of the same symptoms or behaviors[6] among toddlers that Western observers link to PEM. These are summarized in non-technical language at the top of Figure 1: fretfulness, crying, frequent sickness, often ending in death.

What meaning people give to these behaviors, however, varies considerably. There are two first choices to be made – whether to call the behaviors "normal" or "abnormal," and whether to conclude that "something ought to be done" to change them. Three relevant alternative structures[7] flow logically from these first decisions:

1. The behaviors are normal for this age and nothing need be done about them.
2. The behaviors are abnormal and something ought to be done to alleviate or eliminate the root cause(s).
3. The behaviors are perhaps not wholly desirable but are certainly common, i.e., normal, and the decision to respond must be decided contextually.

When these primary cognitive structures are enriched and specified by the addition of other knowledge, cultural expectations, and environmental variables, they yield distinctive world-view positions. Four of these – some distinctly at odds with one another – are summarized in Figure 1.[8]

The two world-view positions most relevant to our discussion are the *Activist* and *Adapter* positions. Those who associate these toddler behaviors with a biomedical organic disease called PEM *and* believe that something can and should be done to alleviate it fall under the *Activist* rubric; they label these toddler behaviors as problematic, neither normal nor "right."

The *Adapter* position is more complex and subsumes a greater range of variation of opinion as well. Many Adapters might agree that these toddler behaviors *are not desirable in an ideal world*, but would argue that the world is not ideal and that the behaviors are normal, at least in the sense of being commonplace. They would very likely want to take a second look before deciding that change was necessary because they would tend to interpret that *what is commonplace is probably serving some useful purpose*, and is therefore something that ought not to be manipulated without full knowledge of the larger socioenvironmental system. In short, they would probably emphasize the *context* in which the behaviors were occurring, advocating change (intervention) sometimes but rejecting it at other times.

Another way of summarizing these differences highlights the decision

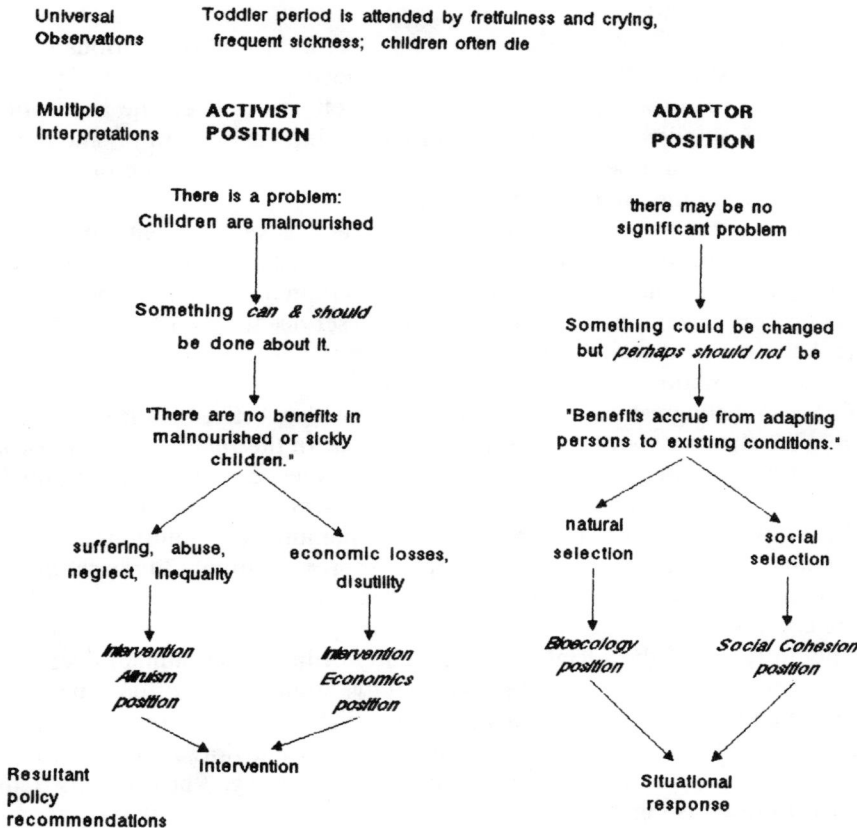

Fig. 1.    Four worldviews relevant to understanding development intervention to alleviate
toddler malnutrition

processes used: Adapters tend to be relativistic and pragmatic (or "instrumental"), while Activists emphasize authority and precedent, and are often
impelled by moral beliefs independent of the situation at hand.

It is clear from this summary that actual persons having these different
perspectives and utilizing such different decision modes would have considerable difficulty communicating. The stage would be set for conflict – and for
intervention failure – were these differences not understood and adjusted for.

But do real people hold these views in the real world? The next two
sections provide evidence that both the Activist and Adapter positions do
summarize cognitive orientations held by actual people.[9]

## The Activist Positions

Since the mid-twentieth century the wealthier, industrialized nations of the world have assumed the task of extending "development" aid to the poorer nations. An important rationale guiding this effort has been the perception that poverty entails suffering, that suffering is painful and dreadful, and that it both can and should be avoided. This altruistic[10] and positivistic rationale is the keystone of the Activist world-view.

Those who carry the development task are activists whose general occupation is that of intervener or change agent; today most of them work directly or indirectly within the vast network of international, national, and private voluntary organizations that have grown up to service the development task.[11] The Activist world-view is briefly analyzed in this section; critical discussion follows presentation of the other world-views.

One can distinguish two subsets within the wider Activist stance, although in real life the two are often closely interwoven. In the *Intervention Economics* position, the societal costs of hunger and sickness are measured mainly in material terms of money and goods, and users are concerned with the *disutility* or *inefficiency* of systems that foster malnutrition. Solutions also tend to be material, emphasizing, for example, improved commodity exchange or production, or income generation and redistribution.

In contrast, in the *Intervention Altruism* position, costs are expressed mainly in terms of the social-spiritual quality of individual human lives, and users worry about suffering and social *inequity*. Solutions are often couched in terms of education to identify to clients both the existence and cause of their suffering and to encourage them to change their behavior. Also offered are various nonmaterial and materials aids (e.g., training, "health huts") intended to decrease inequity.

The Intervention Altruism approach focuses primarily on the individual, while the Intervention Economics approach focuses on impersonal abstractions such as the sector, region, or market. Neither focuses on the society and thus both effectually, if unintentionally, *deemphasize the importance of the community or familial context* in which suffering occurs. However, *it is precisely this social context that has value for many of the Activists' target populations*. Both intervention positions also accept PEM as an organic disease and as a source of suffering. Because of these several beliefs, neither Activist position finds value in malnourished or sickly children.

### Some historical comments

Interestingly, the recognition of PEM as a *disease* is so recent as to be, in effect, a scientific novelty. Current understanding of toddler malnutrition is the result of research done in only a little more than 50 years (counting from Cecily Williams' first major publication, 1933); while the term PEM itself came into common use only after 1970 (Cassidy 1982). The fact that PEM is a "disease" of very recent vintage is often forgotten by interveners who perhaps do not realize that scientific abstractions like "malnutrition" and "organic disease" are not part of the cognitive terrain of nonscientific peoples.

Research into the causes of child malnutrition was originally instigated by the observations of clinicians, most working in colonial settings, who were disturbed by what they perceived as high rates of infant and toddler mortality among village children. We know that toddler malnutrition had existed in earlier periods (e.g., Benham 1981; Cohen and Armelagos 1984) yet before the 1930s it had not provoked a significant helping response. Why not?

Several world-view and politico-economic changes in the nineteenth century seem in retrospect to have laid the foundations for present emphases in international aid, especially to the world's children. For example, traditional Christianity, especially Protestantism, changed from a religion focused on the supernatural to one focused in the world, increasingly defining its mission as one of the alleviating the suffering of less fortunate people (Ahlstrom 1975). This change was influenced and supported by the simultaneous spread of the philosophies of *positivism* and *altruism*. Positivism argued that knowledge of fact is to be based upon the positive data of experience (giving impetus to the growth of science). Altruism was an activist and individualistic theory of conduct that regarded doing good for others as the end of moral action. In the United States, these philosophical orientations found a comfortable home in a nation already characterized as favoring pragmatism, speed, and efficiency, and as trusting in change, youth, and the future (de Crevecoeur 1782; de Toqueville 1835; Thistlethwaite 1961; Hsu 1972; Arensberg and Niehoff 1975).

The nineteenth century also saw the beginnings of an unprecedented growth in wealth and material comfort in Europe and North America, based in large part on the expropriation of the natural resources and labor of colonized areas which became the "underdeveloped nations" of the twentieth century. In America and other new nations, and to a lesser extent in Europe, a growing egalitarian ethos helped to level class distinctions, enabling the poor of these nations to have access to more education and more material goods. The success of nineteenth century scientific and technical production helped to reinforce both the positivist notion of "progress" and the altruistic conviction of the appropriateness of kindly activism.

Toward the end of the 19th century the post-17th century conception of childhood as a vulnerable and necessarily protected stage in the human life cycle (see Aries 1962; Shorter 1977; Fox and Quitt 1980) became vastly popularized. Corresponding to this was a romanticized view of motherhood encoded in the evolving "maternal sentiments" literature (Scheper-Hughes, this volume). These conceptions converged to suggest that infants and children were of central importance to society and to family life, and that mothers were psychologically and biologically predisposed to be loving, indulgent, and self-sacrificing caretakers of their offspring. Zelizer (1985) refers to this relatively new Western ideology as the "sentimentalization" and "sacralization" of childlife. Children, once valued for their (labor) utility to the household economy, were necessarily recast (given the transformation from an agricultural to an industrial economy) as instrumentally useless but emotionally priceless. This ideology of family sentiments, increasingly dominant among the educated and affluent classes, tended to define maternal behavior and "love" in altruistic and class-based terms. It led to an interpretation that women who did not share these values (usually these were poor and less educated) lacked maternal love or *neglected* their children.

This ideology persists. Transferred to the sphere of international development it partially explains the emphatic infant- and child-centered focus of many health and nutrition development efforts, as well as the ready tendency to label Third World parents "neglectful."

The Activist position, characterized by American pragmatism and moralistic sentimentality, can be summarized as the cognitive sequence of "*can* do, *should* do, *shall* do." Jon Rohde, medical doctor and nutrition development specialist, epitomized the Activist position when he said with respect to the implementation of Oral Rehydration Therapy (1984): "You're interested in something that works. And this works. I think that's a good reason to put in ORT projects all over the world."

Although by no means all interveners share this moral pragmatism as their primary approach to human development, the altruistic urge underlies much of the international health and nutrition effort.[12] The following selected quotations indicate the strength of the altruistic position among professional interveners and other spokespersons for international development.

*Emphasis on child survival*
Altruistic thinkers emphasize the welfare of the very young child, even while they recognize that reproducing women, other adults, and school-age children are also undernourished. The small hungry child has (or is perceived by such thinkers to have) more power to motivate the altruistic donor,[13] perhaps because the child is seen as innocent – never the cause of its own plight – and helplessly dependent upon its caretakers. In contrast, adults are viewed as responsible and thus easily culpable – at moral fault – if they do not "appropriately" parent their malnourished children. In this regard consider Chilean activist poet Gabriela Mistral's powerful assessment: "Our worst crime is abandoning the children," which she equates with "neglecting the fountain of life."[14]

This "life" is existence itself, neither necessarily self-aware nor knowledgeable, but a state opposite death, and therefore (for death is suffering, loss, and ending) an unarguable "good." Even when interveners know that the context of the lives they save is miserable, they still want children to live. Child *survival* thus becomes the primary goal, and childhood deaths (perhaps even death itself) are declared "unnecessary." Saouma (1981) argued that "survival is patently the elementary precondition for development," while USAID recently selected "child survival" as the focus linking its various health and nutrition programs (also see Chandler 1984, Cowan and Dhanoa 1983).[15]

Other observers have also commented on this distinctive American survivalist focus, from Mead (1955: 306), who contrasts it to religious systems that
"disallow this tremendous emphasis upon the human lifespan of each individual," to L.F. Newman, who speaks of neonatal intensive care wards as
"creating a cultural construction of fitness resulting from the *requirement to
survive*" (my emphasis; 1984: 3). Levy summarizes the quite striking contrast
between this Activist position and what I call the Social Cohesion position
(below). He describes Americans as putting "individual human life above
social survival and even above human happiness and general well-being," and
contends that "a culture which values the psychic well-being of the kin group
more than the physical well-being of the newborn does not respond well to
demands made upon the group for the benefit of a few non-productive
individuals; it is considered more important to have a harmonious social life
with some infant deaths if necessary" (1962: 159). Imhof analyzes the survivalist focus in historical perspective, tracing the increasing denial of death as
secularization progressed. He notes: "Today, everyone stands for himself,
sets up *his* life work which he has only the duration of his own life to
complete, and must consequently hasten and hurry. Every death is a tragic
event today since it puts an end to a life work" (1985: 21).

*Lack of interest in life context*
The Activist child survival focus is a short-range type of future-orientation;
some present lives are saved, but little emphasis is placed on providing
long-term supportive social, educational, or economic contexts for those
lives. For example, Oral Rehydration Therapy (ORT) is currently popular
because it can both cheaply and relatively easily prevent toddler and infant
deaths from diarrhea. Most often, however, its use is not linked to efforts to
maintain the child once it survives diarrhea, or to prevent recurrent bouts.
UNICEF's present four-part plan to save 20 million preschool lives a year by
encouraging use of vaccinations, breast-feeding, growth charts, and ORT,
does provide a larger context for ORT (See also Pyle 1985). But it is not a
maintenance context, for the plan does not address linked, long-term problems of excess population, underemployment, poverty, lack of educational
facilities, and food scarcity. Or consider a smaller intervention project in a
specific village: Cowan and Dhanoa (1983) documented cases in which certain
children in the households they visited in an Indian village were *unwanted* and
*therefore* malnourished. The interveners nevertheless worked to save these
specific doomed children who had a low chance of ever receiving support
from their social environment.

Outside the media of popular reports, fund-raising letters, or videotapes
designed to activate sympathy in laypersons, altruistic Activists may not
emphasize child innocence or helplessness as a rationale for intervention; in
professional settings they may borrow some of the "pragmatism" of the
Intervention Economics position. For example, in his talk to development

personnel at the U.S. State Department, Jon Rohde (identified above) specifically repudiated purely altruistic reasons for focusing on child survival, and claimed instead that ORT made economic sense and "works." Chandler argues that saving infant lives is cheaper than saving other lives: ". . . lowering infant and child mortality in developing lands offers the greatest opportunity . . . for saving lives at low cost" (1984: 8). He thus argues that it is more economically sound to save infants than their older siblings or parents. Such a claim demonstrates both the short time focus of these Activists and their lack of concern with the context of lives saved, for in actuality the social and economic costs of raising infants are higher than the costs of maintaining already productive members of society.

*Emphasis on unlimited good*
Another idea characteristic of the altruistic position is one I call the "Image of *Un*limited Good." Though the origins of this idea can be traced to the beginnings of the Judeo-Christian tradition (Gregory 1984), continued acceptance of it is surely also linked to the sense that there are unending resources and goods; it is thus also an expression of a "frontier" mentality and of the Activist "can do" or "never say die" position. The Image of Unlimited Good is expressed in defining absolute goals – health for *all*; and the *elimination* or *eradication* of hunger – which translate as expressions of a conviction that the lower end of a distribution can be eliminated:

Health for All by the Year 2000.

Current slogan of WHO and UNICEF

The Right to Food.

"While [increasing production and reducing price fluctuations] are important to overcoming food insecurity, they do not directly address the problem of individual human need. Providing food security for the individual means guaranteeing for every child, woman and man the right to freedom from hunger."

Both quotations from B. Huddleston, Research Fellow, International Food Policy Research Institute, writing for CARE Briefs, 1984

. . . in a decade no child would go to bed hungry, no family would fear for its next day's bread, no individual's potential would be stunted by malnutrition.

(1974 goal of the World Food Conference)

The 1980 Presidential Commission on World Hunger urged that the U.S. 'make the elimination of hunger the primary focus of its relations with the developing world.' The moral and humanitarian reasons for such a policy seem self-evident.

Both quotations from M. McLaughlin, Interfaith Action for Economic Justice 1984: 1, 3

". . . renewal of the commitment for eradicating hunger."
                    U.S. Under Secretary of Agriculture D.G. Amstutz 1984: 2,
                             quoting goals of the World Food Council 1974, 1984.

Though the Image of Unlimited Good has been questioned recently, especially by spokespersons of the ecology movement and the biomedical industry
(Meadows 1972; Meadows and Meadows 1973; Hardin 1972, 1985; Aaron
and Schwartz 1984), the idea that scarcity exists – or at least is a seriously
limiting factor – is still resisted by many altruistic thinkers.

For example, until about the early 1970s, the assumption among those
involved in development was that there was not enough food produced in the
world to feed all the hungry; this assumption fueled the "Green Revolution."
Since then, and as with surprise, Activists have discovered what political
scientists and others have long believed, that is, that people go hungry not so
much because there is not enough food as because food – and wealth – is *not
equitably distributed.*

McLaughlin writes: "What was seen in 1974 as a problem of hunger has
come to be viewed as a . . . problem of underdevelopment, maldistribution
of wealth and income, poverty, social injustice, and, ultimately, of politics"
(1984: 2). Herman (1984: 471) is equally succinct ". . . food production in
Latin America is sufficient to satisfy the nutritional needs of the population.
Poverty, not lack of food, is the root of hunger in the region. . . . Hunger
and, more significantly, malnutrition have unequal distribution of wealth and
income as their primary cause." For development personnel, such observations are still novel enough to require explication. At least one observer
argues that the frustrations of altruistic interveners are directly linked to the
wish that scarcity did not exist: "[A] source of discontent with the market
economy is a vague resentment at often having to pay a material cost to serve
higher values . . . At bottom, and without realizing it, what they resent is the
economic problem – the inexorable fact of scarcity and the need to make
choices" (Yeager, 1984: 11).

At the same time, fundamentally altruistic development experts do define
modified (or, they might say, "realistic", "not naive") positions which again
borrow pragmatism from the Intervention Economics position. Thus, although the overall goal of WHO and UNICEF is "Health for All," in practice
more limited goals are set, and more limited achievements labeled successes.
Success might be declared if child mortality in some locale were reduced from
20% to 5%; similarly success occurs if the governments of the poorest countries
are persuaded simply to spend more of their limited national budgets on health,
as by raising spending from $1 or $2 per person per year to $7 per person-year
(Chandler 1984). My point is not that these altruistic thinkers *can* define such
modified positions, but rather that by repeatedly selecting utopian goals they
force themselves into the position of *having* to do so. Another kind of thinker,
such as an Adapter, would dismiss such goals as unrealistic, yet the occasional
attainments of apparently utopian efforts – such as the virtual eradication of
smallpox – make altruistic thinkers feel justified in their position.

*Altruistic compulsion*
The desire to help, to do good for others, is laudable and common among human beings, but for altruists this desire becomes a need, a compulsion virtually definitional of self. Thus it is often spoken of in moral or religious terms, and the value of intervening to help is felt to be self-evident (see also McLaughlin and Mistral, both quoted above):

Malnutrition should not be attacked because to do so brings utility, but because such a task is morally necessary. What we need to fight for is equity. . . .

C. Shuftan 1983: 134

Unless conscience is dead, we will have to act. 'For God so loved the world that he gave . . .'

S. Mooneyham, International Consultant, 1983: 134

I don't think God will allow the Church to walk away.

G. Gunderson, Administrative Director, SEEDS (Christians Concerned About Hunger), 1984: 13

Alibis for indifference [to world hunger] are defunct.

E. Saouma, Director-General, Food and Agriculture Organization, 1981: 15

. . . I am certain we all share a desire to help [the hungry] in the best ways possible. . . . it is the same small world . . . the same desire for a better life.

J.R. Block, U.S. Secretary of Agriculture, 1983: 2, 7

Note that Shuftan, though accepting Activism, rejects the economic version in favor of a moral (and political) one. U.S. Secretary of Agriculture Block's assumption that "all . . . desire to help" is a natural outcome of the idea that the rightness of eliminating hunger is self-evident. As the powerful language of the quotations indicates, these beliefs are held very strongly: they are *core values* for the speakers and writers. To question their validity, then, is extremely difficult. Altruists who have become aware of the fact that these positions are *not* self-evident to all, may react to this knowledge with emotional desperation, while others, in lower key but still defensive, may find proposed alternatives distressing and "impossible."[16] Thus Levy, speaking of biomedical efforts to save village infant lives, noted: "It is almost impossible for the para-medical worker to voice a dissenting opinion which is usually taken as a Machiavellian desire to see the infant perish" (1962: 160).

Under these conditions of subjectivity, the altruistic thinker may be tempted to assign a pejorative label to non-altruists: "ignorant" if circumstances suggest that the non-altruist hasn't had the opportunity to learn altruistic behaviors, and perhaps "inhumane," "abusive," "racist," or "neglectful" to those who have apparently rejected components of the altruistic world-view. Some of these descriptions have found their way into the development literature; examples are given in Cassidy 1980.

For our purposes, the label of "neglectful" is especialy interesting, for it is often applied by outside observers[17] to any case of childhood malnutrition associated with "harmful" child-care customs, even when the parents feel themselves to be adequate caretakers. Parents might reserve the term to that subset of cases in which they recognized in themselves or in others of their own society indifference to child welfare (Rohner 1975). Given that the two situations may be difficult to distinguish in the real world, the distinction is still unlikely to seem cogent to altruistic thinkers since they find hurtful *any* customs that encourage the development of malnutrition.[18]

However, interveners who recognize neglect as culturally situational (this text; Rohner 1975, Korbin 1981) can attempt to integrate this knowledge into their design plans so as to proceed with "socially sensitive" intervention.

*Intervener view of client population*

A second response, other than the labeling one, seems to be expressed in interveners' preferred view of their client population. The development literature often defines Third World beneficiary populations as "traditional" or "agrarian," terms in rough opposition to "modern" and "urban." The label "traditional" is applied, in general, to rural villagers most of whom engage in semi-subsistence farming using an ancient technology. These villagers have little (Western-style) education and little cash, and are relatively isolated from modernity and the larger market economy. They are materially poor. Malnutrition and other illnesses occur frequently, especially among infants and toddlers, and life expectancy is less than among urban and First World populations. Interveners assume that "traditional" people are dissatisfied with these conditions.

Activists also believe that "traditional" peoples share a distinctive set of attitudes, the most important of which is that traditional – ancestral – ways are best and that there is no need to change. Supposing such perceptions were accurate, one would expect "traditional" villagers to argue that the same child behaviors that interveners link with PEM are in fact typical and "normal." Children are acting as toddlers always do – and always did – and there is therefore no cause for alarm or for change. Intervention projects are therefore not desired.

This position is in many ways a mirror image of the Activist position. Thus, where the Activist finds abnormality, this "accepter" finds normality; where the Activist loves change, the "accepter" is supposed to abhor it; and where the Activist recommends intervention, the "accepter" wants none. The intervener concept of "culture block" nicely expresses this Activist perception of "base traditionalism." A "culture block" consists in one or a set of behaviors defined by outsiders as "harmful" but to which users cling.[19]

Some "culture blocks" are understood to encourage malnutrition; the nutrition intervener hopes to find ways to alter these behaviors. But if clients (appear to) resist, attitudes that interveners first see as being merely *opposite* those of Activists may come to be seen as in *opposition*.

Though there are no doubt individual villagers who think in this rigid manner, I do not know of modern ethnographic sources that describe any *groups* of people whose thinking would conform to this model. Rather, most rural villagers tend to think more like adapters, described below. Indeed, the "traditional" world-view, which one might easily accept as real on the basis of frequent discussion in the development literature, is perhaps better understood as an inversion of Activist values projected onto client populations. It is an early construct of relatively naive (sometimes hostile) Activist intervener efforts to explain client attitudes. Because the interveners did not view their clients as peers, but rather as "troubled people" to whom aid was to be given, they were unprepared – indeed, did not wish – to understand client cultures holistically. Instead, they hoped to manage and manipulate the recipient cultures rapidly and with curative specificity, preferably altering only a few "harmful" customs while leaving the rest intact.

This early Activist image of beneficiary populations has been refined since the 1960s as a result of field experience and the growth of new theory (e.g., cultural ecology, appropriate technology, integrated farming systems). Today many interveners know that cultures cannot easily be fragmented into nonintersecting units, that apparently harmful customs may have adaptive aspects, and that villagers do not uniformly resist change. Nevertheless, the old image is persistent enough that social scientists continue to counter it in print (three recent examples among many: Wylie 1984, Bates 1984, Adams 1985; also see Kahn 1985).

Why might interveners project or cling to an unrealistic image of beneficiaries? First, it seems deceptively familiar because it is a mirror image of the Activist world-view. As mirror image it shares many commonalities with the Activist position, chief of which are the conviction of rightness and the dependence upon authority for knowledge (ancestral in one case, "scientific" in the other). The projection is as linear as its parent, and Westerners have mastered linear thinking. By linear logic, amelioration becomes a task of identifying which attitudes need change, and then of replacing one set of attitudes with another. "Ignorance" will respond to "education."

In contrast, Adapter world-views are more complex and may be difficult for linear thinkers to grasp (see discussion in Jelliffe and Jelliffe 1976). We turn now to a consideration of these.

### The Adapter Positions

Figure 1 identifies two Adapter positions as the *Bioecology* and *Social Cohesion* positions. The first summarizes a position of evolutionary and ecological biologists (but not sociobiologists), few of whom are directly involved in delivering development aid. The second represents the position of Third World rural and poor urban populations, including the main targets of development projects, as interpreted in the research of social scientists.

If we accept, for the moment, that social science efforts to voice the essence of villager world-views have been accurate, it becomes clear that bioecologists and the Third World poor share important perspectives appropriately characterized as "ecological." For example, both focus on the *context* in which the organism finds itself, and ask how the individual organism relates to the larger context. Thus questions of "good" are typically phrased in terms of the *continuity of the group* rather than of the individual, and it is often recognized that what damages an individual organism may paradoxically help maintain the larger group. For the evolutionary biologist this individual organism is an animal (or plant) reproducing in a natural environment, which includes the organism's deme/species and (often) society. For the peasant or traditional villager, the organism is a person functioning as part of the social group. For both, an individual is "successful" if it adapts to *existing* environmental and social conditions.

The future, therefore, is predicated on the present, and can rarely be imagined in either absolute or utopian terms. In addition, time is counted in years or generations rather than in the months characteristic of Activist thinkers. Adapters find that individual survival is relatively unimportant unless those who survive grow to adulthood and take their proper place as productive (reproducing) members of the community (population).

Another reason Adapters tend not to think in utopian terms is that they assume that *scarcity exists*, and that there is never enough to provide an ideal environment for all organisms. Consequently, some competition for resources is inevitable and "normal." For Bioecologists the concept of scarcity is expressed in evolutionary terms. The world-view of peasants was brilliantly summarized by George Foster (1965) under the rubric of the "Image of Limited Good."

Together, these several values mean that Adapters measure the desirability of change against their own twin realities of scarcity and competition, and express "good" in terms of long-term *group* continuity. The large number of interlocking variables that such thinkers perceive and must assess in order to choose between "change" and "preservation" cause their decision-making to be complex and comparatively slow. In the interests of brevity I will not discuss the Bioecology position further (but see Newman 1961; Lisowski 1966; Stini 1971; Robson and Wadsworth 1977; Cassidy 1980).

*The social cohesion position*
This rubric of course actually covers a wide range of culturally distinct positions held by numerous Third World peoples (and some of the poor and "traditional" elsewhere as well), but important commonalities permit a useful grouping. These rural villagers – the developers' typical target populations –

are usually materially poor; scarcity, with attendant hunger, is a constant real threat. Most of their cultural attitudes, as Foster (1965) argued in his explication of the "Image of Limited Good," flow logically from this threat. According to this zero-sum view, the world contains only a finite amount of "good" (resources, energy, goodwill), and one person's gain is necessarily another's loss.

Cultural means to keep scarcity in check take two general forms. The one most familiar to outsiders consists in being cautious about initiating or accepting changes. Since individuals and communities can best persist by establishing and maintaining carefully balanced reciprocal (and cooperative) relationships with one another and with the environment, any changes that seem to threaten this balance are inevitably – and properly – suspect. As noted above, such thinkers do accept some changes, but may resist or reject other changes if, in their experience, such changes could throw into disequilibrium the "good" of the existing system.

A second means to control scarcity consists in distinguishing those groups valued for their productivity from others devalued as less or nonproductive. A traditional community must maintain a high ratio of producers to nonproducers if it hopes to persist, and one way to do this is to deny resources – at least in a relative sense – to those perceived as less productive. The other way is to reward productive membership, such as cooperation in family or community teams. In such a community the *sense of belonging* is a major desired "good," and it may be disastrous to individuals if the social bonds that ensure belonging are cut. (Many intervention projects introduce changes that effactually, even sometimes intentionally, sever such bonds; these are the kinds of changes villagers might predictably resist. For a case analysis, see Howard 1979.)

The most socially, ritually, and economically productive members of such societies are adults. Among the less productive members are children. Many customs and behaviors that interveners have associated with poor child health and lowered chances for survival can be interpreted as societal efforts to decrease the costs of childrearing. This approach might not "make sense" where food is abundant or most children live to schoolage, but where food is scarce and many children die, it does. It is important to note at once, however, that societal efforts to be frugal are typically unrelated to whether or not parents "love" their children.[20] Numerous ethnographic studies (Whiting 1963; Coles 1964–1977; Rohner 1975; Korbin 1981) show that, with few exceptions, poor and village parents *do* love their children and that the quality of their love is not different from that which altruistic parents may offer their children. The patterning and timing of the offer of love may differ, however, specifically favoring ways which *maximize the sense of social relatedness* of the child. In this way the Social Cohesion world-view is taught and made to work.

In some societies children are not awarded "humanness" or "us-ness" at birth,[21] but accede to societal rights only gradually, that is, as they become increasingly socialized and productive. Before such marker events occur, children may receive relatively less attention or care than afterwards. To give but one example, Sargent (this volume) shows how, because Bariba (Benin) people believe that witch-children display oddities of tooth eruption, parents cannot be certain that the child they are raising is human until its teeth erupt normally, and at the usual time, some months after birth. Even then, children are felt to be much like animals until they begin to reason, sometime around age 2. Formal names may not be given until ages 4 or 5. By controlling care according to marker events, parents can avoid forming too close attachments to children who are all too likely to die.

In many societies one sex is preferred over the other, and a child of the devalued sex may be viewed as "socially defective," to use Miller's apt phrase (this volume), increasing the likelihood that it will be underfed and under-stimulated, and that it will succumb to infection, malnutrition, or accident. Girls are often the less valued sex, and this type of social selection is often cited as a main reason why girls in certain areas die at higher rates than boys. In most cases social selection begins at birth, but death comes in the toddler years, which is why observers have denominated these deaths as examples of "delayed," "deferred," or "attenuated" infanticide (Rosenberg 1973; Scrim-shaw 1978; Johansson 1984; see also Gokulanathan and Verghese 1969; Prugh and Harlow 1966). Emphasizing that this social selection represents normal behavior in these societies, Cassidy (1980) has referred to the same phenomenon as "benign neglect" – neither abuse nor malign neglect.

If boys are defined as doing work and having ritual abilities, while girls (apart from helping with younger children) simply "consume resources" until they leave the family at marriage, then such behaviors make a kind of sense. The altruistic Activist thinker might interpret this approach as inequitable and argue that it is unnecessary, but the Social Cohesionistic thinker would probably argue that to spend equally on two children with such different productive potentials is to fly in the face of scarcity, to risk the continuity of the entire social group. Potter (this volume) quotes a Chinese villager (male): "You *must* have a son to carry on the family name. If you don't have a son, you won't have anyone to worship the dead parent's souls. It will cut the generations, there will be no ancestors. You raise sons, sons support you in your old age. It's impossible for the daughters to take care of the aged, because they marry out."

Miller (this volume) describes how contemporary Asian Indian parents use amniocentesis to determine the sex of their unborn children. They then selectively abort female fetuses, apparently preferring to choose against females *in utero* rather than to allow indirect social selection to take its toll slowly at a later date.

Differential valuing can also affect children perceived as "weaker." For example, Scheper-Hughes (this volume) shows how some poor Brazilian mothers may neglect those of their children whom they assess as weaker and less likely to survive. Basing their decision on their perception that life is a struggle, wherein only the stronger survive, these mothers feel that it is necessary to let the weaker die and indeed argue that it is wrong to fight death. Scheper-Hughes describes a mother's grief when such children die as being "as attenuated as her attachment." Ingham (1970) describes a Mexican folk belief concerning moon eclipses: "The moon restores itself to wholeness by eating . . . parts of fetuses – *vulnerable surpluses*" (my emphasis, p. 83).

Yet another form of resource competition that works against small children is preferential food distribution to the most productive, typically the working adults (Cassidy 1980; Dickemann 1984; Pelto 1984).

On the other hand, children who survive such resource competition enjoy steadily increasing social value as they mature and become productive. A four-year-old who can carry and look after a younger sibling is already productive and proportionately more valued. In asking the young child to work, its parent is perhaps acting out of economic necessity but is also, and more importantly, drawing the child closer to valued adult groups and expressing approbation and trust.

### World-view Conflicts Among the Positions

The Adapter and Activist positions summarize strikingly different world-views, each with its own internal logic, each validated by widespread use and measurable "success." Following are two examples of conflict between the positions.

Because persons using the Bioecological perspective can see "benefit" in malnutrition precisely where Activists see "harm," Activists may be tempted to call the Bioecological position "inhumane." Ironically, the deep time sense of Bioecologists suggest to them that Activist interventions are "short-sighted rescue" efforts all too likely to disequilibrate an existing system delicately balanced to accrue benefits to the most people in the long run. This difference in perspective is relevant to intervention even though few Bioecologists are interveners because it offers Activists a "way out" of the single-minded altruistic child-survival ethic. Specifically, based on the biological fact of unequal viability of infants, altruistic Activists might be able to construct a less absolute (and pressured) approach to "saving every life" which might prove widely acceptable. But before such an end could be gained, altruistic Activists would have to be able to view the problem of child survival with some detachment; I return to this subject below.

The Social Cohesion and Intervention Altruist positions seem to be in near opposition: Where the Altruist focuses on individuals, physical health, and longevity, the Social Cohesionist focuses on group robustness. Where the Social Cohesionist fears scarcity, the Altruist hopes it isn't true and the Activist says we can change the world so as to eliminate what we fear. Where the Activist orients toward children, the Social Cohesionist orients towards adults. Worse, when both focus on children they want to raise them quite differently. The Altruist regards children as having an inherent inalienable value, and wants to prepare the child for adulthood by ensuring "optimal" growth and health and by providing time for formal education; parental love is expressed by working to provide such things to one's properly nonproductive, dependent children. The Social Cohesionist also wants to prepare the child for adulthood, but by transforming a currently unproductive nonmember into a productive group member; the loving parent thus integrates its child and makes it useful.

In sum, the two world-views interpret human "good" very differently. To illustrate how this can cause dilemma, consider again the hypothetical four-year-old toting its younger sibling. We have seen how such behavior is valued from a Social Cohesion perspective. An altruistic thinker, however, might find that requiring the child to work *de*values it. As an intervener, such a thinker might wish to eliminate whatever poverty seemed to necessitate the child's working. Yet by relieving the child of its physical burden, such a thinker is also relieving it of some part of its social value and of its sense of belonging. Indeed, this thinker is tinkering with the source of success – the very guts – of the Social Cohesion position, and paradoxically, increasing the chances that the child will experience hunger and malnutrition.

The study of Cowan and Dhanoa (1983), mentioned earlier in this chapter, is worth considering further. Hoping to improve the health of Indian village children, these researchers offered nutrition education to their mothers. Cowan and Dhanoa were able to distinguish four villager valuations of children, from most wanted (first males) to unwanted (mostly late-born females). In a summary paragraph they report: "Success [at achieving children's weights of more than 70% of Harvard Growth Standards] was understandably lower in low priority females, however a success rate of 67% in these unwanted children indicated a significant attitude change [in mothers]. . . . a significant number, while their mothers complied with feeding advice, are still neglected" (1983: 353). The "significant attitude change" refers to interveners' success at getting mothers to feed more and better food to unwanted children, who therefore often survived; clearly it does *not* refer to any change in mothers' valuing of these children, many of whom remained unwanted, with little or no social future in their communities. In this case it seems fair to ask if the altruistic compulsion has succeeded. If the children's equity has not increased, have they been saved any suffering?

## CHANGE AGENT DILEMMAS

What happened in the above examples? It seems that, guided by the perspectives of their own world-view, Activist/Altruist interveners confused or ignored the *social context* of the children's lives and suggested changes that were ameliorative only *in the interveners' own eyes*. Wanting to do good, but defining good from only one perspective, the interveners have done harm.

The adequacy of Altruism as a philosophical orientation depends upon the success with which "doing good for others" can be defined. Problems occur when the alleviation of immediate pain paradoxically ensures future tragedy (for example, when saving child lives results in overpopulation and underemployment), and when the good envisioned by the interveners does not match that envisioned by their clients. The paradox constitutes a central dilemma for altruistic thinkers because, even knowing of the conflict, they *may find it difficult to question components of their own world-view*. The question the concerned intervener will want to entertain is, "Can the altruistic world-view be made responsive to context?" Another way to ask this question is: "Can I, as a change agent, find a way to work in nonaltruistic settings, "doing good" in ways that the non-altruists define, without becoming morally distressed or immobilized?"

Many altruistic thinkers are aware that their helping compulsion is a two-edged sword (discussion in Sims 1981, Kaseje 1985). Many have responded to this realization by developing increasingly sophisticated means to rationalize their needs with those of their ostensible clients. For example, realizing that their priorities may not be those of village clients, change agents have developed methods to help clients identify their own "felt needs" (the commonest term), "priorities," "interests," or "goals." The value of this process has been institutionalized in the form of "social soundness analysis." Considerable attention has also been given to the proper formulation of education and other interventions, so as to make them "sustainable," that is, sufficiently acceptable, culturally and economically, that clients will maintain the new behavior once the project is over. These approaches have been ameliorative; nevertheless, the true context of client lives continues largely unaddressed (also see context discussions in Chafkin 1978; Chen 1983; Korbin 1984; and L.F. Newman 1984).

Another reason why the true context of client lives remains underexamined is structural: the delivery structure of development aid itself limits responses. Western science categorizes and bureaucracies divide themselves into nonintersecting work units, so that most interveners not only expect but are also expected (or even required) to limit themselves to specified areas such as "primary health care," "nutrition education," "family planning," or "employment generation." One who designed an overarching scheme would be unlikely to meet with success, for many colleagues would be unable to comprehend such a scheme. Others (or the agency itself) would argue that it was too ambitious, would take too long, cut across work unit boundaries and cause dissension, give uncertain results, or not be cost-effective. Structural rewards currently accrue to those who get definable results rapidly and within budget; synthetic thinking is neither commonly taught nor rewarded.

A second way in which the delivery structure can be seen to limit the local success of projects is related to the question of deciding who, exactly, the clients are. Organizationally, it makes economic and political sense to maximize the size of the benefited population. Thus interveners may help village-level clients identify "felt" needs but at the same time find they must justify a project by identifying clients' "*unfelt*" needs. The latter may be those of the interveners, those of the sponsoring government or donor agency, or indeed those of any who may benefit directly or indirectly from the intended intervention. Such needs are not only "unfelt" for most villagers, but may even be counter-productive for them.

Two partial solutions to these problems are the "multi-sectoral" and "client-centered" approaches to intervention. In the former, donor agencies try to build bridges between their specialty subdivisions to ensure a wider perspective on problem solving; this approach has been especially popular in the area of nutrition (Hullander 1983; Guerra de Macedo and Daza 1984), but has met with only limited success. In the latter, clients are ideally involved in the design and implementation of intervention, and presumably guide development in directions that *they* perceive to serve their needs (Currey 1981; Pines 1983; Shuftan 1983; Chandler 1984). A potential sticking point is that clients may define needs that the interveners cannot morally accept (such as adult-centered food intervention), or that agencies refuse to fund for political or economic reasons.

In sum, the work context of professional interveners is both philosophically and organizationally complex. Change agents may feel themselves caught in the conflictual, relatively powerless, middle management position, serving one group toward which they feel a moral responsibility, and beholden to another which they represent and which employs them. Pines comments: "Practical realistic planning is rarely neat. It tries to distill something useful from a cauldron filled with the jealousies, weaknesses, power struggles, and aspirations of those responsible for doing something" (1983: 56). Intervener "burnout" appears when interveners, no longer comfortable juggling these many pressures, sense desperation in themselves, become deeply cynical about the helpfulness of their work or of the development "industry," or decide that clients are neglectful, irrational, ungrateful, or frustratingly slow to change.

## RESOLVING THE WORLD-VIEW DILEMMA

Using the model discussed above, it is obvious that interveners have three basic choices. First, they can see the Activist and Adapter positions as mutually exclusive and *withdraw* from further intervention work, feeling it to be useless. Second, they can see the two positions as mutually exclusive and be so convinced of the superiority of their own ethic that they interpret their mission as one of *replacing* the world-view of their clients.

The third choice consists in *recognizing the validity and cogency of both positions* and of seeking commonalities that will permit true communication between intervener and client. The aim is to help clients to engage in ameliorative (*their* definition!) redesign of their own cultures. Based on my assumption that most interveners are impelled by a sincere desire to help, and can recognize the rights of others to believe and behave differently from themselves, I suggest that most professional interveners will aspire to the third of the three possibilities.

However, they will have to be aware that clients might not – might *never* – choose to make decisions like those the change agents favor. Further, to maximize intervention success they will have to modify some Activist and altruist attitudes that presently militate against cross-cultural communication. These are two large demands upon interveners; *they are, however, exactly similar in kind to those interveners ask clients to accept.*

For example, one bias altruists must question is the "Image of Unlimited Good." To a great many people, perhaps especially "traditional" peoples, *scarcity is real.* To them, curative slogans sound like utopian promises waiting to be broken. Small-scale ameliorative projects[22] are infinitely preferable; at least they will seem feasible to beneficiaries.

A related Activist attitude which increasingly is being recognized as needing modification is the attitude that intervention in human affairs can be *fast* and *specific*; as Bates (1984) notes, there are no "quick fixes" where the "human factor" is involved.

A third perception is the positivist focus on science-as-panacea, along with the assumption that its values are self-evident and universal (see Cassidy 1982). For the case in hand, intervener concern with malnutrition and diet, at least at the village level, needs to be replaced by concern with hunger, food, and *the sources of social valuing of people.* In nonaltruistic, nonscientific settings, education will be more effective if it avoids emphasizing scientific or altruistic motivations for change.

The central question for many altruistic thinkers may be to determine how they can practice intervention and work within nonaltruistic world-view settings without becoming morally disturbed. Altruists deeply hope to do good for others. This aim is laudable, and yet when it is rigidly coupled with certain other ideas – child-as-central, child-irreplacibility, short-term survival – it is significantly foreign to Adapter thinkers. When translated into intervention projects, it is also probably not in the best interests of community or social survival. Yet if altruistic interveners hold to this combination of beliefs not as intellectual precepts but as moral compulsions, they *will* be unresponsive to the real context of client lives. Unfortunately, questioning the validity of any part of the compulsion seems to question the whole, draining the personal source of energy of the altruist, and constituting a threat that may be so frightening that, as one reader of this paper stated, the very possibility "provokes defensiveness and prevents activation of the learning mode."

How, then, is the concerned altruistic intervener to begin the process of decreasing the emotional tensions created by the difference between his or her world-view and that of clients? The answer, it seems to me, lies in the practice of dispassion. One must accept the fact that one's reality is not universal, and is not "good" (or, we may prefer to say, useful or functional) in every situation.

It may be helpful to realize that while nonaltruistic world-views character-ize Third World clients, they are also common among Westerners. The "useful child" concept discussed above never wholly died out in the West and is reportedly undergoing resurgence (Zelizer 1985). Both ecological and many economic theories – important to development work – are posited on accepting the reality of scarcity.

The thoughtful intervener will also want to ask him or herself what motivates this desire to "do good." Readers of this paper in the pre-publication stage – all of them interveners – have suggested that they may derive their own sense of self-worth from their sense of "doing good for others," thereby decreasing their own existential pain. The author May Sarton captures the latter idea in one of her poems: "Why do I feel compelled / To answer, day after day, / Answer the stranger at the window? / In the hope that shared pain / Can become healing? / That if I spend myself / Without stint / I shall be made whole? / That the long woe / Will come to an end? / Or the gift come back – / Poetry, forgiveness?"(1984: 34, Stanza 2).

Who is the stranger? Could it be oneself?

Sarton knows her solution lies in changing herself, and she knows it will be difficult: "It is time I heard / My own voice weeping / . . . It is time you let me sleep / the unhealable / Into the dark. / But how to do it? / It would take a pickaxe now / To break through / to the source" (1984: 34, Stanza 3).

And so of course it is difficult for any of us to change. No-one likes to give up cherished assumptions. I do not argue that all altruistic ideals must be abandoned – to do so would be to throw out the baby with the powdered milk! Rather, I argue that the altruistic thinker can learn dispassion, can unravel the strands of thought, can step back and analyze the quality of each, can choose among them, and can construct a new, and moral, theory of good which is *situationally responsive*. I further argue that the altruistic intervener *must* do so if he or she hopes in the long view to truly help the poor and hungry of the world.

### ACKNOWLEDGMENTS

My warmest thanks to the following persons for pre-publication critiques of this paper: Dr. Sandra Callier (Office of International Cooperation and Development, U.S.D.A.), Dr. Phillips Foster (Agricultural Economics, University of Maryland), Dr. Charlotte Leighton (development consultant, health financing), Dr. Elizabeth Meites (development consultant, nutrition), Dr. Nancy Scheper-Hughes (Anthropology, University of California, Berkeley),

Dr. William Stuart (Anthropology, University of Maryland), Dr. Tamara Vega (Nutrition Extension, University of Maryland), Mr. Tom Wilson (USAID), and Ms. Rosalinda Yangas (consultant, primary health care). Oral versions of this paper were presented for discussion to University of Maryland courses on World Hunger and on Philosophy and Public Policy; to the D.C. Women's Group in International Health; and to the 1984 annual meeting of the American Anthropological Association.

## NOTES

1. Both anecdotes date from my fieldwork in Belize in 1973–74. The fieldworker was ill from contact with seeds of the chichem tree. The green gel was a decoction of leaves of the gumbo-limbo tree, a native specific used to relieve chichem poisoning.

2. Intervener, syn: change agent, provider. Intervention client, syn: beneficiary, receiver. The term "interventionist" is in common use but has negative connotations for many and is not used in this paper.

3. Interveners today are quite familiar with characteristics of "traditional" village life that are highly associated with child malnutrition. These have been exhaustively analyzed, and changing explanatory models reflect increasing observer sophistication. The problems thought appropriate for intervention and the methods thought appropriate to alleviate them, both change, reflecting changes in donor agency management or philosophy, in political climate, and in the interveners' technical understanding of their task. For example, the task of alleviating childhood malnutrition, delineated as a distinct problem in the 1950s, has recently become merely a subpart of the task of promoting "child survival." During the same period, Western perceptions of the primary cause of child malnutrition have changed significantly. The major dietary lack, once thought to be protein, is now understood to be energy; the major locus of intervention, once thought to be individual children in hospitals, has become families in communities; the major cause of malnutrition, once thought to be simply food deficiency, is now recognized to be complex and to include food availability, environmental sanitation, rate of infection, lack of access to or misuse of Western-style education or goods, and a plethora of "harmful" cultural behaviors, especially of parents. Even justifications for inducing change are subject to fluctuation; Chafkin [1978], draws attention to how definitions of social equity change with political administrations. Environment-focused analyses of why projects "fail" provoke technical solutions [e.g., the provision of clean water, and immunizations]. Beneficiary-focused analyses produce two distinct types of responses. The ameliorative response is to offer "education" to clients to cause changes that the interveners believe will promote child health and survival. The other response is not so positive: often interveners express disappointment in, frustration with or hostility towards clients who resist or ignore intervention schemes.

4. But see the following for other examples of efforts to unravel aspects of the cognition of world-view or development work: Sims, Paolucci and Morris 1972; Dwyer and Mayer 1975; Jelliffe and Jelliffe 1976; Chafkin 1978; Wilbur 1980; Field 1983; Pines 1983; Shuftan 1983; Gregory 1984; P. Hill 1985; Kahn 1985; and Rifkin and Walt 1986.

5. World-view, a term coined by R. Redfield. Terms with similar meaning include weltan-schauung, paradigm, value system, value orientation. [See Gregory 1984].

6. There is a split between social and natural scientists in use of the word "behavior." I use it in its broader sense to mean any acts – physical, physiological, social, or other – of organisms

7. Besides the three relevant to our discussion, two other structures exist logically. These are: [1] "behaviors are normal, take action" – which doesn't make sense unless "action" is defined as "maintenance" resulting in a structure indistinguishable from "norm no action;" and [2] "abnormal, no action" which is to allow recognized malnutrition, or

abnormality, to continue unchecked, a behavior not consistent with long-term societal continuance. It is possible that the Iᴋ, as described by Turnbull [1972] provide an example of this second reaction. On could also posit a "hard-nose" world-view position in which one group blames another for having "brought it all on themselves" and insists that they "take the consequences." This sort of punitive attitude is not unknown, but for obvious reasons is not common among employable interveners.

8. Other interpretative positions exist. Consider the logical explanatory structures that might be constructed around the problem of childhood malnutrition by Marxist economists, some conservative Christian groups, developmental psychologists, or sociobiologists, to name just a few. Of these, only the Marxist economists and certain Christian groups would be likely to be actively involved in on-going ameliorative efforts in the Third World.

9. It is worth remarking, at this point, on a methodological issue familiar to social scientists, that of the researchers' access to the data. In this paper, the Activists, literate First World interveners, speak for themselves; as researcher I have direct access not only to the documents they produce but also, since I share with them many cultural expectations, to many of their thinking patterns. In contrast, Third World villagers rarely speak to us directly. Instead, their thoughts are relayed through the intermediation of the social scientist. The observations of these scientists are convincing because they are collected systematically and because they report considerable coherence among the views of peoples of similar technological development in terms of their valuing habits. The argument in the second part of my model presentation is based upon secondary social science data.

10. In this paper the concept of altruism is used in the sense of one consciously wishing to do good for another (Funk and Wagnall's Standard College Dictionary [1966]: "selfless devotion to the welfare of others"). It is *not* used in the sociobiological sense of one (animal) instinctively behaving in "selfless" ways that maximize its reproductive potential, nor is there any implication in this paper that human values are or could be genetically encoded.

11. The Activist stance is not limited to the international sphere; it subsumes most "helping professionals" wherever they offer help.

12. Other rationales are also important. For example, the goals of national organizations typically include (besides altruism) concern with maintaining Third World contacts to build markets and to preserve national security. Religious organizations often hope to missionize. Some might argue that underlying many development efforts is First World guilt over past colonial exploitation. The altruistic rationale is, however, the rationale best recognized by the public, most morally acceptable in societies heavily influenced by humanistic philosophies, and most often publicized by donor agencies when seeking public support or reporting on the success of projects.

13. Excerpts from a fund-raising letter from the U.S. Committee for UNICEF, over the signature of Chairman Hugh Downs, February 1984: "In the ten seconds it took you to open and begin to read this letter, three children died from the effects of malnutrition somewhere in the world. No statistic can express what it's like to see even one child die that way . . . to watch the small feeble head movements that expend all the energy a youngster has left . . . to see the panic in a dying tot's innocent eyes. . . . With your help, millions of children will be given the chance of a lifetime – the chance to live – to grow up healthy and strong. Without your help, more children will continue to die painfully, slowly, and needlessly – children like the nine who have died in the past thirty seconds."

14. Line quoted by Gunderson in Seeds [Christians Concerned About Hunger] 1984 from a poem favored by development sources and quoted in full in Marley 1984.

15. Besides defining death as unnecessary, many such sources describe sickness as "tragic" or "disastrous." These conceptualizations differ, for example, from those natural scientists might express concerning the phylogenetic advantages to social groups of the survival of the more fit, or of ontogenic advantages to the individual associated with development of the immune system. They also differ from traditional formulations of Christianity and of other religions, which are relatively accepting of death (see Imhof 1985).

16. Examples of such reactions can be readily evoked during discussions, but are less often written down. Here are some exceptions. As an example of emotional desperation consider Tokyo slum worker and poet T. Kagawa's stanza, in a poem about trying to succor a starving infant girl: "Then do you pity Ishi? / I need your pity, too. / I must help; I must help / *But am helpless*" (1935: 33). As an example of rejecting alternatives consider Bates (1984: 362) who ends his article on appropriate technology by recognizing his own optimism that intervention "must work" and asking: "Indeed, what other alternatives does the world community have?" Similarly, consider article titles that express unilaterality, e.g., "We Can't Walk Away!" (Gunderson 1984) or "The Right to Food" (Huddleston 1984); and the emotionality sometimes associated with critiques of ecological models, e.g., texts edited by Cole 1973 and G. Hill 1973.

17. The distinction being made here, in nontechnical language, is that between what anthropologists call the *etic* and *emic* positions. These terms are often used to distinguish, respectively, between the perspectives of outsiders-to-a-cultural-setting and those of insiders-to-the-same-cultural-setting. Harris (1968) gives formal definitions. The observer (outsider) tends to treat data and persons as objects (as of research or intervention), while the user (insider) tends to see people as subjects; these can therefore also be called the objectivist and subjectivist perspectives. The scientific perspective is generally spoken of as an etic position, as it is intended to be objective, dispassionate, and disinterested. While useful, the insider/outsider distinction breaks down when we realize that the community of scientific observers is not homogeneous but has its own subcultures and ideologies and is therefore often subjectivist (cf., for example, Kuhn 1970, or for a specific case analysis, Harrison and Ritenbaugh 1981). In the present paper, the etic position is represented by those scientists who study and define PEM and its causes but are neither invested in eliminating nor in maintaining/creating it in populations. In contrast, those who apply scientific findings with the *aim* of alleviating malnutrition have priorities separate from and in addition to those of scientist, and must therefore be understood emically (i.e., as representing a distinct and subjective subculture), just as are their Third world clients. This approach is in contrast to that of many Activists, who believe their understanding of PEM to be etic, universal, and culture-free (for further discussion, see Cassidy 1982).

18. One may wonder how often parental neglect is given as the cause of toddler malnutrition when the labelers know that such "neglect" is beyond parental control, since it is due either to ignorance of Western nutrition science or to poverty. The literature suggests that it is quite usual to fuse purposeful and accidental causes of hunger under one label [e.g., "Where so many children were ill or dying as a result of neglect, deliberate or due to ignorance . . ." Cowan and Dhanoa 1983: 344]; but I could find only one actual study of helping professionals' opinions, and this focused on child neglect in the United States (Lena and Warkov 1978). The authors found that a group of 116 Probate Court judges felt that child malnutrition caused by parental dietary ignorance was "neglect" in 18.4% of cases, while malnutrition caused by poverty constituted "neglect" in 8.8% of cases. A group of 614 police, social workers, teachers, and nurses were much more likely to label such cases as examples of parental neglect: for this group 37.3% adjudged dietary ignorance as "neglect," while 22.0% adjudged poverty as "neglect."

19. Jelliffe introduced the concept of "culture block" in a 1957 article which was astute and enlightened for its period. In it, Jelliffe argued that cultural behavior traits could be separated into groups of "beneficial," "neutral," and "harmful" habits regarding child malnutrition, and that interveners might be able to limit their intervention to those which were harmful. This argument was exciting because it indicated that human cultures – which had seemed so amorphous – could be analyzed into easily graspable subparts, and that only a few of these required attention for dietary intervention. Thus intervention became more controllable, more "scientific," for culture seemed to have become manipulable. The argument also seemed to be kind to beneficiaries because they might "keep" most of their culture traits while giving up only a few. In retrospect we can see this argument as fraught

with problems, only one of which was the optimism with which users approached the idea that etic labels could properly be attached to emic categories of behavior. At least another ten years passed before researchers began discussing the limitations of the outsider approach; that discussion continues.

20. The agony of the starving parent is well described in this fragment of a poem by Chinese poet Wang Ts'an, who wrote from 177–217 AD: "A starving woman beside the road / hugs her child, then lays it in the weeds, / looks back at the sound of its wailing, / wipes her tears and goes on alone: / I don't even know when my own death will come – / how can I keep both of us alive?" (in Watson 1971: 35). Recall also abandoned Hagar who, wandering in the desert without water, lays Ishmael under a bush and walks aside, weeping "How can I watch the child die?" (Genesis 21: 16).

21. Of course, Western children also accede to societal rights only gradually even where infants are socially defined as "human" and as "members" from birth. Biologically, on the other hand, it is increasingly recognized that infant humans are born less mature than infants of other mammalian species. Chavez and Martinez (quoted in Ordonez 1984: 181) provide a Western definition of the arrival of humanness relevant to our discussion: ". . . to have the child reach a weight of 8 kg in the first 8 months of life should be the first objective in any preventive intervention in the field of malnutrition. This is what may be called the 'true birth' of the child; it means passing the barrier between what may be called an extra-uterine fetus before reaching that weight, and a true human being with capacities of its own."

22. "Small-scale" must also be measured in terms of the beneficiary community, for Western concepts of small-scale may be vast when translated to a village setting. In a project I was recently involved in, technical assistants wanted to put in a "small" farm of 60 sows, plus baby pigs, in a village of 250 persons. After many days of argument, technical assistants were persuaded to begin with what-they-felt-was-not-a-farm of a mere 6 sows.

## REFERENCES

Aaron, H.J., and W.B. Schwartz
  1984 The Painful Prescription: Rationing Hospital Care. Washington, D.C.: The Brookings Institution.
Adams, J.Q.
  1985 Peasant Rationality: Individuals, Groups, Cultures. World Development (forthcoming).
Ahlstrom, S.
  1975 A Religious History of the American People. Garden City, N.Y.: Doubleday.
Amstutz, D.G.
  1984 Statement of Under Secretary of Agriculture Daniel G. Amstutz before the House Foreign Affairs Committee. Washington, D.C.: U.S. Department of Agriculture. August 2.
Arensberg, C.M., and A.N. Niehoff
  1975 American Cultural Values. In The Nacirema: Readings on American Culture. J.P. Spradley and M.A. Rynkiewich (eds.), pp. 363–378. Boston: Little Brown.
Aries, P.
  1962 Centuries of Childhood: A Social History of Family Life. N.Y.: Vintage Press.
Bates, R.P.
  1984 Appropriate Technologies for Increasing Food Utilization. In Malnutrition: Determinants and Consequences. Current Topics in Nutrition and Disease Vol. 10. P.L. White and N. Selvey (eds.), pp. 355–364. New York: A.R. Liss.
Benham, H.
  1981 Man's Struggle for Food. Washington, D.C.: University Press of America.
Block, J.R.
  1983 Remarks Prepared for Delivery by Secretary of Agriculture John R. Block before the

World Food Council's Ninth Ministerial. Washington, D.C.: U.S. Department of
Agriculture. June 27.

Cassidy, C.M.
nd   Unpublished field research data from Belize village.
1980 Benign Neglect and Toddler Malnutrition. *In* Social and Biological Predictors of
Nutritional Status, Physical Growth, and Neurological Development. L.S. Greene and
F. Johnston (eds.), pp. 109–139. New York: Academic Press.
1982 Protein Energy Malnutrition as a Culture Bound Syndrome. Culture, Medicine and
Psychiatry 6: 325–345.

Chafkin, S.
1978 The Emerging Concern for Human Nutrition and World Hunger. Agriculture and Food
Policy Review Paper. Washington, D.C.: U.S. Department of Agriculture/
ESCS-AFPR-2. September.

Chandler, W.U.
1984 Improving World Health: A Least Cost Strategy. Washington, D.C.: Worldwatch
Paper, no. 59. July.

Chen, L.C.
1983 Planning for the Control of the Diarrhea-Malnutrition Complex. *In* Nutrition in the
Community, A Critical Look at Nutrition Policy, Planning and Programmes, 2nd ed.
D.S. McLaren (ed.), pp. 143–160. N.Y.: John Wiley.

Cohen, M.N., and G.J. Armelagos
1984 Paleopathology and the Origins of Agriculture. N.Y.: Academic Press.

Cole, H.S.D., ed.
1973 Models of Doom: A Critique of the Limits to Growth. New York: Universe Books.

Coles, R.
1964–1977 Children of Crisis, Vols 1–5. Boston: Little, Brown.

Cowan, B., and J. Dhanoa
1983 The Prevention of Toddler Malnutrition by Home-Based Nutrition Health Education.
*In* Nutrition in the Community, A Critical Look at Nutrition Policy, Planning and
Programmes, 2nd ed. D.S. McLaren (ed.), pp. 339–356. N.Y.: John Wiley.

Currey, B.
1981 Fallacies About Famine. Ceres (FAO) 14(2): 20–25.

de Crevecoeur, J.H. St.J.
1782 [1957] Letters from an American Farmer. N.Y.: E.P. Dutton.

de Tocqueville, A.
1835, 1840 [1956] Democracy in America. R.D. Heffner, ed. N.Y.: Mentor Books.

Dickemann, M.
1984 Concepts and Classification in the Study of Human Infanticide: Sectional Introduction
and Some Cautionary Notes. *In* Infanticide, Comparative and Evolutionary Perspectives. G. Hausfater and S. Blaffer Hrdy (eds.), pp. 427–438. N.Y.: Aldine.

Dwyer, J.T., and J. Mayer
1975 Beyond Economics and Nutrition: The Complex Basis of Food Policy. Science 188: 566–70.

Field, J.O.
1983 The Importance of Context: Nutrition Planning and Development Reconsidered. *In*
Nutrition in the Community, A Critical Look at Nutrition Policy, Planning and Programmes, 2nd ed. D.S. McLaren (ed.), pp. 61–78. N.Y.: John Wiley.

Foster, G.M.
1965 Peasant Society and the Image of Limited Good. American Anthropologist 67(2):
293–315.

Fox, V.C., and M.H. Quitt
1980 Loving, Parenting and Dying: The Family Cycle in England and America, Past and
Present. New York: Psychohistory Press.

Gokulanathan, K.S., and K.P. Verghese
   1969 Socio-cultural Malnutrition (Growth Failure in Children Due to Socio-cultural Factors).
   Journal of Tropical Pediatrics 15: 118–124.
Gregory, M.S.
   1984 Science and Humanities: Toward a New Worldview. *In* The Culture of Biomedicine,
   Studies in Science and Culture, Vol. 1. D.H. Brock and A. Harward (eds.), pp. 11–33.
   Newark: University of Delaware Press.
Guerra de Macedo, C., and C.H. Daza
   1984 Regional Strategies for the Improvement of Nutrition in the Western Hemisphere. *In*
   Malnutrition: Determinants and Consequences. Current Topics in Nutrition and Dis-
   ease, Vol. 10. P.L. White and N. Selvey (eds.), pp. 447–455. New York: A.R. Liss.
Gunderson, G.
   1984 We Can't Walk Away. Seeds [Christians Concerned About Hunger] 7(10): 6–13,
   October.
Hardin, G.
   1972 Exploring New Ethics for Survival. New York: Viking.
   1985 Crisis on the Commons. The Sciences 25(5): 21–25.
Harris, M.
   1968 The Rise of Anthropological Theory. New York: Crowell.
Harrison, G.G., and C. Ritenbaugh
   1981 Anthropology and Nutrition: A Perspective on Two Scientific Subcultures. Federation
   Proceedings 40(11): 2595–2600.
Herman, M.
   1984 Socioeconomic Development and Nutrition in Latin America. *In* Malnutrition: Deter-
   minants and Consequences. Current Topics in Nutrition and Disease Vol. 10. P.L.
   White and N. Selvey (eds.), pp. 471–475. New York: A.R. Liss.
Hill, G.
   1973 Madman in a Lifeboat: Issues of the Environmental Crisis. New York: New York Times
   Survey Series.
Hill, P.
   1985 The Gullibility of Development Economists. Anthropology Today 1(2): 10–12.
Howard, M.T.
   1979 Kwashiorkor on Kilimanjaro: the Social Handling of Malnutrition. Unpublished Ph.D.
   dissertation, Anthropology Department, Michigan State University, East Lansing.
Hsu, F.L.K.
   1972 American Core Value and National Character. *In* Psychological Anthropology. F.L.K.
   Hsu (ed.), pp. 241–262. Cambride, Mass.: Schenkman.
Huddleston, B.
   nd[ca. 1984] Confronting World Hunger. CARE Briefs on Development Issues, no. 3.
Hullander, E.L.
   1983 Policy Profiles: AID Drafts Blueprints for U.S. Economic Assistance. Horizons (AID)
   2(7): 33–45.
Imhof, A.E.
   1985 From the Old Mortality Pattern to the New: Implications of a Radical Change from the
   Sixteenth to the Twentieth Century. Bulletin of the History of Medicine 59: 1–29.
Ingham, J.
   1970 On Mexican Folk Medicine. American Anthropologist 72(1): 76–87.
Jelliffe, D.B.
   1957 Social Culture and Nutrition Culture Blocks and Protein Malnutrition in Early Childhood in Rural West Bengal. Pediatrics 20: 128–138.
Jelliffe, D.B. and E.F.P. Jelliffe
   1976 Cultural Interaction and Child Nutrition (Toward a Curvilinear Compromise?). *In*

Nutrition and Agricultural Development. N.S. Scrimshaw and M. Behar (eds.), pp. 263–273. New York: Plenum Press.

Johansson, S.R.
1984 Deferred Infanticide: Excess Female Mortality During Childhood. *In* Infanticide, Comparative and Evolutionary Perspectives. G. Hausfater and S. Blaffer Hrdy (eds.), pp. 463–488. N.Y.: Aldine.

Kagawa, T.
1935 When the Tears Are Mingled. Songs from the Slums. Nashville, Tenn.: Cokesbury Press. pp. 32–34.

Kahn, J.S.
1985 Peasant Ideologies in the Third World. Annual Review of Anthropology 14: 49–75.

Kaseje, M.
1985 Between Science and Common Sense: Nonformal Education for Village Health Workers in Kenya. World Education Inc. Reports no. 25, Summer. pp. 13–14.

Korbin, J.E.
1981 Child Abuse and Neglect: Cross-Cultural Perspectives. Berkeley, Calif.: University of California Press.
1984 Deviance in Child Rearing: Cross-Cultural Issues in Child Abuse and Neglect. Oral presentation at Annual meeting of the American Anthropological Association.

Kuhn, T.S.
1970 The Structure of Scientific Revolutions, 2nd ed. Chicago: University of Chicago Press.

Lena, H.F., and S. Warkov
1978 Occupational Perceptions of the Causes and Consequences of Child Abuse/Neglect. Medical Anthropology 2(1): 1–28.

Levy, J.E.
1962 Response to S. Polgar's article on Health and Human Behavior: Areas of Interest Common to the Social and Medical Sciences. Current Anthropology 3: 159–205 (Levy 186–187).

Lindenbaum, S.
1977 The "Last Course": Nutrition and Anthropology in Asia. *In* Nutrition and Anthropology in Action. T.K. Fitzgerald (ed.), pp. 141–155. Amsterdam: van Gorcum.

Lisowski, F.P.
1966 The Varieties of Man. Journal of Medicine of Ethiopia 4: 71–89.

Lyng, R.E.
1984 Statement of Deputy Secretary of Agriculture Richard E. Lyng before the House Select Committee on Hunger. Hearings on Alleviating Hunger: Progress and Prospects. Washington, D.C.: U.S. Department of Agriculture. June 26.

McLaughlin, M.
1984 Hunger: Interfaith Action for Economic Justice, no. 36.

Marley, D.
1984 Community-Based Health Care. *In* Planning in Managing Primary Health Care Programs. Report of a Workshop Sponsored by the Aga Khan Health Service and Aga Khan Foundation. pp. 45–58. Geneva.

Mead, M., ed.
1955 Cultural Patterns and Technical Change. New York: Mentor.

Meadows, D.H.
1972 The Limits to Growth: A Report for the Club of Rome's Project on the Predicament of Mankind. New York: Universe Books.

Meadows, D.L., and D.H. Meadows, eds.
1973 Toward a Global Equilibrium: Limits to Growth, Collected Papers. Cambridge Mass: Wright-Allen.

Mooneyham, D.
1984 Not Everybody, But Somebody. Traveling Hopefully. Waco, Tex.: Word Books. Reprinted in Seeds [Christians Concerned About Hunger] 7(10): 5, October 1984.

New English Bible
1970 Oxford University Press, Cambridge University Press. Genesis 21: 16.
Newman, L.F.
1984 Fitness and Survival: The High Risk High Risk Spiral. Oral presentation at the annual meeting of the American Anthropological Association.
Newman, M.T.
1961 Biological Adaptations of Man to His Environment: Heat, Cold, Altitude, and Nutrition. Annals of the New York Academy of Sciences 91: 617–633.
Ordonez, L.A.
1984 Nutrition and Behavior: A Review. In Malnutrition: Determinants and Consequences. Current Topics in Nutrition and Disease, Vol. 10. P.L. White and N. Selvey (eds.), pp. 179–185. New York: A.R. Liss.
Pelto, G.H.
1984 Intrahousehold Food Distribution Patterns. In Malnutrition: Determinants and Consequences. Current Topics in Nutrition and Disease, Vol. 10. P.L. White and N. Selvey (eds.), pp. 285–293. New York: A.R. Liss.
Pines, J.
1983 The Community Nutrition Planning Process. In Nutrition in the Community, a Critical Look at Nutrition Policy, Planning and Programmes, 2nd ed. D.S. McLaren (ed.), pp. 51–60. New York: John Wiley.
Pollitt, E.
1973 Behavior of Infant in Causation of Nutritional Marasmus. American Journal of Clinical Nutrition 26: 264–270.
Prugh, D.G. and R.G. Harlow
1966 "Masked Deprivation" in Infants and Young Children. In Deprivation of Maternal Care. M.D. Ainsworth (ed.), pp. 205–225. New York: Schocken Books.
Pyle, D.F.
1985 Growth Charts Don't Cure Malnutrition. World Education Inc. Reports no. 25, Summer. pp. 15–17.
Rifkin, S. and G. Walt
1986 Strategies for Child Survival: Program vs Process. World Education Inc. Reports No. 25, Summer. pp. 9–11.
Robson, J.R.K., and G.R. Wadsworth
1977 The Health and Nutritional Status of Primitive Populations. Ecology of Food and Nutrition 6: 187–202.
Rohde, J.
1984 Current Status of Oral Rehydration Therapy. Oral presentation. Washington, D.C.: State Department. October 18.
Rohner, R.P.
1975 They Love Me, They Love Me Not: A Worldwide Study of the Effects of Parental Acceptance and Rejection. New Haven Conn.: HRAF Press
Rosenberg, E.M.
1973 Ecological Effects of Sex-Differential Nutrition. Oral presentation at the annual meeting of the American Anthropological Association.
Saouma, E.
1981 Food Security in the Face of Crises. Ceres (FAO) 14(2): 15–19.
Sarton, M.
1984 Letters from Maine: New Poems. New York: W.W. Norton. pp. 34–35.
Scrimshaw, S.
1978 Infant Mortality and Behavior in the Regulation of Family Size. Population and Development Review 4(3): 383–403.
Shorter, E.
1977 Maternal Sentiment and Death in Childbirth: A New Agenda for Psychomedical History. In The Medicine Show, Patients, Physicians, and the Perplexities of the Health

Revolution in Modern Society. pp. 67–88. P. Brance, ed. New York: Science History Press.

Shuftan, C.
  1983 Ethics and Ideology in the Battle Against Malnutrition. *In* Nutrition in the Community, A Critical Look at Nutrition Policy, Planning, and Programmes, 2nd ed. D.S. McLaren, ed. pp. 125–141. New York: John Wiley.

Sims, L.S.
  1981 The Community Nutritionist as Change Agent. *In* Community Nutrition, People, Policies, and Programs. H.S. Wright and L.S. Sims, eds. pp. 405–421. Monterey, Calif: Wadsworth Health Sciences Division.

Sims, L.S., B. Paolucci, and P.M. Morris
  1972 Theoretical Model for the Study of the Nutritional Status: An Ecosystem Approach. Ecology of Food and Nutrition 1: 197–205.

Stini, W.A.
  1971 Evolutionary Implications of Changing Nutrition Patterns in Human Populations. American Anthropologist 73: 1019–30.

Thistlethwaite, F.
  1961 The Great Experiment, An Introduction to the History of the American People. NY: Cambridge University Press.

Turnbull, C.
  1972 The Mountain People. New York: Simon & Schuster.

United States Committee for UNICEF
  1984 Fund-raising letter, over signature of Hugh Downs, Chairman.

Vega, T.
  1985 Personal communication (letter), October.

Watson, B.
  1971 Chinese Lyricism, Shih Poetry. New York: Columbia University Press. pp. 35–36.

Whiting, B.B., ed.
  1963 Six Cultures, Studies in Child Rearing. New York: John Wiley.

Wilbur, V.
  1980 Wishful Thinking: The President's Commission on World Hunger. Sojourners [People's Christian Commission] 9: 8–9.

Williams, C.
  1933 Nutritional Disease of Children Associated with a Maize Diet. Archives of the Diseases of Children 8: 423.

Wylie, A.
  1984 Improving International Transfer of Technology. *In* Malnutrition: Determinants and Consequences. Current Topics in Nutrition and Disease, Vol. 10. P.L. White and N. Selvey, eds. pp. 347–354. New York: A.R. Liss.

Yeager, L.B.
  1984 Review: F.A. von Hayak's The Road to Serfdom (1944). The AEI Economist [American Enterprise Institute for Public Policy Research]. November. pp. 10–13.

Zelizer, V.A.
  1985 Pricing the Priceless Child, The Changing Social Value of Children. New York: Basic Books.

NORA J. KRANTZLER

# TRADITIONAL MEDICINE AS 'MEDICAL NEGLECT': DILEMMAS IN THE CASE MANAGEMENT OF A SAMOAN TEENAGER WITH DIABETES

For migrants, maintenance of traditional cultural practices in a new environment may initially ease the transition but subsequently trigger severe conflict. This seems particularly true in two areas, childrearing and medical care, and particularly when migration is from a relatively rural and less technologically-developed setting to an urban one. This chapter will analyze a case example of one such conflict in an American Samoan family who migrated to Honolulu, Hawaii. Six years later, the father, a traditional healer, was charged with 'noncompliance' and 'medical neglect' of his diabetic daughter, and was threatened with her removal from family custody by the State of Hawaii's Child Protective Service. While this case represents an extreme example, it illustrates some crucial issues facing many immigrant populations attempting to maintain their cultural identity in the face of social change. Practices which have represented cultural strengths – and which may in the new environment provide a source of social status and a sense of self-efficacy for members of an otherwise low-status and powerless ethnic group – may place their children at high risk. Indeed, the risk may be not only to children's health but to the integrity of the family unit and the migrant community.

This case example illustrates the difficulty of defining and labelling medical neglect and child maltreatment in a way that is appropriate cross-culturally. As Korbin (this volume) observes, the phrase 'child abuse and neglect' is often used as if it represents a single category rather than a diverse range of behavior. Definitions of abuse and neglect are inconsistent and ambiguous in both theory and practice. The problem is to develop definitions of abuse and neglect which are culturally sensitive, without taking a stance of extreme relativism. Korbin (1980, 1981, 1982) suggests viewing abuse and neglect on three conceptual levels: (1) as cultural practices perceived as abusive or neglectful from the outside (etically) but not from within the cultural group (emically); (2) as idiosyncratic departures from cultural norms of behavior; and (3) as societally-induced harm to children considered beyond the control of individual parents and caretakers. Intent and culpability, as well as physical or emotional consequences, must be taken into account. When cultures with different childrearing practices come into contact, the potential for misconstruing behaviors is great. In a multi-cultural society, protection from misidentification of child abuse and neglect is essential (Korbin 1980). Korbin argues that it is the idiosyncratic departure from culturally acceptable norms of behavior that is most validly considered abuse or neglect.

325

*Nancy Scheper-Hughes (ed.), Child Survival, 325–337.*
© *1987 by D. Reidel Publishing Company.*

With cultural contact, not only may behaviors be misconstrued, but also cognition and affect – expressions of the 'meaning' of sickness to patients and families. Kleinman's (1980) concept of explanatory models (EMs) is useful for deciphering conflicts between patient/family and practitioner perspectives during sickness episodes. The EM includes beliefs about sickness etiology, onset of symptoms, pathophysiology, course of illness, and treatment. As Phillips (1985: 32) has observed, "The difference between EMs of clinician and patient, and the amount of change that occurs in these EMs as a result of the clinical interaction are indicators of the quality of the clinical exchange and may be predictive of patient satisfaction and compliance." Kleinman has developed the EM concept into a procedure that can be used by clinicians: the 'negotiation' model of clinical practice. Using this model, clinicians elicit the patient's EM, present their own clinical EM, compare the two EMs, list the illness problems, and negotiate a treatment plan for these problems. While this model is far from being widely accepted or used, it is "one of the few success stories" in clinically-applied anthropology (*Ibid.*: 32), as it provides an actual procedure for practitioners to use.[1] As this case example shows, use of such a strategy by a physician with a 'transcultural' perspective (in this case, an intuitive one) helped to resolve the conflict between family and 'official medical sector' perspectives which threatened the life of a diabetic teenager.

In discussing this case example, I will focus on both emic and etic interpretations of what happened with this family. The logic informing the family's behavior will be discussed and the nature and rationale of the intervention by the 'official medical sector' analyzed. I will argue that the family's adherence to traditional Samoan medicine, the conflict between family and practitioner EMs, and the family's failure to conform to norms of childrearing behavior of the dominant culture by assigning a 12-year-old to supervise insulin injections resulted in a cultural misconstrual of neglect. In spite of attempts to be culturally sensitive, members of the dominant medical sector used 'cultural differences' to blame the victim. Such accusations may constitute dramatic but self-defeating attempts to socialize immigrant families to cultural norms of childrearing by bringing the force of dominant cultural institutions, medical and legal, to bear on the right of the family to maintain child custody. Both Samoan and biomedical cultural practices – and, more particularly, their interaction – contributed to the progression of severe adolescent diabetes to crisis proportions.

## THE OFFICIAL MEDICAL SECTOR'S PERSPECTIVE

Mary F., a 16-year-old Samoan girl, was brought to the hospital by ambulance after collapsing, semi-comatose, on the sidewalk near her home in a Honolulu housing project. At that point, her illness was 'discovered' and diagnosed as juvenile onset diabetes mellitus. She was initially placed in the Pediatric Intensive Care Unit for 24 hours, then transferred to a pediatric ward for about a week until her diabetes was 'under good control.' She, her parents, and her older sister were taught how to give insulin injections, and Mary was shown how to test her urine for glucose and acetone. She was given a 1-month supply of insulin and other materia medica (alcohol swabs, syringes, etc.). She was further 'counseled' about her diet – told to consume 1900–2000 calories a day and to eat regular meals and snacks. She was then to be followed up with visits to the outpatient clinic. Following the clinic's (unofficial) policy of linking patients with physicians from their own ethnic group, she was assigned to see the sole Samoan pediatric resident, whom the faculty assumed to be an expert on Samoan patients. However, the resident, Dr. A, was very uncomfortable with this status; he had not grown up in Samoa and was not fluent in the very important nuances of the Samoan language. Further, he had developed a sense of both social and cultural distance from the more traditional members of his own ethnic group which rendered their beliefs and behavior inexplicable to him and created feelings of ambivalence and frustration in working with them.

From the official medical perspective, this family was problematic from the start. Neither parent spoke English; Mary and her four siblings at home spoke pidgin English and colloquial Samoan and were moderately literate in English only.

Further, Mr. F. was a traditional healer, calling himself a *foma'i*, or doctor. He was primarily an herbalist and was well-known and respected in the Samoan community and within the housing project as a healer. He was also slightly feared, as he claimed to have access to powerful *aitu*, or spirits (cf. Goodman 1971). Unbeknownst to his medical superiors, Dr. A had previously known Mary's father. As a medical student, he had accompanied Mr. F. on a visit to a woman with mastitis. His recollection of this event reveals his ambivalence:

It was pretty impressive. He told her the reason for her mastitis was that she was arrogant, proud, too show-offy – that's why the demon infected her breast. She was on antibiotics. She was from the Mainland (U.S.). Seeing him was a last resort. They were one of the different types, where *he*, not the physician, was the last resort. He's very proud of the way he treats – boastful. They're all like that. They're very reluctant to say their medicine didn't work. The woman asked me what I thought. I recommended she hang onto the antibiotics, just in case. He used a poultice made with leaves, rubbed it over the breast and massaged, using pressure at certain points. He really wanted to impress me with how his medicines work. We went back the next day and she was much better. It's hard to say whether it was the antibiotics or his treatment, but it was still pretty impressive.

Mr. F. had also treated one of Dr. A's uncles:

My uncle was having bad dreams. Mr. F. showed him pictures of his dead relatives who were responsible; the pictures appeared in bottles. He gave him potions to drive the spirits away. According to my uncle, it worked; he didn't have bad dreams any more . . . People deal with Mr. F. for both spiritual and everyday types of problems.

In this context, Dr. A felt that Mr. F. was competing with him as a healer and admits he "took the family on" reluctantly. He felt he could not "come on too strongly," not only because of the father's competitiveness but also because of the age difference between them. As he said, "I had some respect." He felt that Mr. F. drove the point home to him by calling him "son" in their interactions, indirectly reminding him of the deference owed by virtue of age. The resident noted,

It's a blow to his ego to have Mary sick. He blamed everything on the spirits. They caught her unaware; they drugged her. He also thought the 'dirty blood' in her kept her from getting well. She hadn't had a period. He thought if she'd have her period once, she'd be well. She didn't have her period because it was secondary to the diabetes being out of control.

Over the months following her hospitalization, Mary was seen once in the clinic by a different resident, and then did not appear for her next three appointments. The first time she missed an appointment, her father telephoned to apologize and said Mary was doing fine. During the third month following her hospital discharge, she came to the clinic without an appointment and was seen by a third pediatric resident. Laboratory results showed that her diabetes was again out of control, and she was readmitted to the hospital several days later. She, her parents, and her older sister were again "educated" and "advised about compliance." During the next three months, Mary kept her appointments, "claimed compliance," brought in her daily records of insulin doses and urine sugars, and her diabetes was judged to be under "fair control."

The fourth month after her second hospitalization, Mary came to the clinic with blindness in one eye and diminished vision in the other. She was diagnosed as having cataracts, and Dr. A "again spoke to Mary and her mother about the importance of compliance and the seriousness of the disease." He obtained an agreement from them to bring her into the hospital in two days to have the cataracts removed. Several days later, Mr. F. telephoned saying he refused to admit Mary to the hospital. He was persuaded "after some patronizing," in Dr. A's words, to bring her in for an examination. Dr. A wrote in her chart,

Her diabetes appeared to be very much out of control at that time but I was having a very difficult time with the patient and her father. I showed them how to do the Chem-strip method, which they seemed to be apathetic about. I consented to the father's wishes to have him supplement the insulin with some potion of his that he had prepared especially to control her sugar. Our agreement was to see her again in 2 days. At that time, if her sugar was still high, we would definitely admit her to the hospital. I kept the insulin doses as stated and then (2 days later) I saw them again. This time the father claimed that he had been giving Mary an herbal potion which he claimed would help control her sugar. He had been giving it to her on the morning of this visit and was convinced that her blood sugar would be down. Well, her blood sugar was 878 with a Chem-strip showing 400–800 and acetone of 60. I commented to the father that the diabetes was out of control and there was some severe danger of her going into diabetic ketoacidosis, but at that time he became very angry with me and claimed that he would like to take her from my service and take care of her on his own. He did not believe that there was such an illness which would require daily injections for the rest of one's life and thanked me for my efforts but claimed that he would like to have total control of his daughter's illness at this time. He refused to bring her into the hospital. He did not believe any of the chronicity that I tried to point out with this illness, that all of the manifestations that were now present . . . were related to the diabetes.

That evening, Dr. A arranged to have Dr. B, the only other Samoan physician on the island, take over as Mary's physician. He also contacted the medical director of Child Protective Services (CPS), as "I was concerned it was getting out of my hands and I would probably need assistance from the Child Protective Service." The hospital's final discharge summary concluded that Mary's problems were as follows:

1. Juvenile onset diabetes mellitus, very poorly controlled;
2. Very poor compliance;
3. Severe degree of social disruption and disarray in the patient's life as well as her family situation;
4. Patient needs much guidance and adolescent counseling;
5. A good candidate for Child Protective Service referral, primarily as a matter of medical neglect;
6. Communication barrier . . . because of inadequacies in the English language.

It is noteworthy that only one of the six is a strictly 'medical' problem.

A few days later, Mary's parents took her to a different hospital for cataract surgery following a visit to their home by city police instructing them to do so. After her discharge from the hospital, a nurse visiting the home discovered that it was Mary's 12-year-old sister who was primarily responsible for her insulin shots. Her ability to be responsible enough for this task was questioned by medical and social service staff. This discovery added fuel to the fire, and a petition for 'protective supervision' was filed with Family Court. The petition stated that Mary had been "neglected as to the proper and necessary medical care for her well-being . . . (and) subjected to physical deprivation as a result of the failure of her parents to exercise that degree of care . . . for which they are legally responsible." Thus, Mary was allowed to remain at home only after her parents signed an agreement to comply strictly with physician instructions. The agreement stated that failure to comply would result in Mary's immediate removal from her home and sanctions as ordered by the court.

In summary, from the official medical perspective, Mary's family was judged incapable of caring for her properly because of 'cultural differences.' The diagnosis of 'cultural differences' was, in turn, used as a way of stereotyping and 'blaming the victim' and served to close rather than open the door for further investigation into the family's concerns. Since even the Samoan 'expert' (Dr. A) could not get through to this family, the situation was perceived as hopeless. In fact, Dr. A felt that he had given this family much more "leeway" – bargained with them more – than he normally would have. As Mary's deteriorating health was considered an urgent matter, he believed he had no choice but to force the family into surgery using legal sanctions.

## THE FAMILY'S PERSPECTIVE

Like the physicians at the hospital, Mary's family first became aware of her diabetes when she collapsed and was taken to the hospital by ambulance. Mary had been riding the bus home from school and had become confused; she could not remember where to get off. When she got off the bus, she collapsed on the sidewalk and was subsequently taken to the hospital. This was the family's first experience in a large, modern, technologically sophisticated hospital.

When Mr. F. arrived at the hospital, he spoke with different hospital staff (using a daughter as translator) and was concerned that there was no single physician caring for Mary. (Since it was a teaching hospital, she was seen by residents as well as by attending physicians.) He felt that hospital staff members gave him different interpretations of Mary's illness, including discrepant test results, leading him to perceive her care as experimental and inconsistent. The family also observed a child die while Mary was in the Intensive Care Unit, further reinforcing this perception and instilling fear over Mary's chances of surviving in this hospital. Partly due to language difficulties, they felt they did not get an adequate explanation of her problem over the course of her treatment. When they asked what was wrong with her, their perception was that "everyone said 'sugar.'" What this meant was not clear to the family; they were confused about whether she was getting too much sugar or too little. Mary's mother interpreted the explanations to mean she was not getting enough sugar, so she tried to give her more when she returned home. Over time, confusion gave way to anger, and a basic lack of trust of the hospital and the physicians there developed. The family began to draw on their own resources for explaining and caring for Mary's illness, relying heavily on the father's skills as a healer.

The family's expectations and behavior were logical from the American Samoan perspective. Mr. F. was protecting his right as decision-maker, since he was both head of the household and healer. His expectation that the hospital's social structure would be personal in nature – i.e., that he could negotiate with staff for control over Mary's treatment – was based not only upon the assumption that since her physician was a fellow Samoan, he would understand and respect the father's position. It also made sense from the perspective of one familiar with hospital care in Samoa, where the family plays an important role in caring for the patient and in negotiating care and favors from hospital staff. It is common knowledge there that one fares much better in the hospital if a member of one's *aiga* ('extended family') is on the staff. Although he was also Samoan, Dr. A was socialized to the norms of

American bureaucratic behavior stating that everyone must be treated alike; no one should have preferential treatment.[2]

Other behaviors of the family were grounded in the *fa'a Samoa* – 'the Samoan way' – as well. The hospital in American Samoa does not require appointments, nor does its Pediatric Department have a preventive emphasis. Care is crisis-oriented. Further, in Samoa, Pediatrics includes children up to the age of 12. From the Samoan perspective, a 12-year-old should be relatively independent. Children are expected to do most of the work within the household, including taking major responsibility for sibling caretaking. In this context, it is not surprising that a 12-year-old was assigned responsibility for supervising her sister's insulin injections and recording test results. She was also the child most heavily relied on for translation between her parents and hospital staff. The family expected her level of competence to be high; this expectation was buttressed by the fact that her verbal and written English skills were the best in the family. Interpretation of her role as signifying parental neglect was thus a misconstrual based on cultural differences in childrearing principles and practices.

As the Ritchies (1981) note, Europeans expect parents to maintain control over their children until the end of their second decade; this concept is enshrined in the law and endorsed by the judicial system as well as by 'subjural personnel' such as teachers and social welfare workers. The Polynesian tradition stresses the achievement of physical and social independence at an early age (Metge and Kinloch 1978). However, to non-Polynesians, and especially in new, urban environments, the practice of leaving children to fend for themselves can be dangerous and readily interpreted as neglect (*Ibid.*: 39). This is especially true if the child is seriously ill. In fact, clinical staff in New Zealand hospitals try to keep Samoan children hospitalized until they are judged to no longer need close supervision, because they have found that children discharged earlier often have to be readmitted, having been "immersed in the hurly-burly of family life without a protected convalescence" (*Ibid.*: 39). In this case, the family in some ways treated Mary as if she were much younger than her 16 years – for example, by moving her bed into the living room and trying to do 'special' things for her. Further, both her parents attempted to help with her treatment, by altering her diet and by treating her simultaneously with herbal medicines. While the efficacy of these interventions was problematic, their intent was not. From the family's perspective, the charge of 'neglect' was incomprehensible.

### DISCUSSION

The accusation of medical neglect due to 'non-compliance' reflects the Parsonian orientation that a sick person has a social obligation to seek and cooperate with 'technically competent help' (Trostle *et al.* 1983: 52). Not only does this place an inordinate burden of responsibility on the patient; it also

places restrictively narrow boundaries on the types of resources seen as
relevant to the healing process (*Ibid.*: 53). In this case, traditional Samoan
practices were either demeaned or discounted by hospital physicians; they
represented 'disobedience' rather than attempts to cope with and alleviate
Mary's problems.

As Young (1983: 1210) points out, when the 'official medical sector'
produces high levels of dissatisfaction, this has two important consequences:
the patient and family are not provided with the spectrum of medical services
to which they are entitled, and the dissatisfaction with the medical services
provided may lead them to adopt courses of action which are anxiety-
reducing but ultimately maladaptive from the biomedical point of view. Thus,
the 'costs' of traditional healing can include iatrogenesis and intensification of
the patient's suffering as a by-product of the practices which reduce his or her
relatives' anxiety. In the case of conflict over care in Pediatrics, the child may
not only suffer physically but may also be left confused about the state of her
own health and about who is responsible for ensuring her well-being, and
ambivalent about medical care settings in general (Korbin 1982). The cost-
benefits of traditional healing must not be assumed categorically; success in
providing meaning does not necessarily equal success in healing (Young,
*Ibid.*). While the medicinal plant Mary's father used to treat her diabetes is
cited as useful for diabetes (*suka*) by healers in American Samoa (Office of
Comprehensive Health Planning 1974), its curative efficacy has not been
established.

Within the traditional context, Mary's family acted appropriately. Further,
they had made concessions to 'modern' medicine by hospitalizing Mary twice,
visiting the clinic, and attempting to administer the insulin and alter her diet
at home even though the reasons for doing so were never made clear to them.
In fact, Mr. F. was not averse to the procedure of cataract surgery itself but
rather to having it done at this particular hospital. He felt he was protecting
his daughter. Mr. F.'s reaction to the charge of medical neglect was also
appropriate in the Samoan context. He was bewildered by the accusation and
angered at the coercive tactics employed by the hospital. As the social worker
assigned to their 'case' observed, the family felt their integrity was violated.
Further, since the accusation was a public one, Mr. F. wanted to seek public
exoneration. In the Samoan context, pride is a public emotion (Keene 1978);
one is proud before, and in relation to, others. One competes with others for
the right to be proud. Thus, there is strong disapproval of acts injurious to a
person's (and therefore, a family's) pride. There is also opposition to direct
verbal aggression; and to this end, there are elaborate forms of etiquette and
polite address. Mr. F. felt severe damage to his pride, and he wanted to settle
the conflict in court as a matter of public record.

Mr. F. was persuaded not to take the issue to court by the social worker,
who subsequently recommended that the hospital's charge of medical neglect

be dropped. Many of the issues were resolved as the second Samoan physician, Dr. B, began working with the family.

The pediatric resident, Dr. A, had been caught in a bind between the seemingly conflicting roles of being a 'good Samoan' and being a 'good physician.' A good Samoan treats the whole family – specifically, the head of the family – as the decision-maker in treatment. The *matai* (head of the *aiga*) or the head of the household makes the decisions, especially if he is a healer himself. A good Samoan relies not on rules and regulations imposed externally, but on rules of social interaction based on traditional Samoan values: the pre-eminence of the *matai* or the head of the household, deference of the younger toward the older members of society, and the overriding importance of the *fa'a Samoa*. All such interactions should be indirect and non-confrontational. Unable to reconcile these directives with being a good physician, Dr. A referred the family to another Samoan physician, Dr. B.

Dr. B, while only slightly older than the resident, was able to convince Mr. F. that he was both a good Samoan and a good physician by, first, showing respect. He showed deference to Mr. F. by eliciting his perceptions and beliefs about Mary's illness and working within Mr. F.'s conceptual framework. Mr. F.'s status as a healer was not challenged. Diabetes was described as a 'modern' disease requiring 'modern' treatment. This made sense and allowed Mr. F. to retain his pride. (Mr. F. was not opposed to the idea of 'modern' medicines and was in fact taking some himself for back pain.) Mr. F. was very concerned to understand the pathophysiology of his daughter's illness and had been frustrated with the previous dearth of information given to him. He wanted to know which *organ* was involved and was confused by the focus of previous explanations on 'sugar.' Dr. B was able to explain in Samoan that it was her pancreas (*atepili*, literally, 'liver of the lizard'), and that some people are born with a defective pancreas. He described the making of insulin in graphic and concrete terms to which Mr. F. could relate – slaughtering a pig and grinding up the pancreas.

Dr. B also decided that he needed to see the family in their home environment in order to understand their situation. He began visiting them one day a week. The visits accomplished several goals. First, they enabled the family to remain on their own 'turf,' where they felt comfortable and in control. (As the family did not own a car, travel to the hospital was logistically difficult and time-consuming.) Second, home visits allowed the elaborate social exchanges required for establishing effective rapport to occur. The family was able to establish a social relationship with Dr. B. This was solidified by their ability to show him hospitality; by this means, they could establish an appropriate social balance. Third, visiting allowed Dr. B. to eat meals with the family, to observe their diet and their social interactions in the home. It was through this visiting that he discovered that their misunderstanding of the role of sugar was leading them to exacerbate rather than

TABLE I
Sample evening meals

| | |
|---|---|
| Meal 1: | barbecued chicken |
| | *pisupo* (canned corned beef) and long rice |
| | boiled potatoes |
| | boiled green bananas |
| | cole slaw |
| | fruit punch (sugar-syrup base) |
| Meal 2: | pork chops in gravy |
| | boiled hot dogs |
| | hot dogs in gravy |
| | boiled green bananas |
| | white rice |
| | sugar-based soft drinks |

alleviate the problem. As the Samoan diet is starchy, Dr. B attempted not only to explain which foods are better than others, but to try to find alternative ways of lowering blood sugar such as exercise. This worked well because sports, such as volleyball, are extremely popular among Samoan teenagers. Working within the Samoan dietary framework was much more realistic than attempting to make major dietary changes. Maintenance of the Samoan diet (or variations thereof) was an integral part of family and community life in this housing project. (See Table I for examples of the family's evening meals.)

A final benefit of home visits was the informal teaching about American institutions that could occur in this relaxed setting. For example, when the family expressed hurt and angry feelings about CPS intervention, Dr. B explained to them the philosophy behind the Child Protective Service and the ways in which children are protected from child abuse or neglect in American society. Such education is a much more effective way of socializing patients into the dominant medical care delivery system than are accusations of noncompliance.

Further, the knowledge patients gain from clinical encounters provides a major source of information on biomedicine to ethnic social networks; the clinical encounter is the most important source of information available to ethnic groups on the culture of biomedicine and is often the origin of biomedical knowledge that circulates in ethnic social networks (Harwood 1981). If a prominent traditional healer has experiences he proclaims as catastrophic, this may be expected to have ramifications throughout his social network and to lead others to avoid the biomedical context.

In summary, cultural practices contributing to child morbidity – in this case, to the progression of juvenile diabetes mellitus to life-threatening proportions – may be viewed on several levels. At one level are specific Samoan cultural practices such as the use of traditional medicine to the exclusion of modern medicine, the high carbohydrate-high sugar Samoan diet, and childrearing practices emphasizing early independence. At another level, it is the persistence of these practices in an "alien and rather hostile" environment which may seem to non-Polynesians to be gross parental neglect (Ritchie and Ritchie, *op. cit.*), particularly when the migrant community is characterized by cultural, social, and economic marginality. Expectations of migrant families in such communities may be based on experiences and beliefs which are inappropriate to their current context. At a third level are features of modern biomedicine which also constitute cultural practices contributing to morbidity in this example – such as technical language, the social structure of a large teaching hospital, stereotypic views of ethnic groups, and expectations of patient compliance with overtones of dominance and submission, power and powerlessness. The interaction between practitioners of biomedical and traditional Samoan cultural patterns brought the force of dominant cultural institutions, medical and legal, to bear on members of a marginal social group. While this was effective in accomplishing the biomedical goal of short-term symptom control, it was ineffective for longer-range diabetes control and harmful to the integrity of the cultural group. As Dr. B's strategy demonstrated, considering cultural practices contributing to child morbidity and mortality at several levels of complexity may help in discovering solutions at the microlevel.

### EPILOGUE

Unfortunately, this story does not have a happy ending. Approximately one year following Dr. B's intervention, Mary became comatose at home and was taken to the hospital, where she died. After retiring from his Air Force position, Dr. B had become busy with a new private practice and had stopped visiting the family at home. Instead, he had transferred her care to a physician whom the family liked at the hospital where Mary had had her eye surgery. Dr. B reflected that

She probably was noncompliant. When she felt good, she didn't comply . . . The Child Protective Service question is still there, I think. I think Mary knew the gravity of her problem. She *was* able to see and measure her medication. Part of the culture is still involved. Her father still thought he could solve the problem, though he was not still treating her. But it gave false hope to Mary. . . .

Feeling better, or feeling well, has been cited, more generally, as one of the most common reasons for medical 'noncompliance' (Haynes, Taylor and Sackett 1979). In this case, bridging the gap between explanatory models of official medical practitioners and the family required continuous support and educational efforts in the family's home – monumental effort for a physician working within the current structure of 'modern' medical practice. That this physician made home visits at all was unusual; as these visits were 'after hours,' in the evening following a full day's work, they demanded considerable sacrifice.

While most physicians may be unable or unwilling to visit patients in their homes – particularly on a long-term basis – teaching medical students to adopt a 'transcultural' stance in patient care might help alleviate problems caused by ethnocentrism in defining and labelling problems such as child neglect. Indeed, experimental programs have begun to teach physicians by having them visit alternative healers (Scott 1983) or patients at home with chronic illnesses (Sankar 1986). In most cases, new understanding of the patient's perspective emerges with such experiential learning. Teaching medical students a 'negotiation' model, exploring and working with patient EMs, has also helped encourage a transcultural approach (Berlin and Fowkes, *op. cit.*). A similar form of 'cultural assessment' has been developed for nurses (Tripp-Reimer *et al.* 1984) and would be useful for social workers and others involved in cases of alleged child abuse or neglect, particularly through the CPS.

As Hughes [this volume] points out, and as this example demonstrates, the role of CPS may be extremely problematic where major cultural differences exist. Deciphering the child's 'best interests' may be a complex task requiring creative solutions. In this case, an *initial* approach that was transcultural and negotiation-oriented might have averted the ultimately lethal conflict that began during Mary's first visits to the hospital. However, whether or not Mary's diabetes could ever have been permanently controlled within this alien social and medical context is an unresolved issue.

ACKNOWLEDGEMENT

Supported by N.I.M.H. Postdoctoral Training Grant in Medical Anthropology No. T 32 MH 14614, John A. Burns School of Medicine, University of Hawaii at Manoa, HI.

NOTES

1. A similar model is the LEARN mnemonic developed at Standford University, which aids providers in eliciting and working with patient EMs by spelling out the steps: Listen; Explain; Acknowledge; Recommend; Negotiate (Berlin and Fowkes 1983).
2. As American Samoa modernizes, Western institutions are imposed precariously onto traditional Samoan social structure, causing conflict in many realms other than medical care. For example, an airline pilot who flies between islands in American Samoa angrily recounted his arguments with the woman who runs one of the small airports. He discovered that she had lied to him about the weight of her family's baggage and was enraged because the planes are small and, from his perspective, it was important to be accurate. She, however, was caught between the demands of her *matai* and the demands of her job. She had to please the *matai* by giving him preferential treatment, but the demands of her job required her to treat everyone alike.

REFERENCES

Berlin, Elois Ann and William C. Fowkes
    1983 A Teaching Framework for Cross-Cultural Health Care. Application in Family Practice. The Western Journal of Medicine 139(6): 934–938.

Goodman, Richard
1971 Some Aitu Beliefs of Modern Samoans. J. Polynesian Society 80(4): 463–479.
Harwood, Alan,ed.
1981 Ethnicity and Medical Care. Cambridge, MA: Harvard University Press.
Haynes, R.B., D.W. Taylor, and D.L. Sackett
1979 Compliance in Health Care. Baltimore: The Johns Hopkins University Press.
Hughes, D. Michael
1985 When Cultural Rights Conflict with the 'Best Interests' of the Child. A View from Inside the Child Welfare System. This volume.
Keene, Dennis T.P.
1978 Houses Without Walls: Samoan Social Control. Unpublished Ph.D. Dissertation, Department of Anthropology, University of Hawaii at Manoa, Honolulu, Hawaii.
Kleinman, Arthur
1980 Patients and Healers in the Context of Culture. Berkeley: University of California Press.
Korbin, Jill
1980 The Cultural Context of Child Abuse and Neglect. Child Abuse and Neglect, Vol. 4: 3–13.
1981 Introduction. In Jill E. Korbin, ed., Child Abuse and Neglect: Cross-Cultural Perspectives. Berkeley and Los Angeles: University of California Press. pp. 1–12.
1982 Steps toward Resolving Cultural Conflict in a Pediatric Hospital. Clinical Pediatrics 21(5): 259–263.
1985 Deviance in Child Rearing: Cross Cultural Issues in Child Abuse and Neglect. This volume.
Metge, Joan and Patricia Kinloch
1978 Talking Past Each Other. Problems of Cross-Cultural Communication. Wellington, New Zealand: Victoria University Press.
Office of Comprehensive Health Planning, Department of Medical Services, Government of American Samoa
1974 Samoan Medicinal Plants and their Usage. Unpublished report.
Phillips, Michael R.
1985 Can 'Clinically Applied Anthropology' Survive in Medical Care Settings? Medical Anthropology Quarterly 16(2): 31–36.
Ritchie, James and Ritchie
1981 Child Rearing and Child Abuse: The Polynesian Context. In Child Abuse and Neglect: Cross-Cultural Perspectives. Ed. Jill E. Korbin. Berkeley: University of California Press. p. 186–204.
Sankar, Andrea
1985 Out of the Clinic, Into the Home: Control and Patient-Physician Communication. Social Science & Medicine 22 (9): 973–982.
Scott, Clarissa S.
1983 Medical Student Fieldwork in Alternative Healing Systems. Paper presented at the 82nd Annual Meeting of the American Anthropological Association.
Tripp-Reimer, Toni, Pamela J. Brink, and Judith M. Saunders
1984 Cultural Assessment: Content and Process. Nursing Outlook 32(2): 78–82
Trostle, James A., W. Allen Hauser, and Ida Susser
1983 The Logic of Noncompliance: Management of Epilepsy from the Patient's Point of View. Culture, Medicine and Psychiatry 7: 35–56.
Young, Allan
1983 The Relevance of Traditional Medical Cultures to Modern Primary Health Care. Social Science and Medicine 17(16): 1205–1211.

NANCY SCHEPER-HUGHES AND HOWARD F. STEIN

# CHILD ABUSE AND THE UNCONSCIOUS IN AMERICAN POPULAR CULTURE*

## THE 'DISCOVERY' OF CHILD ABUSE

During the 1960s child abuse and neglect, long grappled with as a vexing and chronic social problem by generations of child welfare and social workers, was suddenly "discovered" and expropriated by a more powerful profession: medicine. When C. Henry Kempe and his associates (1962) at Colorado General Hospital created a new diagnostic entity – the "Battered Child Syndrome" – the American public finally sat up and took notice.[1]

With the mantle of medical legitimacy now thrown over the old problem of child maltreatment, the nation mobilized in a frontal attack on assaultive parents. Into this newly created social space appeared: state reporting laws,[2] new sources of federal funding, programs, and professionals. The National Center for the Treatment of Prevention of Child Abuse was established in 1974, and a whole research industry flourished with specialized journals, research centers, national and international societies and conferences all focused upon child abuse and neglect. National incidence studies, begun in the 1970s, reported sharp increases annually in the reports of maltreatment. Between 1976 and 1981, the total number of reports documented nationwide has more than doubled (the American Humane Association 1983). Social and behavioral scientists rushed in, often with premature casual explanations based on retrospective studies of poorly defined abusers and abused.[3] Research instruments and procedures were designed and implemented for the early detection of "high risk" parents (i.e. *mothers*) at public hospitals. Welfare patients, especially single mothers, were observed throughout labor, delivery, and the hours postpartum for signs of inadequate attachment to their newborns (*see* Kempe and Kempe 1978: 62–63). Based on inferences from this brief period of observation, "problem" mothers were targeted for early intervention programs that included home visits by nurses, clinical social workers, and child welfare workers.

Not suprisingly, the "discovery" of child abuse and the consequent development of interventional strategies also resulted in a proliferation of child abuse experts – researchers, educators, clinicians, therapists, and social workers – occupying newly created positions as members of child trauma teams in hospitals, on child abuse "hot lines", as facilitators in self-help "parenting" and stress management groups, and in emergency shelters and treatment programs for the abused. Child Abuse Prevention (CAP) workers visited schools, clinics, and day care programs in order to alert teachers, doctors and child care professionals to the covert signs (i.e. the distress and agitation) thought to be symptomatic of "sexually abused" children. In addition, they

339

*Nancy Scheper-Hughes (ed.), Child Survival, 339–358.*
© 1987 by D. Reidel Publishing Company.

hold classes to educate even young toddlers, with the use of "anatomically correct" puppets and dolls, about the difference between "good" and "bad" touches by parents and other adult caretakers.[4] This was said to be part of the process of "empowering" children.

Meanwhile, the media (newspapers, television, radio, films, popular books) played an important role in sensitizing the American public to some of the more bizarre and sadistic examples of child maltreatment. The magazine stories and "docu-dramas" broadcast into homes across the nation created a social climate and consensus that allowed for a very dramatic increase in public interventions in the private lives of citizens.

On one level it appeared that we, as a nation, were finally coming to terms with the ways in which children were being used by their parents as receptacles in which to discard the worst remnants of their own childhoods. On another level, however, there is a note of hysteria in the protest and the outrage, somewhat out of proportion to the extent of, and long history of, the problem of child abuse. It seems that we need to raise another question: Why now? Why did it take so long to bring to consciousness and to respond to the problem? Why did public awareness await the *medicalization* of abuse?

This chapter is an attempt to answer these questions, and to explain the "choice" of child abuse as a key (or master) social problem of our times by applying a critical analysis to aspects of the cultural "collective unconscious". In taking a psycho-historical approach to the problem of child maltreatment we are not going to concern ourselves with the issue of whether there is, in fact, more abuse now than in earlier decades or other historical periods. Anthropologists, demographers, social- and psycho-historians have amply documented that children have been killed, exposed, beaten, exploited, severely neglected, and sexually molested throughout the ethnographic and historical records (see deMause 1974, 1982; Hippler 1978; Stein 1978, 1980; Korbin 1981; Shorter 1975; Stone 1977; Scheper-Hughes 1979, 1984; Hausfater and Hrdy 1984). As for the present time, good (i.e. valid, reliable) statistics that could support or deny the allegations of an "epidemic" or a "rising tide" of child abuse are lacking. Child Protective Service Agencies get only the cases that a community will allow it to receive. Meanwhile there is little professional agreement on the definitions of child abuse, neglect, sexual exploitation (*see* Giovanni and Becerra 1979) and on what, in fact, constitutes the "Best Interests of the Child" (*see* Goldstein, Freud, and Solnit 1973; Hughes, this volume).

Here we are concerned with exploring the contemporary meanings and functions of child maltreatment in terms of the unconscious role it seems to play in American life at the present moment. We are attempting what Foucault and his associates call a "history of the present". In taking a strong social constructionist stance, however, we do not mean to imply that child maltreatment is a figment of the imagination, nor do we mean to underestimate its lethal effects on the health and wellbeing of American children.

Along with child welfare professionals we, too, would like to see the cycle of family pathology that contributes to child abuse and neglect broken. But we also know that even the most benevolent and altruistic of motives can sometimes disguise unconscious aggressive and hostile impulses against the poorer and more vulnerable segments of society that most often deviate from dominant patterns of social life and cultural mores (*see* Gaylin, Glasser, Marcus, and Rothman 1978; Pivan and Cloward 1971; Geiser 1973; Prescott 1981). We can see this quite clearly in the Moral Majority rhetoric on women who choose to have abortions, and in the villification of alleged child abusers in the media, and in public intervention programs, and in the courts.

We suggest that the choice of child abuse as an official social problem, and the timing of its occurrence (1960s–1980s) cannot be explained solely in terms of the phenomenon of child maltreatment itself. Rather, the emergence of child abuse as a key social problem concerns, in part, its functions as a generative metaphor, serving to displace other collective unconscious anxieties and contradictions in American society. Specifically, the attention to individual cases of child abuse "out there" masks the complicity (and collective responsibility) in the implementation of local, national, and international policies that are placing our nation's and, indeed, the world's children at great risk. National "guilt" about these hostile policies are displaced by intentifying the "real" abusers as those poor and unfortunate wretches who beat or molest their own children. In this light, the identified, individualized, and *punished* child abusers function as one of our society's official symptom bearers for what is, in fact, a normative pathology. It conceals that extent to which we are an abusive society.[5]

As we approach it here, the social problem of "child abuse" has three distinct aspects which are often merged in practice: (1) child abuse as a description of adult behavior toward children with a value judgement about that behavior; (2) the cultural fantasy – or projective – use to which actual child abuse is put; (3) the acting out of a group fantasy of child abuse through social policies that place children at real risk, thereby actualizing or making real the fantasy. We wish to emphasize that fantasy, here, refers to the unconscious, non-rational influences on thought and decision-making – influences which are out of control precisely to the degree that they are inaccessible to conscious awareness except as mediated by symbol or expressed in action. Often, the occurrence of disturbing or disruptive phenomena in society is both explained and blamed on relatively powerless or marginalized social groups. New England had its witches; late Ottoman Turkey its Armenians; Nazi Germany its Jews, Catholics, and homosexuals. In short, frequently blaming, scapegoating, and stereotyping are frequently involved in the identification, labeling, and proposed solutions to, social problems. Here we will argue that child abuse as a modern social problem is highly contaminated with similar unconscious agendas, a few of which we will try to bring to light in the following pages.

GROUP VIOLENCE AND THE TIMING OF SACRIFICE

We are compelled to argue, somewhat counter-intuitively and against our wishes, that the current outrage against child abusers and the wish to rescue young victims from their adult assailants is an expression of contemporary political culture and is continuous with a larger cultural trend. This cultural trend is expressed in the election into public office of those who have instituted a Draconian social policy toward poor and otherwise vulnerable minorities, including abusive adults and abused children.

Throughout President Reagan's terms of office, beginning in 1980, the progressive social and economic programs put into place during the 1930s through the 1960s with their preferential options for the poor, the unemployed, and minorities (i.e. the Roosevelt, Kennedy, and Johnson programs) were gradually dismantled. Reagan's administration ushered in a new era of belligerent conservatism, and health, social welfare, and educational programs suffered their greatest cuts in the last half century. As a consequence, the vulnerable segments of the population (including mothers and infants, children and adolescents) constituted part of an internal sacrifice.

An understanding of the unconscious dynamic of what deMause calls the present "Time of Sacrifice" (1984: 79) in American popular culture, helps to account for the apparent paradox that *the time of greatest public outcry against child abuse is also the time of the widespread, official planning of sacrifice of children in public policy*. Americans, while giving their consent to abusive social policies, simultaneously expressed renewed horror against child abuse, and exercise a grim moralism toward individuals suspected of harming their children and toward women who have abortions. The 1960s and the early 1970s that were an era of self-indulgence and pleasure-seeking (see Lasch 1978) have given way to the era of dour moralism and punishment in the late 1970s and 1980s. This has contributed to the economic conservatism, and to the victim-blaming that has only exacerbated the problems of the poor. From his analysis of the unconscious content of themes in political speeches and in the media, deMause has argued that during the 1980s,

in accordance with the basic family drama in our unconscious reality, in the deaths of real children. . . . when cuts were proposed for Aid to Families with Dependent Children, school lunches, child care, food programs, food stamps, child abuse programs and dozens of other government activities directly affecting the welfare and lives of children, few spoke up, and those few who did were puzzled by the impotence of their cries (1984: 79). . . . article after article was written during the winter of 1981–2 on the rise in infant mortality in areas hardest hit by budget cutbacks and unemployment, on the over one million additional children on the poverty rolls, or the six million children who had lost health coverage . . . of the half million children who lost health services because of the closing by the government of 239 community health centers. . . . *What had happened to the guilt?* (1984: 80).

The answer, deMause suggests, is that we have displaced the guilt onto selected "criminal" scapegoats so that righteous anger is spent in punishing these "bad" individuals, rather than in providing jobs and health care and social welfare programs that could reduce "poor peoples' crimes" (including domestic violence), and thereby increase the survivability of minority infants and babies. In so doing Americans ignore and deny the institutionalized forms of child abuse which they are supporting in public elections, local and national. What is being repudiated, as well, is a whole century of insight which western culture had gained from the psychoanalytic revolution, including a denial of unconscious motivation in adults *and* in children, and in their actions, thoughts and behaviors toward each other. This has resulted in a ruthless punitiveness toward "sleazy" child abusers and child molestors, unrelieved by compassion and understanding. We have, then, a classic case of victim-blaming. "The more children Reagan sacrificed," writes deMause, "the more local newspapers discovered . . . 'an epidemic of child abuse sweeping the city' [*New York Post*, October 5, 1981, p. 3] (1981: 82).

Contributing to, and informing, the new social conservatism is the resurgence of social Darwinism. This has various facets, a few of which bear directly on public attitudes toward child abuse and child abusers. There is, for example, the renewed interest in the 'natural' and the biological dimensions of human behavior, and a consequent belief that society should, insofar as possible, model itself after certain biological imperatives. Motherhood and 'maternal sentiments' are seen as universal, natural attributes, and those who depart from contemporary, middle class interpretations of *proper* maternal behavior are seen as 'un-natural' as well as 'un-fit' mothers. As Schreir, chief child psychiatrist at Children's Hospital in Oakland, has recently pointed out with reference to national anxiety about child maltreatment, and sexual abuse in particular:

Some of the reactions to child sexual abuse is fueled by anxieties created in other social arenas. Many people are threatened by the increased number of women working, children in day care, abortion rights, and the so-called 'sexual liberation' of the past two decades. Some see the sexual abuse of children as an out-growth of these changes. The ideological and political battles that surround these issues are growing more intense. (1985: 59).

In other words, the anxiety about child abuse is, in part, the displaced expression of anxiety about the many changes our society has undergone with respect to sex roles, sexuality and family life. There is a growing tendency to question the wisdom of these changes and to attribute social problems to them. There is a fear that we, as a nation, have moved too far and too fast in refashioning the family, and that the 'epidemics' of child abuse and incest are the unfortunate, but somewhat predictable, consequences.

Another aspect of the new Social Darwinism that bears on our attitude toward the poor and the vulnerable, is the current focus on individual and group 'fitness'. Stein and others have documented the burgeoning of the "fitness" and "wellness" movements of the 1970s and 1980s (*see* Stein 1982a, 1982b, 1982c; Crawford 1977, 1980, 1985; Pollitt 1982; Whorton 1982) which have been interpreted as having as much to do with a "toughening up" of the national fibre and 'stock' as with promoting health. In attitude and ideology the wellness movement articulates a Darwinist ethos: those individuals or vulnerable social groups that will not or cannot "shape up" will simply lose and drop out of the future. Health and fitness are increasingly defined as an *achieved* rather than as an *ascribed* status, one involving free will and choice, conforming to competitive notions of the *self-made* man or woman. Fat, weak, or unhealthy individuals are morally culpable: they obviously did not eat well, care for themselves properly, or exercise sufficiently. The weak, the poor, and the sick have made that "choice" for themselves, and have only themselves to blame. In all, health and fitness have become new commodities in the bustling, impersonal marketplace of American society, and commodities, as usual, more accessible to some segments and classes than to others. Smugness about one's fiscal and, now, physical fitness are joined with an appalling lack of compassion toward vulnerable and twice stigmatized social groups.

The ethos of personal fitness and toughness expressed in the "self-health" and wellness movements of the 1970s and 1980s is also found in a heightened militancy as the new conservatism comes to bear on public policy. The larger cultural trend includes an internal sacrifice that is itself part of a larger, and largely unconscious, preparation for war and toward a readiness for the sacrifice of the young, especially young pubescent males (*see* Biesel 1985; Coleman 1984, 1985; deMause 1984; Stein 1982b). Americans acting "as if" preparing to go to war – expressed in the fitness movement and in a fascination with war games, toys, and dress – can weep sentimentally over the fetuses of the unborn while *readying to arm their own children for combat in a war that will spell the end to all life and all generativity.* (See Daube 1983).

The American national mood – one which underlies various cultural expressions of pugnacity and a lust for violence – is exemplified in the 1984 Olympic nationalistic fervor and celebration of physical superiority; the "heroism" of Bernhard Goetz, the subway vigilante who brutally shot his teenage assailants in cold blood in New York City in late 1984; in the cyclical popularity of G.I. Joe dolls, paraphernalia, and breakfast cereal; the popularity in young women's fashion of shaved and short hair, neutered dress, and shoulder-padded jackets, emphasizing a more muscular, "aggressive" and "masculine" body image; the on-again, off-again popularity of army surplus, khaki fatigues, and camouflage dress among youth and adolescents. It is within this popular culture emphasizing toughness and militarism that the outrage against child abuse is taking place.

Part of the tragic dynamic of this current strengthening of the national fibre is that it is purchased by the weakening of the already frail and vulnerable, as if the latter must always be singled out and sacrificed in order that the social body and the body politic feel strong and renewed once again. Rationalized by the presumed moral superiority of 'wellness' and 'strength', one need not flinch nor suffer twinges of social conscience at the neglect, if not abuse, of the weak. The burden of guilt is projected onto the classes of "bad" people who are kept in constant public view in the media and under the surveillance of police, teachers, doctors, therapists, and social workers.

It is into this arena that child abuse is introduced as a cultural morality play. The sense of tragedy, of unwitting collusion by family and community members, the many unconscious forces in child victim and adult abuser alike – these are all banished from the lived-out drama. In this way, the field is cleared for the "abusers" (who, God knows, are real enough) to come to bear the entire burden of the public's displaced guilty conscience about the institutionalized abuse of the weak, the young, and the vulnerable to which they, too, are party. There is also suggestions of the projection of a fantasy – the wish to abuse, to hurt, to torture the weak and vulnerable that is concealed in the aggressive tracking down of the "evil" perpetrators of the "crime." In seeing abusers and molestors hunted down and severely punished, members of the social mainstream are able to experience a symbolic sacrifice and thus feel themselves cleansed, stabilized, and whole. The collective fantasy-use of the American child abuse drama is akin to the projections of political and religious "conspiracy theories": e.g. what *we* wish to do, and what *we* feel guilty for having done (or "thought in our hearts" about doing), we accuse *others* of doing. Within the drama of played out role expectations, labeling, and counter-labeling the accused often act out their crimes at *our* own behest and in *our* behalf. Accused and accuser are needed to complete the task, to play out the drama.

## VIOLENCE, REBIRTH AND CHILD SACRIFICE

Summing up over a decade of psychohistorical research by David Beisel, Lloyd deMause, Henry Ebel, Stephen Ryan, Casper Schmidt, and Howard Stein, as well as others, Beisel writes:

Understanding how and why groups regress to earlier ways of thinking and feeling has become a major task for psychohistorians. Much is now known about that process. . . . Accompanying . . . primitive fantasies of sacrifice, suicide, and wishes for death is longing for rebirth. Whatever the psychobiological foundations of fantasies of birth and rebirth might be, no one can deny their widespread existence in history. There is solid evidence that birth and rebirth fantasies cluster at a particular time in a group's life. They appear whenever group regression has reached the point at which its members' aggressive impulses are bubbling to the surface and the group is feeling the need to act them out (1984: 135).

The rebirth is always effected through violence, during which one kills off the bad parts of oneself (those one feels to be the unlovable parts) and revives or restores the good parts (so that one feels cleansed and therefore lovable again). In a paper entitled "Nuclear Politics in the 1980's," Coleman writes that

Child sacrifice existed in many cultures. In Carthage, where whole cemetaries of sacrificed children exist, "their own parents offered them and fondled their children just before they were killed so that they might not be sacrificed in tears" [Tertullian 1984: 31]. A more modern way of sacrificing children is spending money for useless, redundant nuclear weapons while there is a "Sharp Rise in Poor Children" [The New York Times, 4/29/83, p. A12], and we see headlines telling us "Hunger a Severe Problem" [The New York Times, 3/11/84, p. 46] (Coleman 1984: 126).

Under the fantasy of the political sacrifice and rescue of children, it is the "bad" (i.e. impulsive, lazy, aggressive, sexual) children who are being disciplined and purged (to a great extent representing the young members of already stigmatized and therefore suspect and vulnerable ethnic, racial and class minorities), and it is the "good" (i.e. the innocent, a-sexual) children who are understood as being rescued. The splitting into two "kinds" of children corresponds, of course, to the idealized and devalued portions of the adult's own self-image. Likewise we can detect a splitting between two "types" of adults. There are the "bad" adults who abuse or molest their innocent children. These tend to cluster in the poorer and marginalized social groups and classes. One thinks of the grossly stereotyped images of the incest-prone Appelachian hillbillies, or the brutal and abusive alcoholic working class Irish father, or the sexually active and maternally immature and neglectful Black teenage mother that one sees portrayed in media dramatizations of child abuse. Conversely, there are the "good" adults, especially the investigative reporter, the dedicated child welfare worker, the tough District Attorney who are the champions of children's rights, and who are portrayed as rescuing and redeeming victimized children. These are the "Child Savers" (see Prescott 1981), the new American "culture-heroes".

To use a dramaturgical metaphor these four distinct psychological "types" constitute the players on the cultural stage: the larger dramaturgical context – the audience, director, script, etc. – is occupied by the wider mainstream culture, including the official policy makers whose elected job it is to crystallize group fantasies into doctrine.

### UNCONSCIOUS FACTORS IN CHILD ABUSE

It is surprising how often people who seek analytic treatment for hysteria or an obsessional neurosis confess to having indulged in the phantasy: 'A child is being beaten.' S. Freud, "A Child is Being Beaten," 1919.

Recently, several books have appeared (among them: Finkelhor 1979; Rush 1980; Herman 1981; Masson 1984) which, collectively, have built a case for psychiatry's denial of the reality of child abuse, especially the sexual abuse of young girls. They suggest that the timing of the recent 'discovery' of child abuse has to do with the uncovering of the 'truth' of allegations of abuse and sexual molestation. Jeffrey Masson's *Assault on Truth*, the most celebrated of the recent attacks on psychoanalysis from this perspective, contends that

Freud was unable, or chose to ignore the actual occurrence of sexual assault in the life histories of his female patients in preference for the analysis of the unconscious reworking of early events. It is not our intent in this chapter to argue with the feminist analyses of *Freud's* unconscious (including his own apparent inability to deal with *real* individual and family aggression/violence), nor even less to deny the valid point that has been made in these writings. Rather, we wish to suggest another dimension of unconscious defenses at work in the national obsession with child abuse and rescue: the national collective unconscious fear/wish that a "child is being beaten" "a girl is being molested". (Chase 1975). We will explore, through themes in popular and political culture, what happens when the actual occurrence of child abuse coincides with group fantasy.

Hollywood has, of late, produced a genre of science fiction films that portray big, bad, corrupt adults who harm, and sometimes kill, childlike, innocent creatures. In the film, *Close Encounters of the Third Kind*, benign aliens from space are the heroes: infantile, neotonous, fetus-like creatures who communicate with simple souls (the pure of heart) through a lilting melody, a lullabye. Likewise in Spielberg's vastly popular film, *E.T.: The Extra-Terrestial*, good and wise children do battle with an uncomprehending adult world. Adults and children are pitted against one another, with adults representing a society corrupted by materialism and an alienating technology. But these films have their counterpart in other films depicting children as evil, satanic, and seductive, such as: *Rosemary's Baby*, *The Bad Seed*, *The Omen*, and *The Exorcist*. Again we have the splitting of good and evil images.

In all there is a rejection of moral subtlety or ambiguity, and a wish for decisive action, a simple definition of the problem, and clean solutions. The popular fantasy is enacted in the characters of Indiana Jones, Crocodile Dundee, the survivalist hero of *Mosquito Coast*, Rocky, Rambo, the heroes of Star Wars, and so on, where the will to immediate action is the key. As Erikson noted (1959: 28), in times of cultural crisis, the American public endeavors to set things right by wiping the moral slate clean.

A second theme in American popular culture concerns ambivalence toward reproduction and generativity, played out in the dialectical fantasy between rescue and adoption versus murder and infanticidal themes. On the one hand we have the adoption and rescue impulse expressed in the Save-the-Child organizations, as well as in the movement to adopt Third World children, especially Southeast Asian and Central American children whose lives, families, and homes have been disrupted, in large part, by North American aggression and militarism. While school lunch programs and food stamps are cut in American cities, while infant mortality in Detroit and Oakland equals that of some Third World countries, we have an outpouring of sympathy and famine relief aid for mothers and children in Africa. Again, guilt and displacement of guilt, always at a safe distance.

A darker, more obsessive side of the adoption/rescue/infanticide fantasy can also be witnessed in the "Cabbage Patch" doll mania that swept the nation in the early 1980s (Beisel 1984). The Cabbage Patch dolls, fetus-like in appearance, are advertized as abandoned (can we think they are possibly aborted?) infants in search of good homes and the "right kind" of parents. The dolls are extravagantly expensive to adopt, so that poorer families can shelter a cabbage patch kid only at a great personal sacrifice. The dependent dolls come with "authentic" adoption papers and with a proper name. During the 1985 Christmas season a new line of orphaned dolls was introduced – a "Rice Paddy Baby", described as a "squeezable Asian doll that comes with a British passport and a voice that coos: 'I want to immigrate. Will you sponsor me'"? (*Newsweek Magazine*, 12/16/85: 49). From the 1983 Christmas season through Christmas 1986 these Cabbage Patch type dolls have been highly sought after, even fought over, in department stores throughout the United States in an altogether appalling display of consumer fetishism and bad taste on the part of the public. While Asian baby dolls were evidentially highly prized, others were not. In New York City, for example, during the 1985 pre-Christmas "rush" on Cabbage Patch dolls, the only ones still available the week before Christmas at May's Department store in Queens, New York were either damaged or black.

A journalist, writing for the North Carolina *Independent* in 1985 concluded the following:

Life's real facts are that adoptable babies usually come out of somebody's sorrow. And we know that there are a lot of real orphans out there in the world: in Lebanon, Vietnam, Nicaragua, and in El Salvador. And some of them are half-American. . . . Some of us deal with this good-heartedly by posting a monthly check to Foster Parents . . . It's even cheaper and easier to buy our kid a Cabbage Patch orphan. [We feel better] . . . and Coleco collects the cash, a lot of cash. (Collier 1985).

A distorted and misplaced altruism (and some real confusion) contributed to a massive give-away of Cabbage Patch dolls to the children of America's poor, sick, and needy during the Christmas season of 1985, sponsored by *Women's Day* magazine. One thousand dolls were distributed to children beset by a multitude of domestic tragedies. The following excerpts from letters to *Women's Day* concerning the Cabbage Patch give-away are illustrative of the social blindness of the kind-hearted donors: (Garbarini and Pascoe 1985):

The doll will go to one of the patients at Kaiser Foundation Hospital who has been diagnosed as having approximately one year to live. . . .

[Another] child reaping the benefit is an eight year old girl from a one-parent home with a handicapped brother. Her mother walked off and left the children when the girl was two years old. The father is unemployed.

. . . . A ten-year old member of our church, whose Dad had a heart problem and is unable to work will receive a [Cabbage Patch] doll for Christmas.

What we have here is the adoption of dolls for some of the United States' own dispensible and "throw-away" children, those for whom government support and many social services have been greatly attenuated.

Cabbage Patch dolls are serious business, occupying a special niche in American popular culture. The reverse side of the dolls' lovability and their innocence and of the adult's wish to extend solicitous care and protection through the fantasy of rescue and adoption, are barely disguised fantasies of abuse, mutilation, cannibalism, and infanticide. Commenting on the national mood in the 1980s, Lloyd deMause commented:

Sometimes our cannibalistic wishes come close to breaking through into consciousness in their most regressed form – that of eating babies – as we, through such popular comedians as Johnny Carson, made jokes on TV about how much fun it would be to hack up, boil, and eat Cabbage Patch dolls, which children that Christmas had taken to adopting by the millions (1984: 160–161).

A contemporary form of child sacrifice is the spending of money for genocidal and redundant nuclear weapons while there is a sharp rise in the numbers of poor, disadvantaged, malnourished, and illiterate children in the United States. At least one political cartoonist captured the infanticidal motif, and the contradiction between the politics of rescue and the politics of destruction with his juxtaposition of Cabbage Patch dolls and military weapons:

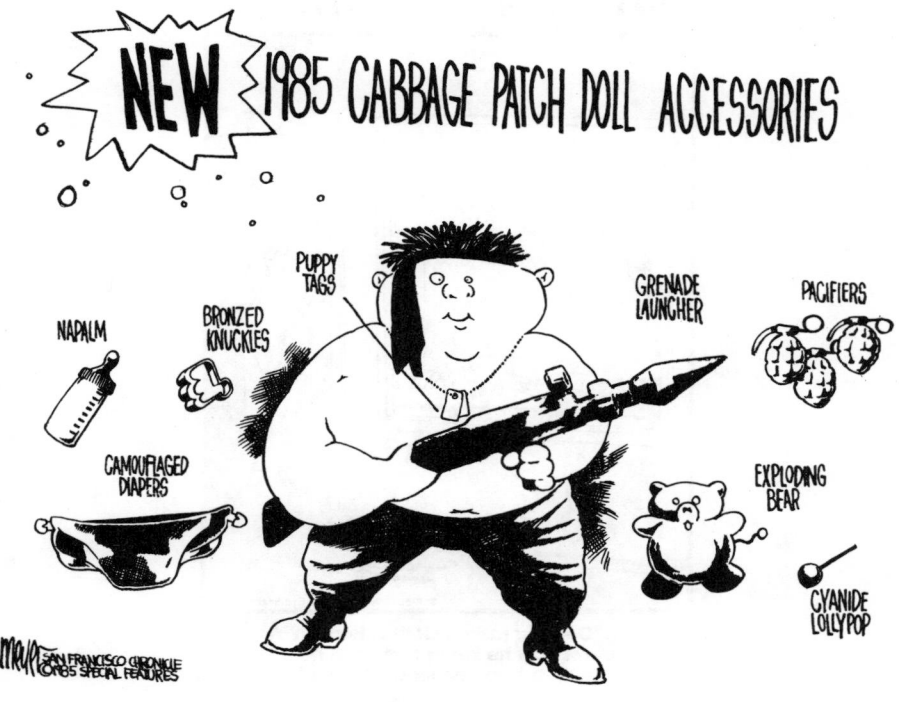

Fig. 1.  *San Francisco Chronicle* December 2, 1985: 53.

Sadistic, infanticidal jokes and commentary directed against the Cabbage Patch dolls has entered into popular discourse. During a TV talk show interview, for example, a rock music star complained that her Mexican-American maid refused to enter or clean the daughter's room because she was afraid of the girl's Cabbage Patch doll. The maid said that the doll was "evil". One of our neighbors told of having bought her daugher a Cabbage Patch doll for Christmas which turned out to be damaged, its arm was torn. The woman wrote to the manufacturer asking for a replacement for the expensive doll. The company responded by issuing the mother *and* her daughter a death certificate for the original doll, and promised that a search was underway to locate a more acceptable adoptive baby doll. One can only imagine the barely suppressed hostility toward children that was involved in the toy manufacturer's death certificate fantasy. The incident is reminiscent of the penultimate bad taste of the cyclically popular and in vogue "dead baby jokes" which Alan Dundes (1979) has linked to cycles in the national anxiety about and obsessive fascination with, abortion. Infanticidal humor has not escaped the attention of Gary Larsen who, from time to time, has indulged in the pastime of uncovering new risks to the newborn as in the following cartoon:

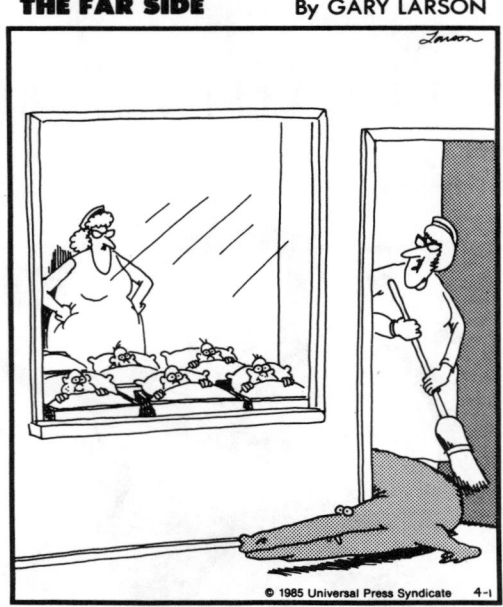

**THE FAR SIDE**     By GARY LARSON

"Get, you rascal! Get! . . . Heaven
knows how he keeps getting in here,
Betty, but you better count 'em."

Fig. 2.   "A Previously Hidden Dimension of Childhood Mortality Finally Comes to Light"
(Reprinted with permission. All Rights Reserved.)

Infanticidal fantasies lead guiltily to counter-phobic fantasies of rescue that are played out in the responses to harm wrought to real children by our own domestic and international policies. We set up rescue missions to undo the damage to those we have placed in jeopardy in the first place.

To reiterate our thesis: the children who are being championed and – albeit few – rescued are seen as the victims of child abusers who are viewed more as criminals to be punished than as tragic, sometimes pitiful characters who need compassion if they are to be helped to change. Child abusers, then, serve as a delegate group (Sterlin 1974) to embody the disavowed evil impulses of mainstream America, while children serve as a delegate group both to embody projected innocence (especially sexual innocence) of childhood, and to serve as group sacrifices. Child abuse, of course, began as a fact, and not as the product of a group fantasy. However, as it has become fueled by unconscious wishes, projections of endangerment and rescue, it has become inseparable from the collective unconscious which has used child abuse toward its own collective ends. If there is a prevalent fantasy that "a child is being abused", "a girl is being molested", then whatever the actual incidence or prevalence of such occurrence, we must also address and understand the combined fear *and wish* that such occurrences take place. In his epochal paper, "A Child is Being Beaten": A Contribution to the Study of the Origin of Sexual Perversions" (1919), a quote from which opens this section, Freud was talking about neurotic patients' sado-masochistic fantasies about child-beating. Here we are talking about what happens when the actual occurrence of child maltreatment coincides with a group fantasy/obsession.

Probably the most disheartening aspect of the de-responsibilitization for child abuse and neglect in this country is the search-and-destroy mission directed at the "bad" parents (especially mothers) who are held individually responsible for the maltreatment of children. We might point, for example, to the vigorous medical-legal campaign to uncover sexual abuse presently being waged in the courts, in schools, and in doctors' offices throughout the country. This campaign has lead to such institutionalized and professionalized forms of sexual abuse as the suggestion to introduce vaginal inspection of little girls by pediatricians during routine medical exams (Cantwell, in press; Krugman 1986) and the often inappropriate use of anatomically correct (SAC) dolls in clinics, social welfare offices, and nursery schools with pre-school aged children for the purposes of sexual abuse "screening" (*see* White, Strom, and Santilli 1985). Due to the number of false allegations of sexual abuse resulting from the indiscriminate use of such experimental and highly questionable investigative measures several class action suits on behalf of the falsely accused are currently in litigation (*see* L. Coleman 1986; Dolan 1984; Goodwin, Sahd and Rada 1978; Green, n.d.). Among their claims are violations of civil rights, the poor scientific status of the criteria in use for verifying suspected cases of sexual abuse, and the eroticization of children by aggressive and suggestive questioning, and use of the SAC dolls by poorly trained police, social workers, teachers, nurses, and doctors. In short, the "child saver" investigators are themselves suspect of playing out a child molestation fantasy. In all, the national focus and obsession with physical and sexual violence toward children serves to divert attention away from the more endemic and more life-threatening problem of child *neglect*.

### THE NEGLECT OF CHILD NEGLECT AS A SOCIAL PROBLEM

To date, national attention and public outrage and response has been directed, almost exclusively, at those "criminal" or "psychopathological" parents who either batter, sexually molest, or otherwise physically abuse their children. However, recent surveys and analyses of national child abuse reporting indicate quite clearly that child battering and sexual molestation are neither the most frequent, nor the most potentially fatal assaults against children. The American Humane Society's analysis (1983) of all officially reported child maltreatment cases in the United States for 1981 indicated that physical injury accounted for less than one-third of all reported cases of child maltreatment for 1979 through 1982, and for approximately 34% of all fatalities (American Humane Society 1983: 12). Sexual abuse accounts for 7% of all reported cases of child maltreatment and for no fatalities. The greatest threat to child well-being and survival in our society today is from neglect, which is broadly defined in child welfare discourse as the "deprivation of necessities", or, in other words, poverty. The intentionality of the "neglectful" parent (usually the mother) is not necessarily taken into account, and even a loving and well-intentioned, but poor, parent raising her child in a

TABLE I
Substantiated maltreatment – percent

| Type | 1979 | 1980 | 1981 | 1982 |
|---|---|---|---|---|
| Major Physical Injury | 4 | 4 | 4 | 2 |
| Minor Physical Injury | 15 | 20 | 20 | 17 |
| Physical Injury (Unspecified) | 3 | 3 | 3 | 5 |
| Sex Abuse | 6 | 7 | 7 | 7 |
| Deprivation of Necessities* | 63 | 61 | 59 | 62 |
| Emotional Maltreatment | 15 | 13 | 12 | 10 |
| Other | 9 | 8 | 12 | 10 |
| Number of cases (in thousands) | 226 | 268 | 236 | 332 |

* failure to provide shelter, nourishment, health care, education, supervision, clothing and failure to thrive, as defined by the states.

*Source*: Compiled from *Highlights of Official Child Neglect and Abuse Reporting*, Annual Reports, 1976–1980, American Humane Association

sub-standard environment of poor housing, insufficient food, inadequate clothing, education and medical care can be reported for child neglect (see Stack 1984; Hughes, this volume). By far the most pervasive, costly, intractable, and potentially fatal risk to American children today is that of child neglect, not child abuse. Neglect accounts for 60% of all child abuse reporting and for 56% of all related fatalities. Yet, child neglect has been ignored by the media, and in the national hysteria about child maltreatment. This, too, must be accounted for.

In its final section on the policy implications of the Humane Society's analysis of official report statistics, the report includes:

A significant issue is that the majority of children (60 percent) seen by CPS [the Child Protective Service] were reported as experiencing deprivation of necessities, or neglect. It is commonly thought that neglect is less 'serious' than other forms of maltreatment. Consequently, at a time when CPS agencies are being forced to limit their responses to cases perceived as the most serious, *neglect cases are likely to be among the first ones screened out*. This poses a serious dilemma. It is clear that in its present form the CPS cannot accommodate all children reported as maltreated, so perhaps it is necessary to screen cases out. However, it was neglect that was the most frequently indicated type of maltreatment for fatalities. . . . [The findings also] support the notion that there is a strong association between the stresses of poverty and the inability to adequately care for children. The problem is that the CPS system is neither equipped nor intended to alleviate poverty. . . . The reporting data revealed that the predominant service type was casework counselling; specific support services were indicated much less frequently. (1983: 23)

Finally, the report concludes with the injunction that, in general, the focus of child welfare policies in this country be "broadened to incorporate the reality of poverty" (*ibid*). We could not agree more fully with this assessment. The point, relevant to our particular analysis, is that the "choice" of child abuse as a master social problem of our times, also includes a strong "choice" for only certain forms of child abuse – battering and sexual abuse – and a *selective inattention* to other forms – specifically, poverty-related neglect. This selective inattention is a consequence of the need to deny the role of our punitive public policies in contributing to the "feminization of poverty", and to the problem of childhood mortality in our inner city, minority neighborhoods. Far less anxiety-provoking is to continue our pursuit of the "bad", out-of-control, assaultive parents. This "choice" in the popular construction of the real problem of child maltreatment was brought home to one of us (NS-H) who was recently interviewed for a televised news series examining child abuse and neglect in California. A taped half-hour interview was reduced to a five-minute segment that comprised a response to the reporter's incessant questioning about child molestation. Clearly, the much longer discussion of child neglect and poverty in California (and the childhood mortality rate in Oakland) were neither sufficiently "sexy" nor *violent* enough for popular consumption. Moreover, who is there to blame, who is there to punish when a child goes to bed hungry? (While we *know* who to blame and punish – or think that we do – when a child has been beaten, or a young girl molested).

## CONCLUSION

What George Devereux spoke of as a "vicious cycle of pathology" (1980: 19) can be seen in the social psychological dynamics and drama of the child abuse problem. As the actual abuse of children is more defined as a social and medical problem, public outrage has led to an increasingly punitive policy toward identified abusers. This, in turn, leads to a diminished sense of social relatedness and responsibility for the problem, and to further reductions in social and economic support for parents with vulnerable and dependent children. This leads to increased stress, and frequently to increased abuse and neglect in those families at greater risk, who are seen as intrinsically bad. Hence, at least some of the child maltreatment that is observed, diagnosed, and treated is actually *created*, and those forms of institutionalized maltreatment reproduced in our social policies and enacted in our popular culture, remain below consciousness, and therefore unrecognized and untreated. If we are to avoid this tangle of absurdities, it is essential to un-mask the contradictions in our behavior. At that time, and not before, we will be prepared to solve, rather than use, the problems of child abuse.

### NOTES

\*  This chapter is dedicated to the memory of George Devereux, who died 29 May, 1985.
1.  A similar process of "medicalization" is now occurring with the attempt to create a new diagnostic category for sexual abuse: the "Child Sexual Abuse Accommodation Syndrome" (Summit 1983) and the "Sexually Abused Child's Disorder" (Corwin 1985). The essential diagnostic features of the latter include a child's displays of age-inappropriate ". . . *awareness* of differentiated sexual behaviors as demonstrated by *specific knowledge*, emotional or behavioral reactions to direct questions about parts of the body" (1985: 8). In other words if a child displays "age-inappropriate" *knowledge* about sexual anatomy and function s/he might be suspect as a victim of sexual molestation. The fact that classes and ethnic groups, rural v. urban children differ with respect to such cultural information is nowhere recognized in this diagnostic check-list for clinicians.
2.  To date (1985), forty-two States have centralized registers for reports of child abuse and neglect. The information kept in these files varies, however, as do State rules on sealing, destruction, and access to, and confidentiality of, these records (Federal Register 1985: 32771).
3.  For a critique of a portion of this literature see Cicchetti and Aber 1980.
4.  While directing a team field research project on professional and community definitions of child abuse and neglect in Taos County, New Mexico in the summer of 1985 (see Scheper-Hughes 1987), one of us learned that a Sexual Abuse Prevention worker gained permission to hold a workshop on sexual abuse with Pueblo Indian children attending a community Head-Start program. Using the Colorado format, children there were told to distinguish "bad" touches as "anywhere the bathing suit covers the body," despite the fact that these children do not use bathing suits in their ritual ablutions in the stream that runs through the Pueblo community. Moreover, anxiety was raised by the suggestion that co-sleeping with parents and cross-sex siblings is "not good", although these celebrated "apartment-dwellers" have lived for more than a thousand years in preferred domestic arrangements of close physical intimacy that includes co-sleeping of parents and childrens and of siblings.
5.  Precisely how, and how subtly, this occurs, can be discerned from the following "micro-analysis": A number of medical colleagues are ardent child advocates (e.g., "The worst sin is

to harm a child"; "I can't imagine why someone would abuse their child."). They work zealously in their clinics, hospitals and community agencies to ensure that abused children are identified, taken to shelters if necessary, receive proper treatment, and that the parents are reported to child welfare. Many of these same clinicians, however, have in recent years developed a caustic humor toward poor and Welfare patients and their families, accept or wish to accept in their practices only paying or third-party insured patients, express a diminished sense of personal responsibility toward patients while heightening their sense of biomedical responsibility toward them, and in their humor about abusive parents reveal a vindictiveness toward them without much tempering compassion (i.e., identifying wholly with the child as victim). Questioning the need for AFDC, Food Stamps, WIC, subsidized school lunches, etc., they often seem to wish upon others the deprivation they once had, or perhaps feel they themselves deserve.

## REFERENCES

American Humane Society
  1976–80 Highlights of Official Child Neglect. . . Denver: A.H.S.
  1983 Highlights of Official Child Neglect and Abuse Reporting. Denver, Colorado: American Humane Society.
Beisel, David R.
  1984 Thoughts on the Cabbage Patch Kids. The Journal of Psychohistory 12(1): 133–142.
  1985 The Vietnam War: A Beginning Psychohistory. The Journal of Psychohistory 12(3): 371–393.
Cantwell, H.
  1983 Vaginal Inspection as it Relates to Young Girls. Child Abuse and Neglect 7: 171–176.
Chase, Naomi
  1975 A Child is Being Beaten. New York: McGraw-Hill.
Cicchetti, Dante and Lawrence Aber
  1980 Abused Children – Abusive Parents: An Overstated Case? Harvard Educational Review 50(2): 244–255.
Coleman, Lee
  1986 False Allegations of Child Sex Abuse: Have the Experts Been Caught With Their Pants Down? Forum (January–February): 12–20.
Coleman, Mary
  1984 Nuclear Politics in the 1980s. The Journal of Psychohistory 12(1): 121–132.
Collier, Carol
  1985 Toys That Bear Watching: The Cabbage Patch Conspiracy. The Independent, December 6–19: 2.
Corwin, David L.
  1985 Sexually Abused Child's Disorder. Draft #3, October 14. Children's Hospital, Oakland, California.
Crawford, Robert
  1977 'You are Dangerous to Your Health': the Ideology and Politics of Victim-Blaming. International J. of Health Services 7: 663–680.
  1980 Healthism and the Medicalization of Everyday Life. International Journal of Health Services 10: 365–388.
  1985 A Cutural Account of 'Health' – Self-Control, Release, and the Social Body. In J. McKinlay, ed. Issues in the Political Economy of Health Care. New York: Methuen.
Daube, David
  1983 Black Hole. unpublished manuscript. Boalt Hall, School of Law, University of California, Berkeley.
deMause, Lloyd
  1974 The History of Childhood. New York: The Psychohistory Press.

1982 Foundations of Psychohistory. New York: Creative Roots, Inc.
1984 Reagan's America. New York: Creative Roots, Inc.
Devereux, George
1980 Basic Problems of Ethno-Psychiatry. Chicago: University of Chicago Press.
Dolan, M.
1984 Molest: False Allegations on the Increase. Los Angeles Times July 16, Part 1, p. 1.
Dundes, Alan
1979 The Dead Baby Joke Cycle. Western Folklore 38(3): 145–157.
Edgerton, Robert
1981 Foreword. *In* Jill Korbin, ed. Child Abuse and Neglect: Cross-Cultural Perspectives. Berkeley: University of California Press.
Erikson, Erik
1959 Identity and the Life Cycle: Selected Papers by Erik H. Erikson. New York: International Universities Press.
Federal Register
1985 Office of Human Development Services: "Child Abuse and Neglect Prevention and Treatment Proposed Research Priorities for Fiscal Year 1986", Vol. 50, No. 157: 32769–32771.
Finkelhor, David
1979 Sexually Victimized Children. New York: Free Press.
Freud, Sigmund
1959 (1919) "A Child is Being Beaten": A Contribution to the Study of the Origins of Sexual Perversions. The Complete Freud 17. London: Hogarth Press.
Garbarini, Alice and Elizabeth Jean Pascoe
1985 Does Anybody Out There Care? Yes! Women's Day, December 3: 52, 56.
Gaylin, Willard, Ira Glasser, Steven Marcus, and David Rothman
1978 Doing Good: the Limits of Benevolence. New York: Pantheon.
Geiser, Robert
1973 The Illusion of Caring. Boston: Beacon.
Giovanni, Jeanne and Rosina Becerra
1979 Defining Child Abuse. New York: Free Press.
Goldstein, Joseph, Anna Freud, and Albert Solnit
1973 Beyond the Best Interests of the Child. New York: Free Press.
Goodwin, J., D. Sahd, and R. Rada
1978 Incest Hoax: False Accusations, False Denials. Bulletin of the American Academy of Psychiatry and the Law 6(3): 269–276.
Green, Arthur H.
n.d. Did He or Didn't He? True and False Allegations of Sexual Abuse in Child Custody Disputes. Unpublished paper available from the author at the Presbyterian Hospital, BH 616–622 West 168th Street, New York, New York 10032
Hausfater, Glenn and Sarah Blaffer Hrdy
1984 Infanticide: Comparative and Evolutionary Perspectives. New York: Aldine.
Hefler, Ray E. and C. Henry Kempe
1978 Child Abuse and Neglect: the Family and the Community. Cambridge, Massachusetts: Ballinger Publishing Company.
Herman, Judith
1981 Father/Daughter Incest. Cambridge, Massachusetts: Harvard University Press.
Hippler, Arthur E.
1978 A Culture and Personality Perspective of the Yolngu of Northeastern Arnhem Land. Part I: Early Specialization. The Journal of Psychological Anthropology 1(2): 221–244.
Kempe, C. Henry, et al
1962 "The Battered Child Syndrome", Journal of the American Medical Association 181: 17–24.

Kempe, Ruth and C. Henry Kempe
  1978 Child Abuse. Cambridge, MA: Harvard University Press.
Korbin, Jill
  1981 Child Abuse and Neglect. Berkeley: University of California Préss.
Krugman, Richard D.
  1986 Recognition of Sexual Abuse in Children. Pediatrics in Review 8(1): 2–7.
Lasch, Christopher
  1978 Haven in a Heartless World: the Family Besieged. New York: Basic Books.
Masson, Jeffrey
  1984 The Assault on Truth: Freud's Suppression of the Seduction Theory. New York: Farrar,
    Strauss, and Giroux.
Pivan, Frances and Richard Cloward
  1971 Regulating the Poor. New York: Vintage.
Pollitt, Katha
  1982 The Politically Correct Body. Mother Jones (May): 66–67.
Prescott, Peter S.
  1981 The Child Savers. New York: Alfred Knopf.
Rush, Florence
  1980 The Best Kept Secret: The Sexual Abuse of Children. New York: Prentice-Hall.
Ryan, William
  1971 Blaming the Victim. New York: Vintage.
Scheper-Hughes, Nancy
  1979 'Breeding Breaks Out in the Eye of the Cat': Sex Roles, Birth Order and the Irish
    'Double-Bind'. Journal of Comparative Family Studies, X(2): 207–226.
  1984 Infant Mortality and Infant Care: Cultural and Economic Constraints on Nurturing in
    Northeast Brazil. Social Science and Medicine 19(5): 535–546.
  1987 The Best of Two Worlds, the Worst of Two Worlds: Reflections on Culture and
    Fieldwork Among the Rural Irish and Pueblo Indians. Comparative Studies in Society
    and History 29(1) (January).
Schreier, Herbert
  1985 Child Sex Abuse Laws Too Rigid? Open Forum, San Francisco Chronicle Thursday,
    October 24: 59.
Shorter, Edward
  1975 The Making of the Modern Family. New York: Basic Books.
Stack, Carol
  1984 Cultural Perspectives on Child Welfare. New York University Review of Law and Social
    Change.
Stein, Howard F.
  1978 Judaism and the Group-Fantasy of Martyrdom: the Psychodynamic Paradox of Survival
    Through Persecution. The Journal of Psychohistory 6(2): 151–210.
  1980 An Ethno-Historic Study of Slovak-American Identity. New York: Arno Press/New
    York Times Press.
  1982a 'Health' and 'Wellness' as Euphemism: the Cultural Context of Draconian Health
    Policy. Continuing Education for the Family Physician 16(3): 33–43.
  1982b Neo-Darwinism and Survival Through Fitness. The Journal of Psychohistory 10(2):
    163–187.
  1982c Wellness as Illusion. Delaware Medical Journal 54(11): 637–641.
Sterlin, Helm
  1974 Separating Parents and Adolescents: A Perspective on Running Away, Schizophrenia,
    and Waywardness. New York: Times Books.
Stone, Lawrence
  1977 The Family, Sex, and Marriage in England, 1500–1800. New York: Harper and Row.

Summit, Roland C.
   1983 The Child Sexual Abuse Accomodation Syndrome. Child Abuse and Neglect, 7: 177–193.
Tertullian
   1984 Quoted in "Child Sacrifice in Carthage – Religious Rite or Population Control?" Biblical Archeological Review X(1).
White, Susan, Gerald Strom, and Gail Santilli
   1985 Clinical Protocol For Interviewing Preschoolers With Sexually Anatomically Correct Dolls. Available from the senior author at the Department of Psychiatry, Case Western Reserve University, Cleveland, Ohio 44109.
Whorton, James
   1982 Crusaders for Fitness: the History of American Health Reformers. Princeton: Princeton University Press.

DON HANDELMAN

# BUREAUCRACY AND THE MALTREATMENT OF THE CHILD: INTERPRETIVE AND STRUCTURAL IMPLICATIONS

This paper discusses how social-welfare officials interpret an instance of the suspected maltreatment of a child; the ways in which such interpretation is structured in a bureaucratic context in order to construct a case; and the implications of interpretation and of the emerging structure of the case for the practice of child-welfare. The venue of discussion is the child-welfare division of the public Department of Social Services in the city of St. John's, Newfoundland.[1]

## 1. LACUNAE AND PREMISES

During the past two decades the maltreatment of children has come to be recognized as a salient social problem in Western nation-states. The horrific record of hard-core cases of child-abuse and neglect is well-documented, and its evidence is unequivocal. However, my remarks are directed toward those instances that may be called potential or possible suspicions of maltreatment, where there is uncertainty either as to how something untoward happened to a youngster or whether this might occur in the future. The wider penumbra of such instances of suspicion (*cf.* Steele and Pollack 1974: 90) likely produces a higher incidence of cases than does the core of unequivocal instances of maltreatment (*cf.* Scott 1969, who develops this position with regard to the bureaucratized treatment of a disability).

There are two gaping lacunae in research into instances that I am calling ambiguous. The first is the lack of explication of how the identification of maltreatment is done (*cf.* Light 1973: 571; Parke and Collmer 1975: 7). The second is the lack of information on the contexts of work in which investigation is done. Both of these kinds of information have salient significance for the value of the conclusions and the intervention of child-welfare investigators.

The investigation of instances marked by uncertainty is pervaded by psychologistic thinking in which emphasis is laid less on how parents do behave toward their children, but more on their presumed intentions and motivations, and on the psychopathologies that may underlie these (*cf.* Gil 1973: 119; Gelles 1974; Davoren 1974: 136; Renvoize 1975: 39, 167; Morris and Gould 1963: 32).[2] Investigators rely on their perceptions of the minds and psyches of the possible perpetrators in order to establish what did happen, why this happened, and what may happen in the future.

Therefore it is incumbent on the researcher to understand how investigators perceive and proceed in their work, in order to comprehend how they carry this out. A verdict of maltreatment not only signifies what may have

359

*Nancy Scheper-Hughes (ed.), Child Survival, 359–376.*
© *1987 by D. Reidel Publishing Company.*

happened in the world of the client household, but also what has occurred during the process of investigation, in the world of the investigators. The identification of maltreatment is, first and foremost, a social process that is informed by considerations of ideology, by conditions of work, and by the sorts of organizations within which such work is carried out. The first lacuna in research is that discussions of these crucial aspects of how investigation is done are virtually absent in studies of maltreatment, and in reports by practitioners. These begin from the premise that the identification of mal-treatment and its perpetrators has been done successfully; and so their primary focus is then treatment and prevention. But, in point of fact, how the identification of maltreatment is done in numerous instances that are ambi-guous is highly problematic and questionable (Handelman 1978, 1979, 1983).

In the Western nation-state much of the work of identifying, evaluating, and dealing with offenders is done by public and private welfare agencies, by the judicial apparatus, and to a degree by children's departments of hospitals. In other words, bureaucratic organizations are essential to the processes whereby damage to children is defined officially as maltreatment. These bureaucratic contexts inform the perceptions and the procedures of child-welfare workers as they go about their routine practices. The second lacuna in research is that information on such contexts also is conspicuous by its absence in the literature on maltreatment. There is almost no mention of how such bureaucracies do their tasks, of how they deal with inbuilt problems of definition and validation of ambiguous instances of suspected maltreatment, and of the untoward consequences that their procedures may have for the households that are investigated.[3]

At issue, then, is the manner of work of child-welfare officials who are employed in bureaucratic organizations. Bureaucracies are pervasive in mod-ern life, but this does not mean that the logic of their operations should be taken-for-granted as known and understood. Anthropologists in particular should be cognisant that the idea of bureaucracy that we live with is itself a fairly recent cultural construct of the Western nation-state (Handelman 1981: 6–12), and not a natural fact of life. Therefore it is necessary to reiterate briefly certain of the premises of bureaucratic organization. Bureaucracies are goal-directed: they exist in order to define, to classify, and to solve or to expedite problems. Ideally they are invested with well-defined powers, arro-gated to positions of authority, that are delineated in universalistic terms. Bureaucrats are armed with explicit laws, rules, and regulations with which to make rational decisions. As Weber (1964: 330–339) noted, rational bureau-cratic purpose depends on the application of rules to particular instances through the special knowledge that such officials command.

Yet the application of rule to instance, of idea to action, cannot proceed without the intervention and the mediation of the notion of "interpretation." This refers to the search for meaning, for the likely significations that are stressed by phenomenal elements (viz. the "facts") in the course of building a case of maltreatment. The very term, "case", one that is native to helping-bureaucracies, rests on the premise that the elements of its composition are together because they make sense in this kind of causal configuration. In other words, that together these elements signify some pattern of meaning that is of direct relevance to the organization concerned, but that also accurately represents the contours and the dynamics of a social problem that is native to the world outside the organization. The manner of reasoning itself may be termed configurational: the uncovering of elements that apparently have some affinity to one another; and the interpretation of these affinities to establish whether or not their connections are lineal. In other words, whether these connections have a relationship of cause-and-effect that is necessary to "make a case" that separates the suspect instance from the flow-of-life, and that gives it a distinct ontological status that requires intervention.

The notion of "interpretation," although it is part of the stock-of-knowledge (Schutz and Luckmann 1973) of investigating officials, often is uncodified, and is tacit and common-sensical. Common-sense interpretation is at once flexible and final, open-ended and foreclosing. Therefore officials have difficulty in consciously scrutinizing and evaluating the implications of how they do interpretive work: for it is "common sense" or it "makes sense" in ways that should be evident to other members of the same organization. In terms of this perspective the outcome of "interpretation" should not require further explication. Consequently, and regardless of their efforts to be systematic, objective, and consistent, investigating officials rarely realize fully what their own contributions are to such outcomes.

## THE IDEA OF "CASE"

In the child-welfare division that I studied, it is in the investigation of a specific instance of suspicion that the process of interpretation intersects with the context of bureaucratic work to produce the emerging structure of a case. The building of a case begins with a report of suspicion of maltreatment. A case, like the bureaucratic organization that gives it life, is explicitly goal-directed. It is put together by assembling the "facts" from relevant persons in order to establish the status of the allegation. The aim of a case is to arrive at the truth. As the facts are interpreted, logical connections are made among items of information. From such connections the structure of case comes into being.

But here I am referring to two kinds of structure. One is a causal accounting of the facts, as these are arranged lineally, through time. In other words, this is the plot or story-line of the case, one that is easily accessible for review, although it may have its murky moments. Nonetheless, this story-line lies quite close to the surface, as it were, of the context of work, and it can be discussed routinely by officials as a continuous chronological sequence of occurrences. Yet there is another structure to an emerging case, one that is

more hidden from the common-sense interpretations of child-welfare officials. This "deeper" structure is predicated on a simple opposition between
punition and rehabilitation of the offender/client, and on the mediation of this
dualism. Therefore there is a more structuralist dilemma that is embedded in
the construction of case, one that is partially independent of the problem of
interpretation, but that has significance for the manner in which a case is
conducted. I will return to this deeper structure during the discussion of the
case-example itself.

A developed case is a construct that is brought into existence to establish or
to invalidate a causal link between person and event, in the sense that a
person caused the event to occur, whether by commission or omission. The
appearance of a case – the perception of its surface manifestation – is treated
as real by childworkers. But I must stress that, since the appearance of a case
is understood as real, it is the construct itself that has an impact on the lives of
people. This is so, even though the deeper structure of case may put into
question the causal inference of its appearance.

In the child-welfare division that I am discussing, there is an inbuilt tension
between bureaucratic directives to investigate allegations of maltreatment
and the lack of guidelines as to how to do this. According to the Newfoundland Child Welfare Act of 1972, the reporting to the authorities of suspected
neglect and abuse is mandatory. But the Regulations of the child-welfare
division state only that:

> Every Welfare Officer, at some time in his career, will have brought to his attention a child who is
> not receiving the care and upbringing considered necessary for his proper development. This
> child for some reason, or for a number of reasons, may be considered a neglected child. Every
> such complaint or report of neglect must be investigated to determine its authenticity and the
> extent of the neglect (Section 221).

The above is the *only* reference in the Regulations about what a childworker
should seek in checking the validity of a suspicion. The remainder of the
Regulations describe procedures that are relevant only after the childworker
has decided that the instance is one of maltreatment.

Article 2, Subsection (p), of the Child Welfare Act of 1972, provides
twenty criteria according to which a child (under the age of sixteen) can be
considered "neglected." But these criteria are summations that denote that a
decision already has been reached. Thus the criterion used most frequently
for the apprehension of a youngster (Article 2, Subsection (p) (iv)) states that
a neglected child is one, ". . . whose parents, or surviving parent, or guardian
or other person in whose charge he may be, cannot by reason of misfortune,
disease or infirmity properly care for him, or are unfit to have charge of him,
or refuse to maintain him." The questions of how to understand, for example,
"misfortune", or "are unfit to have charge of him," are left initially to the
interpretations of the childworkers.

When the decision is one of maltreatment, the offspring in question can be apprehended without a warrant, and held in the care of the Department of Social Services for a maximum period of ten days without a court hearing. If legal proceedings are initiated, there are four possible kinds of decision. The family-court judge may dismiss the case. He may leave the child within the household, but instruct the Department to supervise. He may make the child a "temporary ward" of the Department, to be placed in a foster home or in an institution for an initial period of one year. Or, the child may be made a "permanent ward" of the Department – then the youngster is removed from the household for an indefinite period, and under certain conditions he may become eligible for adoption. Although the family court usually is loathe to rule for either of the latter two options, the decision by the Department to intervene in a household is fateful for the family concerned.

## INTERPRETATION, OPPOSITION, AND MEDIATION IN CASE-CONSTRUCTION: AN INSTANCE FROM CHILD-WELFARE

When elements that are to become a case begin to accrue, their collection resembles what structuralists term "bricolage." These elements are shuffled in various combinations, as caseworkers search for likely logical connections among them. In this early stage there is no necessary or deterministic patterning (See Handelman 1979). Yet, given the goals of the of the investigation, such a configuration can emerge quite quickly. As this occurs, the emergent case acquires what I have called here the more "surface" structure of lineal directionality and incipient causality. This structure becomes real for the investigators. In turn, this reification of the case becomes the medium through which the investigators continue to interpret new elements that are added to it.

The first element of the instance of suspicion discussed here came to the Department in the form of a letter from a neighbor of the family, whom I call Fort. The letter alleged that, with the husband, Mr. Fort, in a tuberculosis sanitorium, his wife enjoyed the company of other men, leaving her three young children unattended.[4] The investigation was assigned to the child-worker in whose geographical sub-region the household was located.[5] The ensuing investigation found the three children neatly dressed, and the apartment clean and tidy. There was no evidence of physical neglect. As a matter of routine, a file was opened on the family in the child-welfare division. This complemented their file in the social-assistance division. Mr. Fort, the bread-winner, was often out-of-work and received monthly welfare payments. But the social-assistance file was quite ordinary, and the family was not seen as problematic. Some months later Mr. Fort left the sanitorium. He complained several times to the Department that his wife drank heavily, stayed out at night, and did not care for the children. He then left her and requested that the three children be placed in a foster home.

Another investigation followed. Mrs. Fort admitted the caseworker, but

refused to discuss her own behavior. Again there was no evidence of maltreatment. On a subsequent visit, Mrs. Fort told the caseworker that, "Welfare interferes with other people's lives." The caseworker responded: "If she
wouldn't let me help her then I would have to go to court to make the
children temporary wards. Apparently she didn't believe me and shut the
door in my face." Mr. Fort and the family's landlord agreed to testify that
Mrs. Fort often was drunk, and that she brought men home. The caseworker
informed Mrs. Fort of the date of the court hearing, but pleaded with her to
be permitted to aid the family. "I said we didn't need to go to court if only she
would talk to me and let me *help* her keep the family together. She then said I
could take the children now but she would not go to court. I told her we didn't
want the children but only to *help* her. She still wouldn't listen and shoved the
children over to me and kept screaming for them to go". The caseworker left
with the two older children, aged four and five. Mrs. Fort would not part with
the youngest, Mandy, then aged one year. Mr. Fort was not the father of
Mandy; and Mrs. Fort referred to the infant as her "love child."

According to the criteria of the Department there was no *prima facie*
evidence of child-neglect here. To the contrary, children and dwelling were
well looked-after. But what did become an issue was Mrs. Fort's behavior
toward the caseworker. The caseworker saw her own task as one of "helping." Mrs. Fort utterly rejected intervention, and so too this beneficence.
Therefore this rejection was understood to say something about her character
(and not about the mandate for intervention). The configuration of meaning
that the caseworker began to construct related Mrs. Fort's behavior toward
her to the allegations of her husband. In the caseworker's interpretation, the
issue speedily became one of the character of the mother, and therefore one
of what she *might do* to her children, but not what she had done or what she
was doing.

It is apparent that this inference was questionable, and that it was beyond
the official mandate of the child-welfare division. But, according to this
pattern of meaning, there was here an instance of neglect, one that would be
real in its consequences for the children involved. The caseworker proceeded
as if this inference were valid, and it did become real in its consequences for
Mrs. Fort. The *potential* for maltreatment replaced the absence of actual
neglect as the object of the caseworker's endeavors. As the caseworker
continued to press Mrs. Fort, so the latter more adamantly objected. The
next development in the emerging story-line of the case confirmed the
caseworker's interpretation. Mrs. Fort threw two of her children to the
childworker, signifying that she cared nothing for them. Given the plot being
developed, it was not relevant whether she did so because she indeed was
indifferent to their welfare or because she was badgered into an ill-measured
response. Her motivation in doing so already was accounted for in the
caseworker's interpretation of her character. She had shown neglect toward
her offspring. That the immediate cause of this may have been the case-

worker's attempts at intervention also was not relevant: from the perspective of the child-welfare division, the caseworker was uncovering the facts, not interpreting their creation.[6]

On behalf of the child-welfare division the caseworker petitioned the family court to have all three children made temporary wards for one year. The judge reasoned that Mrs. Fort had demonstrated toward her two older children an indifference that was tantamount to neglect, and ordered them made temporary wards. But he found no evidence of neglect with regard to the youngest. He ruled that she would remain with her mother who, in the future, would be subject to the supervision of the child-welfare division.

This decision outraged the childworkers. The case had been interpreted as one of neglect, a label that was to apply to all three children. Therefore the court should have ordered all three removed. Instead the mother kept the one child she cared for deeply. This questioned the bureaucratic story-line the caseworker had put together. She did not doubt her reification, but she did question the validity of the verdict; and she wrote to the Director of Child-Welfare: ". . . We are at a loss to explain how the judge could declare two children neglected and yet the third, who was subjected to the same type of treatment, was not made a ward. We are convinced that not just two but all three children involved were being neglected and the youngest child, while she is allowed to remain with her mother, will continue to be neglected . . ."

In his reply the Director recommended that the caseworker increase her household visits to twice-weekly, and added: ". . . In situations such as this it is our responsibility to maintain as much supervision as possible and when necessary to present such cases to court." The childworkers were to watch Mrs. Fort until they uncovered evidence of the neglect that had yet to occur. Then her third could be taken.

The severity of the departmental reaction to the court verdict illuminates a significant aspect of how such emerging cases are structured through time. This is less readily apparent if the case is understood solely as a lineal sequence of interpretation. It may also help to explain, in part, why child-workers voiced an immense dislike of maltreatment cases. When the construction of a case points to the presence of maltreatment, the sequence of its emergence incorporates an official decision – a court verdict or a departmental directive – to take remedial action. Such action either removes the child from the home or institutes departmental supervision of the household. As the case emerges through time, it develops a dual form. The first phase of this duality may be termed one of investigation and punishment. This is followed by a phase that may be termed one of "rehabilitation." Under the supervision and tutelage of the caseworker, the offending parent is expected to show an improvement in attitude and behavior that would warrant either the return of the child or the removal of the supervision.

For caseworkers the shift from being a punitive agent to one of rehabilitation, toward an offender who has become a client, is a most difficult one.

Some caseworkers who have concluded what I call the punitive phase are unable to switch roles to the rehabilitative. Others are unable to complete the punitive phase. As one put it, "Either you take one side or the other, or you get torn apart." Another added, "My God, we're the biggest threat . . . Imagine how a mother feels when we come to take her kids away." Sometimes a caseworker will recognize the punitive attitude that is inherent in contacts with potential offenders, even if there was only a hint of suspicion. For example, the most experienced of the childworkers once said of a young couple: "I felt that I should drop in and see them occasionally for their own protection, in case we should receive complaints – and that they should cooperate for their own good."

The two case-phases, of punishment and rehabilitation, are opposed to one another, along various dimensions, as indicated below.[7] This dualism, inherent in the composition of such cases, is their deeper structure that I referred to earlier.[8] But these phases are not only opposed to one another: they must be also complementary if the entire case is to be brought to a satisfactory conclusion, one that is marked by the rehabilitation of the offending parent. The problem of bridging these two structural phases is crucial. Therefore, in line with structuralist thought, one would expect to be able to uncover here an implicit mediator of phase-opposition.

Dimensions of opposition in the emergent structure of developed cases

| Dimension | Phase 1 | Phase 2 |
|---|---|---|
| goal | investigation | rehabilitation |
| outcome | punition | help |
| temporal orientation | past/present | future |
| duration | brief | lengthy |
| attitude of childworker | suspicion | sympathy |
| behavior of childworker | coercion | accomodation |

The mediator that I think operates here is the idea of "cooperation", the evidence of which is expected of the offender/client. This idea rarely is accorded explicit recognition by the childworkers: therefore it would appear to be a structural mechanism. On the other hand, the meaning with which this idea is invested suggests that it rests still on the interpretation of behavior. Therefore it is not only a structural mechanism, but is also subject to reification.[9] Nonetheless, the childworkers' expectations often are phrased in terms of various kinds of "cooperation" that the offender should evince in order to demonstrate rehabilitation. Here the idea of "cooperation" is not a psychological notion, but a social one. What is all important is the presentation of self on the part of the offender/client. For it is from this that the childworkers infer what they understand as the psychological state (the motivations and attitudes) of the client.

Although its epistemological status is not clear, the presence of this mediator may be a location in case-construction at which interpretation itself requires mediation. This mediation then itself fills a structural position, one that is more-or-less coterminous with the shift from punition to rehabilitation. Nonetheless, the structural form of the emerging case remains strongly dependent on interpretation in order to bring itself to satisfactory completion, in bureaucratic terms.

The cooperation of the offender/client indicates to the caseworker that her interpretation of maltreatment does have validity – for the former shows understanding and appreciation of the goals and efforts of the latter. But should the client reject, oppose, or defy the caseworker, this suggests that the latter's interpretation may be incorrect. Thus threatened, the caseworker then is likely to become more coercive and punitive toward the client, in order to drive her to accept the validity of this interpretation. From the perspective of child-welfare, the idea of cooperation often projects a sense of joint effort and consensus between caseworker and client, and so it should lead to a meeting of minds and points of view. But the more implicit ontological status of the idea of cooperation, one that is bared in instances of defiance, is that of hierarchy, authority, and coercion.

Therefore, often in tacit ways, the idea of cooperation conveys the priority of the authority and power of the state, as this is represented by welfare personnel. It is to this authority that the offender/client must submit, and it is this that establishes the correct order of hierarchy in the relationship between state and citizen. Thus, in terms familiar to structuralist thought, points of mediation are loci of the frequent production of symbols and symbolic acts. This is so with regard to behavior that the idea of cooperation requires of clients. The implementation of cooperation demands of the client acts that are highly symbolic of submission, of subordination and penance, in which the most private of familial domains crumble before representatives of the state.[10]

In the Fort case the judge's verdict was anomalous to the line of interpretation of the childworkers; and so it prevented the case from shifting smoothly into its rehabilitative phase. Mrs. Fort kept the one offspring she cared for; and this took from the child-welfare division the major resource with which to seek her cooperation. Therefore the case itself became anomalous, and the caseworker was trapped in her own construction of its punitive phase. Later, the childworkers' attempts to escape the punitive phase through coercion eventually succeeded, but in doing so they thwarted the rehabilitative aim of the case.

The caseworker made her twice-weekly visits, but Mrs. Fort rarely admitted her to the dwelling. With time this childworker was followed in succession by two others. On the rare occasion that they gained entry they reported that the child was well-cared for. Still, they were certain that evidence of maltreatment eventually would turn up.

For the next two years Mrs. Fort persisted in her implacable refusal to cooperate with the child-welfare authorities. If they harbored any reservations about her presumed maltreatment, this evaporated in the face of her defiance. Indeed, one may say that their certainty of "neglect" was elicited in large measure *because* she rejected their "help" in learning how to care for the child. She could escape their continued presence and pressure only by accepting the character they had prepared for her in the case. The more she resisted submitting to this, the more anxious they became that she do so, in order to complete the temporal-structural form of the case, and so also their own tasks.

During the following year a fifth childworker took over the case. There still was no evidence that the youngster was neglected, but the surveillance continued, off and on. When this latest caseworker tried to visit Mrs. Fort, "She told me not to come back and slammed the door in my face."[11] This childworker later stated: "She cannot be approached as she refuses to let a worker inside the door. This woman is antagonistic and *rebellious* to the point of being dangerous."

A few weeks later, and some three years after the two older children were removed, an incident occurred that once again convinced the childworkers that they were justified in perceiving Mrs. Fort as an unfit mother. One morning a neighbor telephoned the child-welfare division, saying that Mrs. Fort had beaten her daughter the previous night. Two childworkers, accompanied by two police detectives, rushed to the address. Mrs. Fort denied beating Mandy, but one childworker announced that there were four bruises on the child's legs. While one worker telephoned a hospital, Mrs. Fort locked herself and Mandy in the kitchen. The detectives ordered her to open the door or they would break in. If they did so, she replied, she would stab the child, or scald her with boiling water. After a lengthy argument Mrs. Fort acceded, and the detectives found the youngster under a table, barricaded in by chairs. Her mother stood with a kitchen knife in hand and with a kettle nearby. At the hospital the examining physician stated that the girl had not been ill-treated in any way. He added that she was a healthy child.

Finally Mrs. Fort had filled the role assigned to her in the case. Her hysterical reaction and her threats were interpreted as evidence of her true character, not as the culmination of lengthy periods of pressure by the childworkers, nor to their sudden appearance with the police. The childworkers thought the apprehension of the child an error only in that she showed no evidence of ill-use – her mother still was thought of as a *potential* cause of harm to the youngster.

The childworkers placed two conditions on the return of the child to her mother: first, that Mrs. Fort permit the caseworker to visit the household every two days, to help her become a proper mother; and second, that she undergo a psychiatric examination. Mrs. Fort submitted, and this evidence of "cooperation" seemed to shift the case into its second structural phase, that of rehabilitation. On the basis of a single interview the psychiatrist found Mrs. Fort to be of limited intelligence and, in his opinion, quite "paranoid." She expressed her fears: that the child would be taken from her, which was why she had reacted as she had during the apprehension; that her telephone was bugged; and that her letters were stolen. All this, she claimed, was the search for evidence that would justify the removal of Mandy. On the other hand, he found the girl to be a "bright normal child", to whom there was no danger so long as her mother accepted the supervision of the childworkers and psychiatric treatment.

The diagnosis of paranoia solidified the story-line of the case. In retrospect this diagnosis validated all of the Department's efforts to make the mother accept guidance. Since the perception of the case was causal, with its roots in Mrs. Fort's psyche, the condition of paranoia explained her motivation in continuously rejecting the childworkers. It was not, nor could it be, a reaction to the coercive pressures that she had withstood for a lengthy period. Her condition was wholly her own responsibility, and it demonstrated just how much she was in need of help.

Mrs. Fort missed her psychiatric appointments; she said her phone was monitored; and she insisted that the caseworker, skulking in a variety of disguises, followed her whenever she went out. The caseworker turned for advice to the psychiatrist. Although he had seen the mother only once, the psychiatrist described her as one of his most paranoid patients. The following day he wrote to the caseworker that Mrs. Fort apparently was at times "psychotic", and that her condition seemed to be deteriorating. He added that she was a potential danger to her daughter, and that it probably would be best if the child were taken away. He concluded that this in itself might make Mrs. Fort so acutely ill that she would have to be hospitalized.

One should note again the counterpoint of the developing structure of the case and the achievement of its bureaucratic goal. Structurally, the case was put together as a sequential unfolding of two phases, in opposition to one another, but mediated by the idea of cooperation. On a more surface level, the case was invested with meaning through lineal interpretation aimed at finding a solution that would evince cooperation. Thus, at the juncture of the two phases of the case, the lineal progression of interpretation and the deeper phase-structure of the case became highly dependent upon one another, in order to complete the synthesis of the case as a diachronic composition.

The case still was stuck between its punitive and rehabilitative phases. Mrs. Fort's degree of cooperation was minimal, but as yet there was no substantive evidence that she had maltreated her daughter. Supervisor and caseworker concluded that, "Although there was no physical abuse evident in this case, there was 'emotional abuse' in the sense that it was inevitable for Mandy to develop abnormally under her mother's care." Trapped within the teleological effects of causal construction, the childworkers did not recognize the paradox that they had helped to create. Over three years before their interpretation had pointed to Mrs. Fort as an unfit mother, for all three of her offspring. They scrutinized her lifestyle and behavior, but their expectations did not materialize. She saw them as a threat, and limited contact to the best of her ability. When they seized the child, in an abrupt display of power and coercion, they pushed the mother into a hysterical reaction. For the child-workers this was proof that their interpretation of the case was correct. For Mrs. Fort this may have been the cutting-edge of her persecution by the childworkers.

Following the diagnosis of paranoia, attempts at intervention were intensified. Not surprisingly the childworkers uncovered further evidence of Mrs. Fort's mental instability, much of it associated with keeping her daughter from them. If three years before it was inevitable that the mother would mistreat her daughter, it was now inevitable that the child would develop abnormally because the mother was paranoic. If the causal logic of the case initially was indeterminate, it now had the solidity of predetermination. For the childworkers, in retrospect, Mrs. Fort had been mentally-disturbed for years, and this explained her irrational refusal to cooperate with them. A case that began with the problem of how to save mother and child was discovering its resolution in the destruction of the mother in order to save a child who apparently needed no succour.

The childworkers knew that the family-court judge would not agree to wardship on the grounds of hypothetical emotional-abuse. But if the child could not be removed from her mother, then perhaps the mother could be separated from her child. Caseworker and supervisor considered this alternative: to commit Mrs. Fort for observation in a mental hospital. In this they had the support of the psychiatrist, who wrote that: ". . . it was possible for Mrs. Fort to be a potential danger not only to her child but also to herself as well." To accomplish the commital the caseworker would make a deposition to the court, declaring that Mrs. Fort was apparently insane. The court would issue a warrant to arrest Mrs. Fort, which would be executed by the police. Then a psychiatric examination, by two court-appointed psychiatrists, would determine whether commital was warranted.

The caseworker was uncertain whether to proceed, for now she felt driven to a step of conscious coercion. The following day she conferred with the supervisor and the Regional Administrator, who was in charge of the field operations of all of the social-service divisions within a region that included the city of St. John's. She was reminded that although Mrs. Fort was sincere in her love for her daughter, if she would not voluntarily accept psychiatric treatment (here another euphemism for cooperation), she had to be forced to. The caseworker still hesitated: "They were pushing me hard to take a decision, and have her committed. Finally (the Regional Administrator) came right out and said it – 'You had better take some action this afternoon, because if something happens to that child in the meantime, and (the head of a local citizen-rights group) gets ahold of it . . .' So who do you think would get shit piled on shit? All on me, that's who. Because if anything happened to that child while I was diddling, it would be my responsibility. So I went down to the court and did it."

The Department of Social Services existed among other organizations, to whose pressures it was sensitive. When the caseworker vacillated, she was admonished that the interpretation of the case had to be compatible with the aims of the bureaucracy; and that, on occasion, it had to answer to outside audiences (cf. Jehenson 1973: 226–227). She also was encouraged to accept that the commital of Mrs. Fort was a neat solution to a bureaucratic problem, and one that was compatible with the reality of Mrs. Fort as a person.

Later that day, some six weeks after Mandy was mistakenly apprehended, three policemen, the caseworker, and Mrs. Fort's social-assistance welfare officer, all went to the Fort apartment. The police entered and returned shortly with mother and daughter. The caseworker was struck by Mrs. Fort's lack of resistance: "It was very interesting, that this time she didn't cause a scene but was very mild and docile." She was examined at the jail, and both psychiatrists recommended her commital for a thirty-day period of observation. With Mrs. Fort incarcerated and unable to care for her daughter, the child-welfare division had grounds on which to request temporary wardship for the child for a duration of twelve months, and to place her in a foster home for this period. As she prepared the request for wardship, the caseworker reiterated the more structural dilemma of the child-welfare division: "If Iona (Mrs. Fort) had only recognized that all we wanted to do was *help* her, this probably wouldn't have happened."

## IMPLICATIONS

The implications of my argument for practitioners of child-welfare are three-fold. First, although processes of interpretation in bureaucratic contexts often are those of implicit knowledge, they can be made more "reflexive" on the part of practitioners. The self-critical awareness that reflexivity denotes is not restricted to one's sense of self and other as psychological beings, but extends equally to the structures and processes within which one lives and works. In no sense does the "social construction of reality", which is connoted by an emphasis on interpretation in case-building, argue that the maltreatment of children is a fictitious issue. But, by elevating implicit features of organizational life to conscious inspection and evaluation, it does insist on degrees of self-critical awareness that often are downgraded, or are lacking, in routine bureaucratic work (*cf.* Scott 1970).

Reflexive awareness demands not only the scrutinization of why certain steps are taken, but also the laying bare of their underlying premises – in other words, it demands an epistemology of casework that is less mildly philosophical in intent and is attuned more harshly to the practics and practice of child-welfare. So, for example, this requires the unpacking of what is

signified by organizational and occupational glosses like those of "cooperation" and "help". The recognition of the centrality of interpretive processes
will invalidate the position that rules are applied in mechanistic fashion to
particular instances. So too, such an awareness will negate the premise that
the childworker is simply a rational instrument that uncovers the objective
"facts" of an instance of suspicion, as these truly exist out there in the world
of the client.

The rationalization of the client-as-object denies that the childworkers
themselves are implicated in the kinds of cases that they put together. To the
contrary, the building of a case is so often a joint, if conflictual, effort by both
officials and clients; and it is this that bureaucratic and professional realities
frequently deny (*cf.* Handelman 1976, 1980). Yet it is this sense of social
structure, its production and reproduction, that anthropologists and sociologists are especially able to elicit. And welfare officials who reject this knowledge will continue to be dumbfounded by the ways in which cases do not
develop in accordance with their expectations – as were the officials who dealt
with Mrs. Fort.

There is a further point to be considered here. Social structures, whether
large or small-scale, are reproduced in part through processes of interpretation. In Western societies these processes are understood to be located within
individual beings, in their perceptions and motivations, and so forth. Therefore critical awareness at least contains the potential to change perception and
interpretation. It is as grave an error to attribute human action solely to
normative constraints as it is to picture the person wholly as a psychological
puzzle. True, at times this will pit the practitioner against other bureaucratic,
research, and psychologizing personnel – and at potentially high personal
risk, as Mrs. Fort's last caseworker realized. But the alternative, to succumb
wholly to the expeditious common-sense lineaments of a task, is inevitably to
stultify, and to become incapable of recognizing in others the humanity and
frailty that we accord to ourselves.

The second implication derives from the structural view of case-
development taken in this paper. The identification of phase-opposition and
its mediation points to a level of structure more implicit than that of the
interpretational. How this level operates to structure cases must lead one to
examine more seriously how mediators, like the idea of cooperation, tend to
gloss and to obscure the harsh visages of hierarchy, coercion, and submission.
But beyond this, one must recognize that the particular structural disjunction
discussed in this paper, that between punition and rehabilitation, and the
kinds of problems it creates, are themselves bureaucratic and occupational
constructs. Therefore, so long as organizations similar to the Department of
Social Services value such ideational distinctions, they will be difficult to
resolve and will produce anomalies like that of the case of Mrs. Fort. In other
words, the eradication of deeper structural disjunctions requires changes in

the very logic of organization of a bureaucracy, and not simply surface alterations in, for example, the education of childworkers, their attitudes, or the size of caseloads.

This leads directly to the third implication. This relates to oppositions between social-structural principles that are embedded in the fabric of the wider society, and therefore that encompass particular organizations, that themselves may be established to deal with the consequences of such more ramified disjunctions. Thus certain pervasive dilemmas in the relationships between state and citizen, between officials and clients, may themselves be more surface manifestations of still deeper oppositions, disjunctions, and anomalies. Positivist-oriented social-planners frequently argue that social problems can be solved through the application of instrumental solutions: larger budgets, more expertise, the rationalization of service and delivery systems, a more "humanistic" approach to clients, better-defined techniques of intervention, and so forth. Permit me to close on a more pessimistic note.

It is incumbent on us to ask whether the state and its organs can really substitute for the members and services of what is understood in Western society as an organic family unit (cf. Gaylin et al. 1978) – for example, as surrogate parent for a child removed from a family, or as a compensator through commodities for family-members who are absent or who have died (cf. Shamgar-Handelman 1981). Or, whether such and other intervention brings to the fore principled structural oppositions and disjunctions, of value and substance, between relationships that are perceived as "natural" ones and those that are brought into existence by man-made edict (cf. Schneider 1968). There are numerous examples of such disjunctions that seem to be generated by the need to map relationships of state and citizen onto those of kinship and family.[12] The resultant tacit structural anomalies may well have no solution, short of radical social change. When they are treated as soluble, in rational common-sensical terms, this merely leads to the growth and expansion of bureaucracies that themselves reproduce these structural oppositions and disjunctions. In turn, the latter continue to generate anomalies and conflicts that are mediated and are as-if resolved through the application of the might of the state to family situations. As in my little example of Mrs. Fort, there likely are no panaceas. Perhaps the best one can hold out for is an informed critical awareness, on a number of levels, that just might avert some tragedies.

### NOTES

1. Data were collected during 1973–1974, as part of a wider study of the Department of Social Services in St. John's, Newfoundland. The study was supported by a research fellowship in the Institute of Social and Economic Research, Memorial University of Newfoundland.
2. The implications of this position are criticized elsewhere (Handelman 1978: 18–24, 1983: 6–9).

3. One would expect anthropologists especially to be sensitive to such issues. Yet these are quite disregarded, for example, in the recent volume edited by Korbin (1981), where some of the contributions deal with bureaucratized societies.

4. This case is discussed at greater length, although from a different perspective, in Handelman 1983: 21–31.

5. The St. John's urban area is divided into a number of sub-regions, each of which constitutes the jurisdiction of a child-welfare official. Within such a sub-region all matters that pertain to the welfare of children are the responsibility of the same childworker, whether this be adoption or maltreatment. The child-welfare division employed nine caseworkers and a supervisor. Holding constant the length of time they served in the division, not all of the childworkers were equally experienced with instances of maltreatment. Reports of maltreatment that reached the division were concentrated heavily in poorer and more congested neighborhoods of the city. The Forts lived in one of these, whose residents had the reputation in the Department of being antagonistic to welfare officials of any stripe. The incidence of reports of maltreatment was linked strongly to social class. As well, anonymous allegations were used to settle scores among kin and neighbors. Other reports came from hospital clinics and emergency rooms used more often by poorer residents. In addition, in congested areas, the noises of crowded living-quarters reached more easily the ears of others.

6. I see this as a problem of welfare bureaucracy that has a wider cachet, beyond the contexts of Newfoundland. More generally it is related to the recasting of the focus of investigation as "object" rather than as "subject." As "object" the client, of course, is objectified, and so becomes an autonomous entity who is independent of any intersubjective consequences that derive from his relationship with a welfare bureaucracy (cf. Handelman 1976).

7. See, for example, Michael Hughes' discussion (this volume) of the conflicts he felt between care and coercion, between control and compassion, and between being an investigator and a social worker.

8. Where, as in this child-welfare division, the same caseworker is responsible for the implementation of both punition and rehabilitation, I would expect the opposition between the two phases to be excacerbated.

9. In other words, like the surface appearance of interpretation, the deeper structure of the case may also be a product here of bureaucratic inventions of procedure. Nonetheless, the opposition between punition and rehabilitation is found in other structures of the wider society, as is the opposition between state and family. The particular form of phase-opposition discussed in this paper may be a product of the Newfoundland welfare bureaucracy, but the kinds of conflicts this signifies have wider and deeper relevance.

10. Such symbolism clearly is in evidence, for example, in the visits of welfare officials to the dwellings of their clients. Not only have they the right to gain entry, and to check the quality of living within by sight, touch, and smell (in that order of importance), but once within they may enter the most intimate regions of the household.

11. During this period the two older children were made permanent wards of the Department of Social Services (Handelman 1983: 24–26). The child-welfare division wanted to place them for adoption, but Mrs. Fort refused to sign the necessary documents. This is what this caseworker was trying to obtain on this visit.

12. The inculcation of a hierarchy of relationships, in which the state comes to supersede the family, may begin early in the life of the child. See, for example, Shamgar-Handelman and Handelman 1986.

## REFERENCES

Davoren E.
    1974 The Role of the Social Worker. In Ray Helfer and Harry Kempe (eds.), The Battered Child (Second Edition). Chicago: University of Chicago Press.

Gaylin, W., I. Glasser, S. Marcus, and D. Rothman
    1978 Doing Good: The Limits of Benevolence. New York: Pantheon.
Gelles, Richard J.
    1974 Child Abuse as Psychopathology: A Sociological Critique and Reformulation. *In* Suzanne Steinmetz and Murray Straus (eds.), Violence in the Family. New York: Dodd, Mead.
Gil, David G.
    1973 Violence Against Children: Physical Child Abuse in the United States. Cambridge: Harvard University Press.
Handelman, Don
    1976 Bureaucratic Transactions: The Development of Official-Client Relationships in Israel. *In* Bruce Kapferer (ed.), Transaction and Meaning: Directions in the Anthropology of Exchange and Symbolic Behavior. Philadelphia: Institute for the Study of Human Issues. pp. 223–275.
    1978 Bureaucratic Interpretation: The Perception of Child Abuse in Urban Newfoundland. *In* Don Handelman and Elliot Leyton, Bureaucracy and World View: Studies in the Logic of Official Interpretation. St John's: Memorial University of Newfoundland. pp. 15–69.
    1979 The Interpretation of Child Abuse: Bureaucratic Relevance in Urban Newfoundland. Sociology and Social Welfare 6: 70–88.
    1980 Bureaucratic Affiliation: The Moral Component in Welfare Instances. *In* Emanuel Marx (ed.), A Composite Portrait of Israel. London: Academic Press. pp. 257–282.
    1981 Introduction: The Idea of Bureaucratic Organization. Social Analysis 9: 5–23.
    1983 Shaping Phenomenal Reality: Dialectic and Disjunction in the Bureaucratic Synthesis of Child Abuse in Urban Newfoundland. Social Analysis 13: 3–36.
Jehenson, Roger
    1973 A Phenomenological Approach to the Study of the Formal Organization. *In* George Psathas (ed.) Phenomenological Sociology. New York: John Wiley. pp. 219–247.
Korbin, Jill E. (ed.)
    1981 Child Abuse and Neglect: Cross-Cultural Perspectives. Berkeley: University of California Press.
Light, R.
    1973 Abuse and Neglected Children in America. Harvard Educational Review 43: 556–598.
Morris, Marian G. and Robert W. Gould
    1963 Role Reversal: A Concept in Dealing with the Neglected/Battered-Child Syndrome. *In* The Neglected Battered-Child Syndrome. New York: Child Welfare League of America.
Parke, Ross D. and Candace Whitmer Collmer
    1975 Child Abuse: An Interdisciplinary Analysis. Chicago: University of Chicago Press.
Renvioze, Jean
    1975 Children in Danger. Harmondsworth: Penguin Books.
Schneider, David
    1968 American Kinship: A Cultural Account. Engelwood Cliffs: Prentice-Hall.
Schutz, Alfred and Thomas Luckmann
    1973 The Structures of the Life-World. Evanston: Northwestern University Press.
Scott, Robert A.
    1969 The Making of Blind Men. New York: Russell Sage Foundation.
    1970 The Construction of Conceptions of Stigma by Professional Experts. *In* Jack D. Douglas (ed.), Deviance and Respectability. New York: Basic Books.
Shamgar-Handelman, Lea
    1981 Administering to War Widows in Israel: The Birth of a Social Category. Social Analysis 9: 24–47.
Shamgar-Handelman, Lea and Don Handelman
    1986 Holiday Celebrations in Kindergartens in Israel: On Relationships Between Represen-

tations of Collectivity and Family in the Nation-State. *In* M.J. Aronoff (ed.), The Frailty of Authority (Political Anthropology, Vol. 5). New Brunswick: Transaction Books. pp. 71–103.

Steele, B.F. and C.B. Pollock
     1974 A Psychiatric Study of Parents Who Abuse Infants and Small Children. *In* Ray Helfer and Henry Kempe (eds.), The Battered Child (Second Edition). Chicago: The University of Chicago Press.

Weber, Max
     (1964) The Theory of Social and Economic Organization. First published 1947. This Edn. edited by Talcott Parsons. New York: The Free Press.

# WHEN CULTURAL RIGHTS CONFLICT WITH THE "BEST INTERESTS OF THE CHILD": A VIEW FROM INSIDE THE CHILD WELFARE SYSTEM

Social scientists and historians have identified a source of crisis in the modern family: a loss of autonomy attendant to the proliferation and influence of child care experts – pediatricians, educators, child psychologists, and especially child welfare workers (*see* Donzelot 1979; Lasch 1977; Meyer 1983). The possibilities for professional and state intervention have multiplied with the dramatic increase in the number of reports of child abuse and neglect processed and investigated by Child Protective Service (CPS) agencies in the United States. It is important to note that these interventions have not always been either randomly or equitably distributed. There are, for example, a disproportionate number of low income and cultural minority families represented in the child abuse and neglect caseloads managed by the child welfare system in the United States.

I begin this paper with two charges: (1) by consistently failing to acknowledge the importance of children's ethnic identities and their cultural traditions CPS (Child Protective Service) agencies and workers have been disproportionately destructive of the family integrity of cultural minorities; (2) CPS agencies and workers have just as consistently failed to attack and to change the root cause of child maltreatment as reported in 58.8% of all cases (U.S. House of Representatives 1986) and implicated in 34% of all child fatalities in this country (National Committee for Prevention of Child Abuse Monthly Memorandum, December 1985) – "the condition of poverty with its attendant psychological stresses and problems in daily living" (American Humane Society Annual Report 1981).

With reference to the first charge I would point to an American Indian association's study conducted in 1976 which indicated that one of every four American Indian children nationally was not living with his or her family at the time of the study (Unger, ed. 1977). Eighty-five percent of these same children were living in non-Indian foster care homes denied access to their nuclear and extended families as well as to their tribal homes and communities. The disparity in foster care placement rates for Indian and non-Indian children in the United States is truly shocking. In the state of Wisconsin during the early 1970s, for example, the risk of an American Indian child being separated from his or her parents was found in the above study to be nearly 1600% greater than for non-Indian children (Byler 1977, cited by Fischler 1980: 342). William Byler, the Executive Director of AAIA, explored the criteria in use and the grounds for the removal of Native American children and the termination of parental rights, and found that neglect

377

*Nancy Scheper-Hughes (ed.), Child Survival, 377–382.*
© *by D. Reidel Publishing Company.*

accounted for a full 99% of all removals (cited by Fischler, *op cit.*). The evaluation of neglect, however, frequently involved judgements based on cultural misunderstanding and the tendency by social workers to pathologize family patterns and child rearing norms that deviate from those of the dominant white culture. Byler cites, for example, cases where children were removed from Indian homes because the circulation of children among blood and affinal kin was viewed as "neglectful", or where traditional permissiveness and lack of physical discipline was viewed as parental abrogation of responsibility [see Hauswald, this volume, for another and highly critical perspective on this point of view].

All too often child neglect is simply conflated with family poverty, and while the symptom (neglect) is "treated" (by removal), the underlying root cause (i.e. poverty of the parents) is left undisturbed. The poverty of the parents was likewise identified as the main grounds for removing children from their homes in a recent report on foster care and adoption in the state of North Carolina (Governor's Advocacy Council on Children and Youth 1978). National incidence surveys conducted by the American Humane Association each year indicate that child neglect occurrs about twice as frequently as all other forms of child maltreatment combined, and that neglect (defined as the deprivation of basic necessities) is really indistinguishable from household poverty in most cases. Hence, children are removed from their parents for reasons that may have very little to do with parental hostility or ineptitude toward the care and development of their children.

Since the late 19th century the "best interests of the child" has been used as a basic standard in deciding child custody disputes in U.S. courts. The "best interests" standard has also been adopted by the CPS system in deciding when children should be removed from their homes, where they should be placed, and the conditions under which they would be returned to their parents or placed for permanent adoption. A new federal mandate for "permanency planning" with respect to child welfare (Public Law 96–272) has increased the pressures on CPS workers to locate permanent placements for children in the custody of departments of social services – whether these permanent placements mean further pressure on natural parents to relinquish their claims to the children so as to expedite adoption proceedings or even when in some cases it means a relatively permanent placement (until age of emancipation) in a psychiatric or other treatment facility. A particularly unfortunate side effect of this well-intended but often misguidedly applied piece of legislation is that permanency planning has tended to decrease the flexibility that CPS workers previously had to maintain poor and minority children within traditional and informal kin networks. The haste to locate a permanent "solution" to child abuse tends to translate into the termination of parental custody, since treatment of the problem family and addressing the root causes of poverty, homelessness, and unemployment require both time and resources not available to most CPS agencies. Adding further insult to injury, termination of parental custody entails for many cultural minority children a permanent separation from wider family and kin ties and a dislodgement from community, class, and cultural milieux.

In recent years American Indian, Hispanic, and Afro-American lawyers, educators and child rights advocates have responded to the disproportionate disenfranchisement of poor and minority children by the CPS bureaucracy in asserting that children have a legitimate *right to culture* – that is, a *right* to grow up in, be nurtured and educated by, and belong to, a community of kinship and shared meanings that is each individual's natural birthright. A right to culture is, with few exceptions, a still largely unrecognized component of the child's "best interests". The Indian Child Welfare Act, passed in 1978 (*see* Barsh 1978) is perhaps the most definitive statement of this point of view, but one which has had its own fair share of critics who feel that this law subordinates children's rights to parental, family, and tribal rights (see Fischler, *op cit*). Meanwhile, politically activist and minority social workers have developed cultural training programs for child welfare workers in order to correct the white bias in traditional social work education [the cultural sensitivity training by Hispanic and Pueblo social work educators at New Mexico Highlands University, Las Vegas, is a model of its kind in this regard].

This chapter raises the question: Can social workers, in conjunction with the U.S. courts, act in the "Best Interests of the Child" (*see* Goldstein, Freud and Solnit 1973, 1979) *without* doing violence to the "cultural rights" of the child, his kin group, and his community? I will identify in the following pages at least one source of contradiction in the bureaucratic structure of the CPS system in the U.S. which perpetuates a kind of double-bind in the implicit mandate to social workers to be both agents of care and agents of social control. This mandate is implicit in the fragmentation of child welfare workers' responsibilities among the welfare agency, the courts, the community, the parents, and the children they are expected to serve. The contradictory injunction to be simultaneously empathic *and* punitive (i.e., "change your behavior or your child will have to be removed") throws the CPS worker into a conflict which is often expressed in the ambiguous and chronic malaise known as CPS worker "burn out".

The following analysis and case studies are based on an "Insider's View" of the CPS system. I am a clinical social worker with more than ten years of experience in the field of child protection. My anthropological "training" has come largely through the course of marriage to, and shared fieldwork experiences with, an anthropological spouse. It was at her urging that I have contributed my reflections on this subject. I have worked in child welfare in four states and culturally distinct regions of the United States: as a CPS worker in a large city in the Southwest; as a Child Abuse and Neglect Assessment worker in a large city in the Northeast; as a CPS Permanency Planning worker in a small city serving a largely rural population in the

Southeast; and, currently, as a clinical social worker with a child protection team at a pediatric hospital on the west coast. I will begin by presenting aspects of three child welfare cases in which cultural (and cultural rights) issues were present – sometimes recognized, sometimes denied. The cases were ones that I managed; obviously all names and other identifying features have been altered. None are current cases.

## CASE NO. 1: "BABY J."

It was a snowy afternoon deep into a brutal New England winter when I was assigned to an emergency call to assess the risk of child abuse to a newborn infant, Baby J., who had just returned home with his mother from the inner city hospital where he was born. Home was a small, over-heated one-bedroom apartment in a run-down public housing project in a notorious "ghetto". The anonymous caller (a neighbor) stated that the young parents in question, Ester and James, had been quarreling and that Ester had been injured. The caller went on to add that James was a heavy and frequent drinker and had been known in the past to batter his wife. In addition to the newborn there was a two year old daughter. I went to investigate the case in the company of an older Black male social worker whose assistance I had requested to negotiate a situation where previous experience had taught me I would be denied entry. [In emergency situations such as these there is no attempt to assign workers to cases on the basis of age, race, sex, or experience where any combination of these might be helpful].

It required a great deal of persuasion before the husband, James, agreed to open the door and let us come into the apartment. Ester's face was swollen and badly bruised; she had difficulty speaking and was in visible pain. James was hostile but sober. Both reacted with shock at our intimation that the baby and his older sister might be in physical danger in the midst of the obvious domestic conflict. James admitted his violence toward his wife, but he adamantly denied that he had ever, nor would he ever, harm one of his children. He said that he posed no danger to them, and his wife concurred. We talked for nearly three hours and finally with James' encouragement, Ester agreed to be taken to the city hospital's emergency room. I accepted the judgement of my older and more experienced colleague, a native of the community, that Baby J. and his sister would be safe with their father for the time being. The responsibility and accountability should anything happen to either child remained mine alone, however, since cases are assigned to individual workers and remain their individual responsibility.

At the hospital X-rays showed that Ester's jaw had, indeed, been broken and she was hospitalized for three days. Following her discharge she refused placement with her children in a shelter for battered women then operating in the city. She insisted that she wanted to return home and to James. I carried the case for forty-five days (the most time that an assessment worker is allowed before the case is either closed or passed on to a treatment worker), and during this time I frequently came into conflict with my supervisor and with medical professionals over the management of the case, particularly with respect to my reluctance to remove the children and place them in foster care. I argued that this should be considered a drastic and ultimate, rather than a usual and proximate, action. I pointed out that the couple had extensive social support in the proximity to James' mother and his brother and sister-in-law who lived in the same project and who helped out daily in child care and shopping and cooking. In addition, James had agreed to enter a counselling group for abusive husbands and he seemed to have been able to stay sober since the crisis. As an additional safeguard, however, I asked Ester and James to accept a live-in homemaker, paid for by social services, and I found an older Haitain woman, herself a nurturant grandmother, to accept the position. She was fully informed of the situation.

I was close to congratulating myself on a skillful management of a complicated case when I was awakened at home by an angry and desperate telephone call from James who said that he did not trust me and that he feared I would take the children away so that he had hidden them where I could not find them. James was verbally abusive, but he interspersed his threats with bouts of uncontrolled weeping. It was clear that he had been drinking, but he swore that the children were safe. I spoke with him for over an hour. For the next two days I went to James' apartment and talked with him, trying to reestablish trust, and never threatening him with a loss of custody. I had, however, reported the situation to my supervisor as was my responsibility to the case and to the "missing" children involved. On the afternoon of the second day, during a home visit, James' mother arrived with the two babies, much to my evident relief. The babies were healthy and being well-cared for by their grandmother. Soon after, my assessment time elapsed and I transferred the case to a CPS treatment worker with the recommendation that the family be helped to stay together in light of James' efforts to stay sober and his participation in group therapy, and given Ester's adamant refusal to consider even a brief separation from the father of her children at this time.

The cultural rights issue embedded in the management of this case hinged on whether or not to trust the viability of the couple's traditional social support system in their extended kin network, rather than to petition the court for CPS custody of the children and their immediate placement in a child shelter followed by temporary placement with a foster family in the city. I did not rely solely on my own judgement in this case, but I continually sought the advice of the older Black male social worker whose sense of the situation was that the children were never in any real danger, although the mother was, and this represented an, at least indirect, risk to the wellbeing of the babies. What complicated the management of the case was the thinly veiled hostility that both James and his mother (and to a much lesser extent, Ester) expressed toward me as a relatively young (at that time), white, male

CPS worker. The conflict between *care* and *coercion*, compassion and control, between my role as "investigator" and my role as "social worker" was, of course, never resolved (nor, under the present CPS system, is it resolvable) before I had to move on to my next crisis. I was, however, satisfied that in this case I had acted on behalf of my survivalist motto and strategy within CPS work: to do the *least harm* (rather than the overly optimistic standard of – to do the most good). The harm that was implicit in *this* situation, and never really mediated, was that of striving to keep together a marriage with demonstrable evidence of wife-battering. However, the placement of the newborn and year-old in a foster home was the greater evil – not only for the babies, but for Ester and James as well. And I acted with the best interests of the family as a whole in mind, trying not to pit the best interests of the infants against those of the adults, since in this situation, their best interests were interdependent.

## CASE NO. 2: "RICKY"

Ricky was a ten year old white, Appalachian boy who became my case while I was a Permanency Planning worker for the Department of Social Services in a Southern state. When Ricky was two years old he fell into the fireplace at home and emerged with severe burns. After his treatment at a Shriner burn treatment center in another state, Ricky was flown home in a private plane through the munificense of a wealthy, private donor – much to the dismay and humiliation of Ricky's "poor but proud" Daddy. Several days later Ricky's father fell into a drunken rage and pulled the burn bandages off his son's arm, yelling obscenities all the while. Ricky was immediately removed from his parents on the grounds of physical and emotional abuse and the boy was placed in the home of a foster mother who was part of Ricky's natural mother's social network in the rural, backwater community. The two women belonged to the same white, evangelical, fundamentalist church.

At the time I was assigned Ricky's case his natural parents (now divorced) had voluntarily released their parental rights over Ricky which made the boy free for permanent adoption. The foster mother who had cared for Ricky for seven years was willing to remain his foster mother on an indefinite, but long-term basis. She was not willing, however, to adopt the boy, at least in part because she recognized the unalienable motherhood or Ricky's natural mother, her neighbor and friend. The foster mother did not understand why the CPS agency was putting pressure on her to formalize her relationship to Ricky through adoption. She believed that her actions toward the boy over the years spoke for themselves. Ricky, for his part, was happy in his present situation. He was attached to his foster mother, made occasional visits to his natural mother and his two siblings who lived in the same general vicinity. Ricky attended local public school where he was placed in a special classroom for emotionally handicapped children since at the time he was diagnosed as a hyperkinesic child. He saw a therapist weekly.

My mandate under Permanency Planning was to pursue *formal* adoption for Ricky although both his therapist and his legal guardian *ad litem* were opposed to this plan. I recommended to the County Attorney that permanency for Ricky could best be achieved through permanent and formal adoption; my supervisor testified in court for the same. We both felt that Ricky was in a relatively disadvantaged situation and that his "best interests" could be served by his adoption into a family better able to supervise his developmental special needs, and to provide for his education after he reached adolescence. The Judge, however, ruled in favor of long-term foster care in his present context, and we did not appeal the court's decision.

In this case I now believe, with some distance and hindsight, that I had failed to recognize Ricky's own ethnic and class identity, and that he, too, had a right to culture and community (and continuity) that was endangered by Permanency Planning guidelines. Informal adoption and fosterage are characteristic of poor, white Southern families as well as of poor, urban Black families (see Stack 1971). In conducting a little self-ethnography (see Stein 1982), I came to realize that I entertained strong biases against Ricky's "red-neck", hillbilly community and foster family. I had wanted to rescue Ricky from his "deprived" (and racist) environment and see him adopted into a more liberal, middle class environment and milieu. In short, Ricky's foster family was too close to the negatively stereotyped "hillbillies" that had populated the poorer section of my own Columbus, Ohio, childhood home.

The "child saver" ethos is strongly inculcated in CPS workers through the moralistic and often class-biased tone of traditional social work philosophy and education. Ironically, this education allows one to be somewhat more suspect of negative stereotypes toward non-white clients than of negative stereotypes toward poor, white clients who are, in fact, closer to the cultural backgrounds of many social workers. The "child saver" mentality must be recognized as a potent psychological force in sustaining the artificial conflict between a child's "best interests" and his or her "cultural" (and class) interests.

### CASE NO. 3: "ROBERT"

Robert was a fifteen year old Black adolescent living with his single mother and two younger sisters on the outskirts of a small, industrial city in the South. He referred himself to the Department of Social Services in that county, alleging that his mother, Donna, had abused him physically. Donna not only denied these charges, she reversed them, saying that Robert had attacked her with a pan of boiling water, and had threatened her on more than one occasion, with a can of mace. The CPA assessment worker was unable to untangle the web of accusations and counter-accusations between mother and son, but she substantiated the charge that Robert was, at the very least, suffering from neglect due to his mother's inadequate parenting skills. Robert was failing in school, he manifested many overt behavior problems, and he acted in a frighteningly aggressive manner both at home and at school. It was decided that mother and son should be separated and that Robert should be placed at a county emergency shelter for troubled adolescents. Before the placement papers were signed, however, Robert ran away and he was reported as a "missing" child.

At this point I was assigned the case as a permanency planning worker for Robert. I carried the case for eleven months and, again, I ran into conflict with my supervisor, the courts, and medical professionals over my efforts to keep Robert in the custody of his extended family and to find, locally, the medical and psychiatric and educational special services that he clearly needed. My first charge, however, was to find Robert. This did not prove difficult insofar as, far from living "underground", Robert had simply gone to live at the home of his mother's brother (his maternal uncle), rather than face placement at the adolescent shelter. Robert expressed a great deal of anxiety about the shelter because it was "so far out in the country" where he didn't know anyone, and because he had heard rumors about homosexual harassment in institutions similar to this one. He begged to be allowed to remain with his uncle until he was able to return home to his mother. I convinced Robert that his best chance of returning home was through treatment at the shelter.

Things did not go well for Robert at the emergency shelter, however. He was diagnosed as incorrigible – an "unsocialized aggressive" adolescent according to the then new criteria of the DSM-111 – after he had physically threatened (but not assaulted) a teacher at the shelter. A clinical psychologist recommended long-term, residential psychiatric treatment. Soon after, Robert was transferred to a highly structured, locked adolescent ward of a local, private, and prestigious teaching hospital near his home community. Once confined there Robert was again diagnosed, this time as having neurological special needs. Nonetheless, the hospital's review board recommended Robert's immediate discharge after his thirty-day insurance coverage was used up. I suspected that it was the lack of insurance that had motivated the decision, and consequently I resisted the decision. Robert's hospital psychiatrist urged the Department of Social Services to take Robert's custody from his mother so that the boy would be eligible for state reimbursed long-term residential treatment care.

I opposed the psychiatrist and conferred with the County attorney. Ultimately I was able to have Robert transferred to the adolescent unit of a nearby state mental health facility from which it was not difficult to facilitate weekend home visits between Robert and various members of his extensive kin network. Even the few visits between Robert and his mother were without serious incident. In the process, however, I had alienated the health professionals and administrators of the private hospital, as well as eroded the trust of my supervisor who had me placed on disciplinary probation for having pursued an independent course with respect to Robert's placement and aftercare. Both the psychiatric staff of the teaching hospital and my supervisors found it difficult to accept my judgement that Robert had a cultural right to remain within his family network, and that within this flexible web of relations Robert's "best interests" would be served.

### DISCUSSION

Children are removed from their families and their cultural milieu for many reasons, not all of them having to do with protecting children from situations that could endanger their health, development or psychological security. Not infrequently children are removed from their homes because their parents are poor or because the CPS system finds it easier to remove children from low-income households than to locate the kinds of economic and social support necessary to maintain the children within the family setting. Sometimes children are removed from their parents because culturally different styles of parenting are viewed as symptomatic of pathology. And sometimes children are removed from their homes because the CPS system under permanency planning is unable to recognize traditional solutions such as *informal* adoption and fosterage. This does not mean to deny, however, that even traditional and normative patterns of child-rearing are sometimes harmful to children's wellbeing, and one does not want to make the opposite error of bending over backward to see the potential "good" in all cultural adaptations [*See* Hauswald, this volume, for a useful corrective to the misuse of cultural relativism with respect to dealing with poorly functioning Navajo families].

There is one kind of abuse that is almost wholly unrecognized by the CPS system, and likely to remain so, I am afraid. I am referring to the harm that occasionally results from the incompetent intrusions of inadequately trained, over-worked and over-extended, and grossly underpaid CPS workers. The street level case worker is sent out to investigate allegations of abuse and neglect that were often not properly screened by the harried telephone intake-worker. He or she often finds himself or herself investigating situations without really understanding the nature of the charges or the motives of the informant. Not infrequently the CPS worker encounters raw hostility, some of it laced with racial and sexual overtones. These same sentiments of hostility and rejection can be projected back onto the vulnerable and defensive parents and children that the worker is supposed to serve. In all, CPS work is inherently stressful, and the individual worker often feels isolated, overly-responsible, and unsupported. S/he must engage in quick and independent decision-making, and must often back up those decisions in court. In relation to the other professionals who deal with child custody decisions – doctors, psychiatrists, psychologists, special educators, lawyers, judges – the child welfare case worker occupies the very bottom rung of the status hierarchy. S/he is frequently blamed for the mismanagement of cases in which a host of professionals actually had a hand. The CPS worker often suffers from a "spoiled" professional identity which hardly facilitates his/her ability to deal compassionately with deviant families also suffering from a stigmatized identity as "poor trash", "drunks", and "child abusers". The present organization of CPS direct practice flies in the face of good social work theory, and is hardly conducive to forging the alliances between social worker, families and communities that is at the heart of social work practice in the best sense of that term.

However, despite these obstacles, some recommendations can be made. All of these concern ways in which "cultural" and "cultural rights issues" might be recognized as part of, rather than opposed to, the best interests of the child. The curriculum and training of direct practice social workers needs to be overhauled. In most parts of the country case work training remains overwhelmingly *psychological* in cast, oriented to case by case analysis of individual, pathological family types. The larger social, cultural, and economic context that impinges on these families is rarely examined or discussed as relevant. In addition, the theories of normative human growth and psychological maturation that are presented in social work textbooks are often class-biased and culture-bound. Insofar as most social work clients are from cultural minority and poor households and communities, it is imperative that social workers be trained in comparative family systems, kinship and marriage, cross-cultural child development by professionals with the appropriate expertise. In the meantime, however, cultural training programs should be part of the usual continuing education of all case workers in CPS social welfare agencies.

Secondly, it would seem that in difficult cases of child custody where many competing professional interests are involved, some effort to solicit and interpret community interests, sentiments, and values should be attempted. Citizens review boards are only a partial response to this need. Finally, in court cases where child custody decisions hinge on the definition and interpretation of abuse and neglect, cultural anthropologists might sometimes be called upon to serve as expert witnesses, helping the courts to untangle normative from deviant patterns of child-rearing in the families of cultural minorities, and to untangle poverty from neglectful parenting in poor families. Anthropologists might also help to identify functioning from disintegrated kinship networks, and traditional from disrupted family adaptations [Again, see Hauswald, this volume]. They could also serve to identify potential but as yet untapped sources of strength and social support within the community.

In conclusion, each child's right to grow up in and belong to a community of kinship and meaning – i.e. a child's right to culture – as well as the right to live free from physical harm, neglect, and the deprivation of necessities are all affirmed in the 1959 United Nations' *Declaration of the Rights of the Child* (Resolution 1386, Principal III, United Nations, General Assembly, 14th Session, November 20th, 1959). It is most unfortunate as well as contradictory for child protective social workers to deny a child's right to culture in the name of acting in his or her "best interests".

## REFERENCES

American Humane Society
  1981 Highlights of Official Child Neglect and Abuse Reporting. American Humane Association, Child Protective Division: Denver, Colorado.
Barsh, Russel Lawrence
  1980 Indian Child Welfare Act of 1978: A Critical Analysis, Hastings Law Journal, 31.
Byler, William
  1977 The Destruction of American Indian Families. In S. Unger, ed. *The Destruction of American Indian Families*. New York: Association on American Indian Affairs, pp. 1–11.
Donzelot, J.
  1980 The Policing of Families. London: Hutchinson.
Fischler, Ronald
  1980 Protecting American Indian Children. Social Work 25(5), September: 341–349.
Goldstein, J., A. Freud, and A. Solnit, eds.
  1973 Beyond the Best Interests of the Child. New York: Free Press.
  1979 Before the Best Interests of the Child. New York: Free Press.
Governor's Advocacy Council on Children and Youth
  1978 'Why Can't I have a Home: A Report on Foster Care and Adoption in North Carolina', Governor's Advocacy Council on Children and Youth.
Lasch, C.
  1977 Haven in a Heartless World. New York: Basic Books.
Meyer, Philippe
  1983 The Child and the State. New York: Cambridge University Press.
Morey, S. and O. Gilliam, eds.
  1974 Respect for Life: the Traditional Upbringing of American Indian Children. Garden City, New Jersey: Waldorf Press.
National Committee for the Prevention of Child Abuse
  1985 NCPCA Leadership Monthly Memorandum, December (mimeo).
Stack, Carol
  1974 All Our Kin: Staregies for Survival in a Black Community. New York: Harper and Row.
Stein, Howard
  1982 The Ethnographic Mode of Teaching Clinical Behavioral Science. In Chrisman and Maretzki (eds.), Clinically Applied Anthropology, pp. 61–82. Dordrecht, Holland: D. Reidel.
Unger, Steven, ed.
  1977 The Destruction of American Indian Families. New York: Association on American Indian Affairs.
United States House of Representatives
  1986 Abused Children in America: A Report of the Select Committee on Children, Youth, and Families. Summary of Findings (mimeo), March 3, 1987.

# LIST OF CONTRIBUTORS

Prof. Claire Cassidy, 6201 Winnebago Road, Bethesda, MD 20816.

Prof. Marten de Vries, Department of Social Psychiatry, University of Limburg, P.O. Box 616, 6200 MD Maastricht, The Netherlands.

Prof. Nelson Graburn, Department of Anthropology, University of California, Berkeley, CA 94720.

Dr Don Handelman, Department of Sociology and Anthropology, Hebrew University of Jerusalem, Jerusalem 91905, Israel.

Dr Sara Harkness, Department of Maternal and Child Health, School of Public Health, Harvard University, 677 Huntington Avenue, Boston, Massachussetts.

Dr Lizabeth Hauswald, 818 Oxford St., Berkeley, CA 94707.

Dr Michael Hughes, Child Protection Team, Department of Social Services, Children's Hospital Medical Center, 747 52nd St., Oakland, CA 94609.

Prof. Jill Korbin, Department of Anthropology, Case Western Reserve University, Cleveland, OH 44106.

Dr Nora Krantzler, 242 Coronado Drive, Aptos, California.

Prof. J.S. LaFontaine, 14 Addington Square, London SE5 7JZ, U.K.

Dr Maria Lepowsky, Department of Anthropology, 5240 Social Science, University of Wisconsin, Madison, WI 53706.

Prof. Barbara Miller, Graduate Group in Demography, University of California, Berkeley, CA 94720.

Dr Dennis and Dr Dorothy Mull, Department of Family Medicine, California College of Medicine, University of California, Irvine, CA 92717.

Prof. Lucile Newman, Department of Anthropology, Box G, Brown University, Providence, RI 02912.

Dr Sulamith Potter, Department of Anthropology, University of California, Berkeley, CA 94720.

Prof. Nancy Scheper-Hughes, Department of Anthropology, University of California, Berkeley, CA 94720.

Prof. Howard Stein, Department of Family Medicine, University of Oklahoma, Health Sciences Center, Oklahoma City, OK 73190.

Prof. Marcelo M. Suarez-Orozco, Department of Anthropology, University of California, San Diego, La Jolla, CA 92093.

Dr Charles Super, Judge Baker Child Guidance Center, 295 Longwood Avenue, Boston, MA 02115.

# INDEX OF SUBJECTS

*The Culture, Illness, and Healing Book Series*

*Editors*

Margaret Lock and Allan Young

Leon Eisenberg and Arthur Kleinman (eds.), *The Relevance of Social Science for Medicine*, 1981, x + 422.

Arthur Kleinman and Tsung-yi Lin (eds.), *Normal and Abnormal Behavior in Chinese Culture*, 1981, xxiv + 436.

Carolyn Fishel Sargent, *The Cultural Context of Therapeutic Choice*, 1982, xii + 192.

Anthony J. Marsella and Geoffrey M. White (eds.), *Cultural Conceptions of Mental Health and Therapy*, 1982, xii + 414.

Noel J. Chrisman and Thomas W. Maretzki (eds.), *Clinically Applied Anthropology*, 1982, viii + 438.

Robert A. Hahn and Atwood D. Gaines (eds.), *Physicians of Western Medicine*, 1985, ix + 346.

Ronald C. Simons and Charles C. Hughes (eds.), *The Culture-Bound Syndromes*, 1985, xv + 516.

L. L. Langness and Harold G. Levine (eds.), *Culture and Retardation*, 1986, xv + 212.

Craig R. Janes, Ron Stall, and Sandra M. Gifford (eds.), *Anthropology and Epidemiology*, 1986, ix + 350.

John G. Kennedy, *The Flower of Paradise*, 1987, xii + 268.

Nancy Scheper-Hughes (ed.), *Child Survival: Anthropological Perspectives on the Treatment and Maltreatment of Children*, 1987, x + 396.

## DATE DUE

| | | | |
|---|---|---|---|
| APR 1 8 2000 | | | |
| | | | |
| MAY 0 4 2000 | | | |
| | | | |
| | | | |
| | | | |
| | | | |
| | | | |
| | | | |
| | | | |
| | | | |
| | | | |
| | | | |
| | | | |
| | | | |
| | | | |

Printed
in USA

HIGHSMITH #45230